DELIBERATE PRACTICE IN

EMOTIONALLY FOCUSED COUPLE THERAPY

Essentials of Deliberate Practice Series
Tony Rousmaniere and Alexandre Vaz, Series Editors

Deliberate Practice in Child and Adolescent Psychotherapy
Jordan Bate, Tracy A. Prout, Tony Rousmaniere, and
Alexandre Vaz

Deliberate Practice in Cognitive Behavioral Therapy
James F. Boswell and Michael J. Constantino

Deliberate Practice in Dialectical Behavior Therapy
Tali Boritz, Shelley McMain, Alexandre Vaz, and
Tony Rousmaniere

Deliberate Practice in Emotion-Focused Therapy
Rhonda N. Goldman, Alexandre Vaz, and Tony Rousmaniere

Deliberate Practice in Emotionally Focused Couple Therapy
Hanna Levenson, Sam Jinich, Alexandre Vaz, and
Tony Rousmaniere

Deliberate Practice in Interpersonal Psychotherapy
Olga Belik, Jessica M. Schultz, Scott Fairhurst, Scott Stuart,
Alexandre Vaz, and Tony Rousmaniere

Deliberate Practice in Motivational Interviewing
Jennifer K. Manuel, Denise Ernst, Alexandre Vaz, and
Tony Rousmaniere

Deliberate Practice in Multicultural Therapy
Jordan Harris, Joel Jin, Sophia Hoffman, Selina Phan,
Tracy A. Prout, Tony Rousmaniere, and Alexandre Vaz

Deliberate Practice in Psychedelic-Assisted Therapy
Shannon Dames, Andrew Penn, Monnica Williams,
Joseph A. Zamaria, Tony Rousmaniere, and Alexandre Vaz

Deliberate Practice in Psychodynamic Psychotherapy
Hanna Levenson, Volney Gay, and Jeffrey L. Binder

Deliberate Practice in Rational Emotive Behavior Therapy
Mark D. Terjesen, Kristene A. Doyle, Raymond A. DiGiuseppe,
Alexandre Vaz, and Tony Rousmaniere

Deliberate Practice in Schema Therapy
Wendy T. Behary, Joan M. Farrell, Alexandre Vaz, and
Tony Rousmaniere

Deliberate Practice in Systemic Family Therapy
Adrian J. Blow, Ryan B. Seedall, Debra L. Miller,
Tony Rousmaniere, and Alexandre Vaz

ESSENTIALS OF DELIBERATE PRACTICE SERIES
TONY ROUSMANIERE AND ALEXANDRE VAZ, SERIES EDITORS

DELIBERATE PRACTICE IN
EMOTIONALLY FOCUSED COUPLE THERAPY

HANNA LEVENSON   ALEXANDRE VAZ

SAM JINICH   TONY ROUSMANIERE

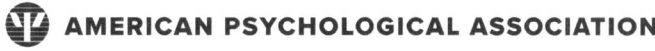 AMERICAN PSYCHOLOGICAL ASSOCIATION

Published by
American Psychological Association
750 First Street, NE
Washington, DC 20002
https://www.apa.org

Order Department
https://www.apa.org/pubs/books
order@apa.org

Typeset in Cera Pro by Circle Graphics, Inc., Reisterstown, MD

Printer: Gasch Printing, Odenton, MD
Cover Designer: Mark Karis

Library of Congress Cataloging-in-Publication Data

Names: Levenson, Hanna, 1945- author. | Jinich, Sam, author. | Vaz,
    Alexandre, author. | Rousmaniere, Tony, author. | American Psychological
    Association.
Title: Deliberate practice in emotionally focused couple therapy / Hanna
    Levenson, Sam Jinich, Alexandre Vaz, and Tony Rousmaniere.
Description: Washington, DC : American Psychological Association, 2025. |
    Series: Essentials of deliberate practice series | Includes
    bibliographical references and index.
Identifiers: LCCN 2024024491 (print) | LCCN 2024024492 (ebook) | ISBN
    9781433842962 (paperback) | ISBN 9781433842979 (ebook)
Subjects: LCSH: Couples therapy. | Emotion-focused therapy.
Classification: LCC RC488.5 .L46 2025 (print) | LCC RC488.5 (ebook) | DDC
    616.89/1562--dc23/eng/20241107
LC record available at https://lccn.loc.gov/2024024491
LC ebook record available at https://lccn.loc.gov/2024024492

https://doi.org/10.1037/0000436-000

Printed in the United States of America

10 9 8 7 6 5 4 3 2 1

With abundant gratitude, we dedicate this book to the creator of Emotionally Focused Couple Therapy.

Dr. Sue Johnson
1947–2024

Her groundbreaking work focusing on love has illuminated the path to understanding the essential role of connection in our lives.

Contents

Part III   Strategies for Enhancing the Deliberate Practice Exercises   245

Series Preface

Tony Rousmaniere and Alexandre Vaz

We are pleased to introduce the Essentials of Deliberate Practice series of training books. We are developing this series to address a specific need that we see in many psychology training programs. The issue can be illustrated by the training experiences of Mary, a hypothetical second-year graduate school trainee. Mary has learned a lot about mental health theory, research, and psychotherapy techniques. Mary is a dedicated student; she has read dozens of textbooks, written excellent papers about psychotherapy, and receives near-perfect scores on her course exams. However, when Mary sits with her clients at her practicum site, she often has trouble performing the therapy skills that she can write and talk about so clearly. Furthermore, Mary has noticed herself getting anxious when her clients express strong reactions, such as hopelessness, skepticism about therapy, or becoming very emotional. Sometimes this anxiety is strong enough to make Mary freeze at key moments, limiting her ability to help those clients.

During her weekly individual and group supervision, Mary's supervisor gives her advice informed by empirically supported therapies and common factor methods. The supervisor often supplements that advice by leading Mary through role-plays, recommending additional reading, or providing examples from her own work with clients. Mary, a dedicated supervisee who shares tapes of her sessions with her supervisor, is open about her challenges, carefully writes down her supervisor's advice, and reads the suggested readings. However, when Mary sits back down with her clients, she often finds that her new knowledge seems to have flown out of her head, and she is unable to enact her supervisor's advice. Mary finds this problem to be particularly acute with the clients who are emotionally evocative.

Mary's supervisor, who has received formal training in supervision, uses supervisory best practices, including the use of video to review supervisees' work. She would rate Mary's overall competence level as consistent with expectations for a trainee at Mary's developmental level. But even though Mary's overall progress is positive, she experiences some recurring problems in her work. This is true even though the supervisor is confident that she and Mary have identified the changes that Mary should make in her work.

The problem with which Mary and her supervisor are wrestling—the disconnect between her knowledge about psychotherapy and her ability to reliably perform psychotherapy—is the focus of this book series. We started this series because most therapists experience this disconnect, to one degree or another, whether they are beginning trainees or highly experienced clinicians. In truth, we are all Mary.

To address this problem, we are focusing this series on the use of deliberate practice, a method of training specifically designed for improving reliable performance of complex skills in challenging work environments (Rousmaniere, 2016, 2019; Rousmaniere et al., 2017). Deliberate practice entails experiential, repeated training with a particular skill until it becomes automatic. In the context of psychotherapy, this involves two trainees role-playing as a client and a therapist, switching roles every so often, under the guidance of a supervisor. The trainee playing the therapist reacts to client statements, ranging in difficulty from beginner to intermediate to advanced, with improvised responses that reflect fundamental therapeutic skills.

To create these books, we approached leading trainers and researchers of major therapy models with these simple instructions: Identify 10 to 12 essential skills for your therapy model where trainees often experience a disconnect between cognitive knowledge and performance ability—in other words, skills that trainees could write a good paper about but often have challenges performing, especially with challenging clients. We then collaborated with the authors to create deliberate practice exercises specifically designed to improve reliable performance of these skills and overall responsive treatment (Hatcher, 2015). Finally, we rigorously tested these exercises with trainees and trainers at multiple sites around the world and refined them based on extensive feedback.

Each book in this series focuses on a specific therapy model, but readers will notice that most exercises in these books touch on common factor variables and facilitative interpersonal skills that researchers have identified as having the most impact on client outcome, such as empathy, verbal fluency, emotional expression, persuasiveness, and problem focus (e.g., Anderson et al., 2009). Thus, the exercises in every book should help with a broad range of clients. Despite the specific theoretical model(s) from which therapists work, most therapists place a strong emphasis on pantheoretical elements of the therapeutic relationship, many of which have robust empirical support as correlates or mechanisms of client improvement (e.g., Norcross et al., 2019). We also recognize that therapy models have established training programs with rich histories, so we present deliberate practice not as a replacement but as an adaptable, transtheoretical training method that can be integrated into these existing programs to improve skill retention and help ensure basic competency.

About This Book

This book in the series is on emotionally focused couple therapy (EFCT), an evidence- and attachment-based couple therapy approach within a humanistic and systemic framework designed to help distressed couples by altering their dysfunctional, inter-active cycles. Guiding partners to take new and often quite vulnerable emotional risks with each other is the primary way for EFCT therapists to restructure attachment bonds from insecure to secure. Although this book focuses on the treatment of couples, it should be noted that EFCT has expanded its client base and can also be used (with modifications) with individual clients (EFIT; Johnson & Campbell, 2022) and families (EFFT; Furrow et al., 2019).

In this book, we adopt deliberate practice methods to support experiential—learn by doing—training opportunities. This experiential focus is consistent with EFCT's training model (Palmer-Olsen et al., 2011). Importantly, this book is not intended to replace core readings, exposure to foundational EFCT theory, and principles of practice. Rather, it is intended to augment the wide diversity of other training components. For more information on these training components, please refer to the International Centre for Excellence in Emotionally Focused Therapy (https://iceeft.com/).

Thank you for including us in your journey toward psychotherapy expertise. Now let's get to practice!

Acknowledgments

We acknowledge Rodney Goodyear for his significant contribution to starting and organizing this book series. We are grateful to Susan Reynolds, David Becker, Elizabeth Budd, Joe Albrecht, and Emily Ekle at American Psychological Association Books for providing expert guidance and insightful editing that has significantly improved the quality and accessibility of this book. We would also like to acknowledge the International Deliberate Practice Society and its members for their many contributions and support for our work.

We wish to thank the greater emotionally focused therapy community of therapists, supervisors, trainers, researchers, theoreticians, and originators whose commitment to this model is inspirational. There are so many couples, individuals, and families whose lives have been fundamentally changed due to their efforts. We also wish to acknowledge the members of our local Northern California Community for Emotionally Focused Therapy (NCCEFT). Their support throughout the years has helped us to become better therapists, better partners, and better people.

We are sincerely indebted to Jamie Bachman whose knowledge and sophisticated perspective greatly improved our exercises. Jay Seiff-Haron and Nalini Calamur gave us insightful consultations during critical phases of the book. We also extend our thanks to Rajika Mehra, who helped get our drafts into proper form.

Our work gained immeasurably with input from our knowledgeable emotionally focused couple therapy (EFCT) colleagues—namely, Robert Allan, Jamie Bachman, Jim Furrow, Natalia Gilabert, Paul Greenman, Paul Guillory, Silvina Irwin, Elana Katz, Lisa Palmer-Olsen, Viveka Ramel, Martiño Rodríguez, Zoya Simakhodskaya, Sandra Taylor, and Senem Zeytinoglu-Saydam.

Finally, to our partners, children, grandchildren, and friends, thank you for your encouragement and the gift of time to devote to this endeavor.

The exercises in this book series have undergone extensive testing at various settings. For everyone who volunteered to "test run" this work and provided critically important feedback throughout the method refinement and writing process, we cannot thank you enough. In particular, we would like to mention:

- Elizabeth Bateson, Nancy Anderson, Lisa Call, Peter Cellarius, Angela Jensen-Ramirez, and Sharon Mead, EFCT Peer Consultation Group, Bay Area, CA, USA

- Jamie Bachman, Jay Foy, Karen Flynn, Emily Kurutz, Daphne Leahy, Reed Malcolm, Charlie Ruff, Julie Tapley, Lourdes Vargas-Bogardas, and Trent Wright, EFCT Consultation Group, Bay Area, CA, USA

- Members of the Northern California Community for Emotionally Focused Therapy, Berkeley, CA, USA

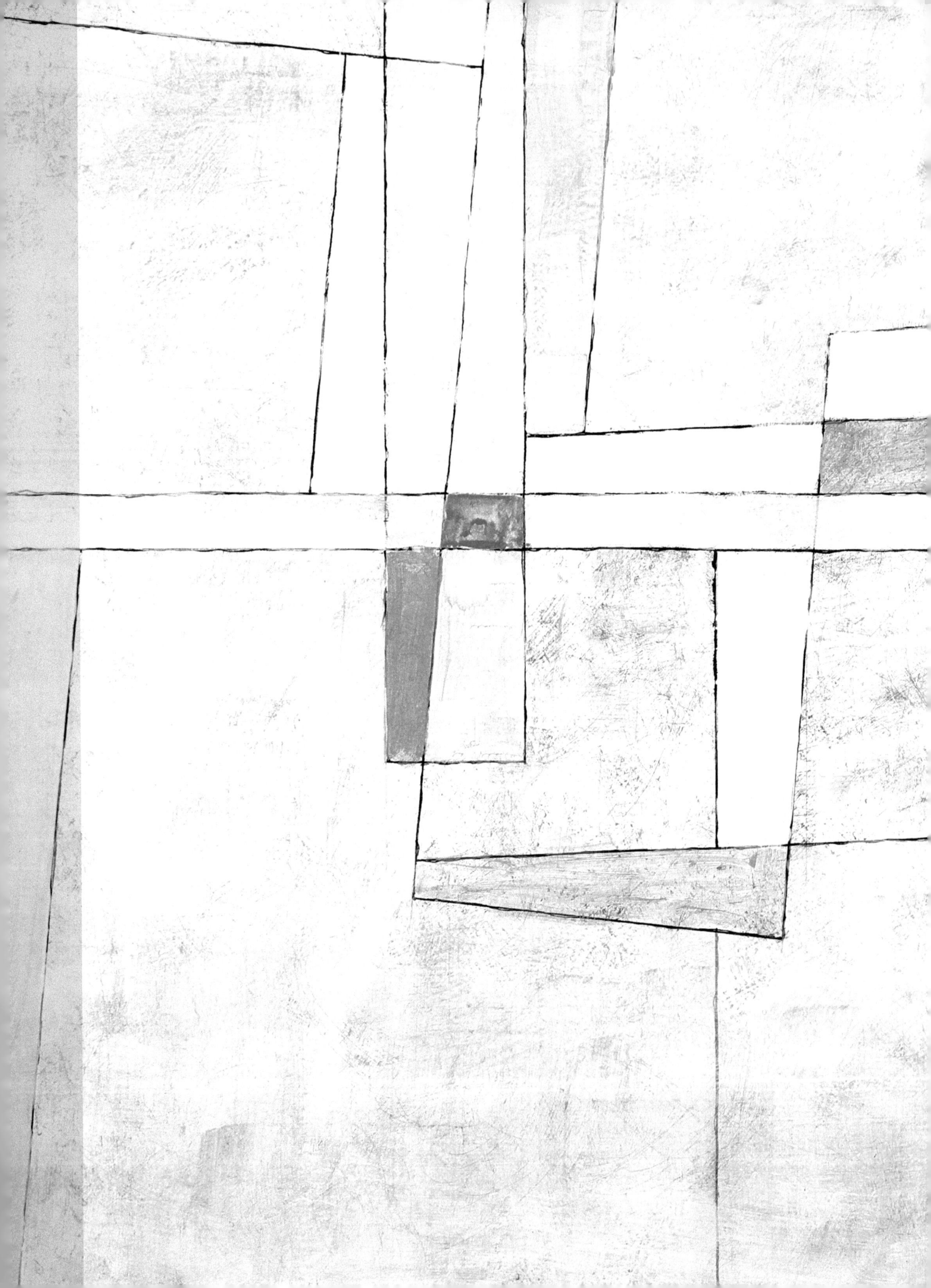

Overview and Instructions

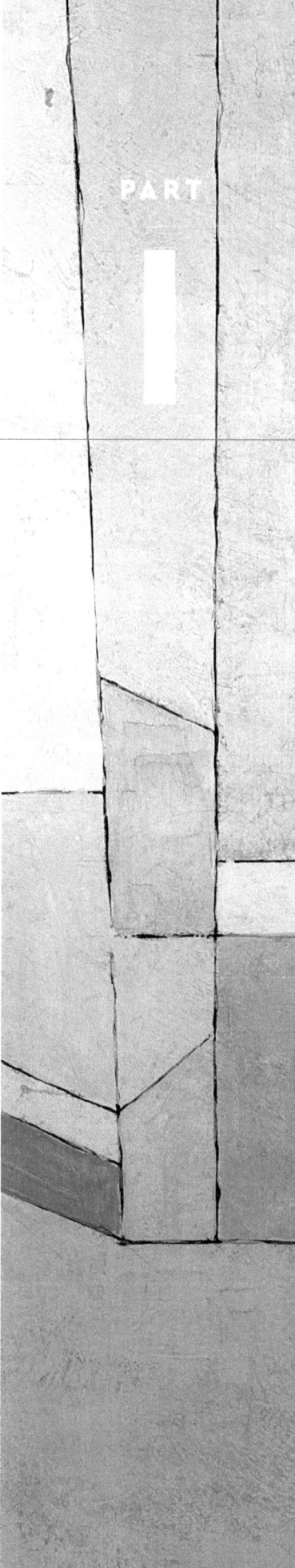

In Part I, we provide an overview of deliberate practice, including how it can be integrated into clinical training programs for emotionally focused couple therapy (EFCT), and instructions for performing the deliberate practice exercises in Part II. **We encourage both trainers and trainees to read both Chapters 1 and 2 before performing the deliberate practice exercises for the first time.**

Chapter 1 provides a foundation for the rest of the book by introducing important concepts related to deliberate practice and its role in psychotherapy training more broadly and EFCT training more specifically. In this first chapter, we present an overview of EFCT, outlining its key principles and processes, as well as some of the research supporting this model. We also individually review the 12 skills from these exercises that are covered by the deliberate practice exercises in Part II.

Chapter 2 lays out the basic, most essential instructions for performing the EFCT deliberate practice exercises in Part II. They are designed to be quick and simple and provide you with just enough information to get started without being overwhelmed by too much information. Chapter 3 in Part III provides more in-depth guidance, which we encourage you to read once you are comfortable with the basic instructions in Chapter 2.

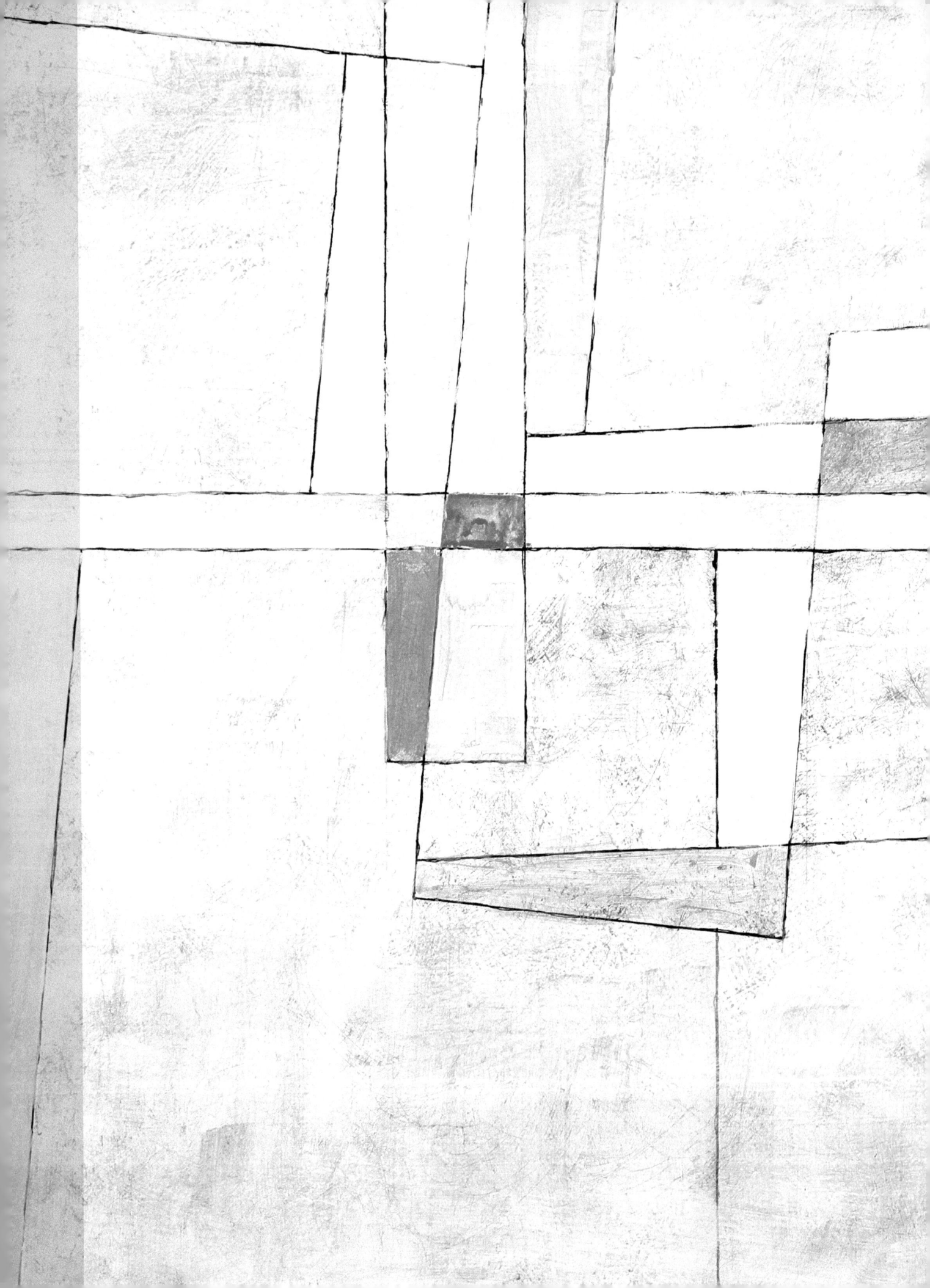

Introduction and Overview of Deliberate Practice and Emotionally Focused Couple Therapy

As a trainer and a supervisor of emotionally focused couple therapy (EFCT), we often hear about the struggles that our trainees go through as they are learning this elegant, straightforward, yet complex model. We hear things like this:

"This is way too complex."
"I don't know if I am doing this right!"
"It sounds so simple when I read about EFCT, but doing it is something else!"
"I never remember what step or stage I am in or what to do next!"
"I never seem to do what I'm supposed to, in the moment, when I need to."
"I watch my tapes and I am embarrassed by how many things I let pass where I could have intervened."
"I keep tracking the negative cycle but don't know how to advance to the next step like exploring the couple's underlying emotions."
"If I just let a few days or weeks pass without reviewing the model, it seems to become fuzzier in my head and I can't seem to remember everything that I am supposed to do."

Perhaps some of you reading this today can identify with one or more of these. We all have been there.

Sue Johnson, in a communication to her EFCT trainer team (personal communication, 2024), suggested that after years of focusing on steps and stages, they should also turn their focus to microskills and macroskills as a more effective and reliable way to help their trainees learn how to create new change events in the couple's work. She shared that her own work improved when she focused on teaching and practicing skills.

Following the growing (but still nascent) trend of using deliberate practice to learn various psychotherapy approaches, we (Hanna and Sam) decided to write this book alongside our colleagues and series editors Tony Rousmaniere and Alexandre Vaz. We realized that we had an advantage applying deliberate practice to EFCT because EFCT has always espoused experiential learning as one of its primary values. However, in the actual training, EFCT has usually relied on open-ended role-plays and watching videos of expert therapists performing EFCT as well as discussion of the concepts and interventions involved.

https://doi.org/10.1037/0000436-001

Deliberate Practice in Emotionally Focused Couple Therapy, by H. Levenson, S. Jinich, A. Vaz, and T. Rousmaniere

In other words, although the training has been rich and effective (Montagno et al., 2011), there has been the absence of deliberately practicing an intervention repeatedly until it becomes "muscle memory." In this book, we take EFCT to the next level of strategically and programmatically focusing on specific skills that can be practiced individually or in combination with other skills to improve performance and confidence in the model.

Twenty years ago, Hanna and Sam met in Ottawa, Canada (although we both lived just a few miles from each other in the San Francisco Bay Area of California). We traveled to Canada to learn EFCT from Sue Johnson and her colleagues in one of their 5-day externships in the early days of their training program. When we returned, we were so impressed by this emotionally focused, process-oriented, humanistic, attachment-based approach to working with couples that we organized a handful of therapists interested in learning the model and, as a group, invited two of the EFCT founders, Alison Lee and Gail Palmer, to come help us learn EFCT in what became the first Core Skills series taught.

In my (Sam's) journey to become an EFCT therapist, I discovered that as time elapsed, I was forgetting what I had learned from the externship and the Core Skills training. As soon as the training was over, things became fuzzier, and I felt like there was something wrong with my ability to learn the model or that there was something uniquely challenging about this particular model. It seemed organic and simple when watching Sue and her EFCT trainers do a live case or watch them on video, but it was quite challenging for the skills to feel like they came naturally to me. I thought perhaps that I just needed more experience. This changed when I became a trainer 9 years later. I often admit publicly that I learned EFCT after I became an EFCT trainer, and I often tell my students that the best way to master the model is to try to teach it. I promise you that by practicing with others, your skills will improve dramatically, your outcomes will improve, and, best of all, you will not feel like there is anything wrong with your ability to learn EFCT.

My (Hanna's) original training was in social psychology and personality theory. So when I became a clinical psychologist several years later, it seemed natural to me that one would look for the social (between) and individual (within) influences on personality, difficulties, and growth. Also, as a researcher and a teacher, I was eager to use models that had an empirical basis. Since I learn best when I am researching something, I (working with two outstanding graduate students) developed a self-report fidelity scale to help practitioners know when they were doing (and not doing) EFCT (Levenson et al., 2009; Montagno et al., 2011). This project developed into a larger research endeavor on the effects of training in EFCT. Long story short, when I found EFCT, it felt like I had a home base that made sense clinically, empirically, didactically, and idiosyncratically. I was hooked.

However, despite EFCT's commitment to learning through experiential exercises, workshops, and training videos, the learning curve was steep, bumpy, uneven, and not always clearly marked. As I became more experienced in the model, first as an EFCT-certified therapist and then as a certified supervisor, I wanted to help my supervisees and colleagues who were struggling how best to learn this powerful model.

Why Are We Writing This Book?

Ostensibly we are writing this book to help you learn how to do EFCT more effectively and efficiently. But we want to do more than that: We would like to inspire you! First, we would like to embolden you to harness the energy behind this powerful model so that you can have an increased ease and enthusiasm as you work with distressed couples. Second, we would like you to appreciate your own capacity to learn and even master skills— a capacity that perhaps you didn't even realize you had—through deliberate practice.

Overview of the Deliberate Practice Exercises

The main focus of the book is a series of 14 exercises that have been thoroughly tested and modified based on feedback from EFCT trainers and trainees. The first 12 exercises each represent an essential EFCT skill. The last two exercises are more comprehensive, consisting of an annotated EFCT transcript and improvised mock therapy sessions that teach practitioners how to integrate all these skills into more expansive clinical scenarios. Table 1.1 presents the 12 skills that are covered in these exercises.

Throughout all the exercises, trainees work in pairs or in groups of three under the guidance of a supervisor and role-play as clients and therapist, switching back and forth between the two roles. Each of the 12 skill-focused exercises consists of multiple client statements grouped by difficulty—beginner, intermediate, and advanced—that calls for a specific skill. For each skill, trainees are asked to read through and absorb the description of the skill, its criteria, and some examples of it. The trainee playing the client then reads the statements, which present possible scenarios relevant for EFCT clinical practice. The trainee playing the therapist then responds in a way that demonstrates the appropriate skill. Trainee therapists will have the option of practicing a response using the one supplied in the exercise or immediately improvising and supplying their own.

After each client statement and therapist response couplet is practiced several times, the trainees will stop to receive feedback from the supervisor. Guided by the supervisor, the trainees will be instructed to try statement–response couplets several times, working their way down the list. In consultation with the supervisor, trainees will go through the exercises, starting with the least challenging and moving through to more advanced levels. The group (supervisor–clients–therapist) will have the opportunity to discuss whether exercises present too much or too little challenge and adjust up or down depending on the assessment.

Trainees, in consultation with supervisors, can decide which skills they wish to work on and for how long. In our testing experience, we have found practice sessions last about 1 to 1.25 hours to receive maximum benefit. After this, trainees become saturated and need a break.

TABLE 1.1. The 12 Emotionally Focused Couple Therapy Skills Presented in the Deliberate Practice Exercises

Beginner Skills	Intermediate Skills	Advanced Skills
1. Evocative inquiry: identifying patterns and eliciting attachment fears and needs	6. Tracking the therapist's inner experience	8. Gathering and assembling elements of emotion
2. Evocative reflection: eliciting and heightening emotional experience	7. Providing a rationale for emotionally focused couple therapy	9. Enactments: deepening emotional experience and choreographing engaged encounters
3. Validating partners' experiences and tracking dysfunctional patterns		10. Slicing the risk thinner: helping partners express difficult emotions
4. Attachment-reframed validation		11. Interrupting negative process early in therapy: catching the bullet I
5. Deepening emotions with RISSSSC: speaking simply, slowly, and softly		12. Interrupting negative process later in therapy: catching the bullet II

Ideally, EFCT learners will both gain confidence and achieve competence through practicing these exercises. Competence is defined here as the ability to perform an EFCT skill in a manner that is flexible and responsive to the client. Skills have been chosen that are considered essential to EFCT and that practitioners often find challenging to implement.

The skills identified in this book are not comprehensive in the sense of representing all one needs to learn to become a competent EFCT clinician. Some will present particular challenges for trainees. A short history and description of EFCT and a brief description of the deliberate practice methodology is provided to explain how we have arrived at the union between them.

The Goals of This Book

The primary goal of this book is to help trainees achieve competence in core EFCT skills. The expression of that skill or competency may look somewhat different across clients or even within sessions with the same client.

The EFCT deliberate practice exercises are designed to achieve the following:

1. Help EFCT therapists develop the ability to apply the skills in a range of clinical situations.

2. Move the skills into procedural memory (Squire, 2004) so that EFCT therapists can access them even when they are tired, stressed, overwhelmed, or discouraged.

3. Provide EFCT therapists in training with an opportunity to exercise the particular skill using a style and language that are congruent with who they are.

4. Provide the opportunity to use the EFCT skills in response to varying client statements and affect. This is designed to build confidence to adopt skills in a broad range of circumstances within different client contexts.

5. Provide EFCT therapists in training with many opportunities to fail and then correct their failed response based on feedback. This helps build confidence and persistence.

Finally, this book aims to help trainees discover their own personal learning style so they can continue their professional development long after their formal training is concluded.

Who Can Benefit From This Book?

This book is designed to be used in multiple contexts, including in graduate-level courses, supervision, postgraduate training, and continuing education programs. It assumes the following:

1. The supervisor is knowledgeable about and competent in EFCT.

2. The supervisor is able to provide good demonstrations of how to use EFCT skills across a range of therapeutic situations, via role-play and/or video. Alternatively, the supervisor has access to examples of EFCT being demonstrated through psychotherapy videos. (We have provided a listing of such resources in Appendix C.)

3. The supervisor is able to provide feedback to students regarding how to craft or improve their application of EFCT skills.

4. Trainees will have accompanying reading, such as books and articles, that explain the theory, research, and rationale of EFCT and each particular skill. Recommended reading for each skill is provided in the sample syllabus (Appendix C).

The exercises covered in this book series were piloted in multiple training sites across four continents (North America, South America, Europe, and Asia). This book is designed for trainers and trainees from different cultural backgrounds worldwide. This book is also designed for those who are training at all career stages, from beginning trainees, including those who have never worked with real clients, to seasoned therapists, emphasizing the importance of lifelong learning. All exercises feature guidance for assessing and adjusting the difficulty to target the needs of each individual learner precisely.

Deliberate Practice in Psychotherapy Training

How does one become an expert in their professional field? What is trainable and what is simply beyond our reach, due to innate or uncontrollable factors? Questions such as these touch on our fascination with expert performers and their development. A mixture of awe, admiration and even confusion surround people such as Mozart, Leonardo da Vinci, or more contemporary top performers such as athletes Serena Williams, Michael Jordan, or Caitlin Clark and chess virtuoso Garry Kasparov. What accounts for their consistently superior professional results? Evidence suggests that the amount of or time spent on a particular type of training is a key factor in developing expertise in virtually all domains (Ericsson & Pool, 2016). "Deliberate practice" is an evidence-based method that can improve performance in an effective and reliable manner.

The concept of deliberate practice has its origins in a classic study by K. Anders Ericsson and colleagues (1993). They found that the amount of time practicing a skill and the quality of the time spent doing so were key factors predicting mastery and acquisition. They identified five key activities in learning and mastering skills: (a) observing one's own work; (b) getting expert feedback; (c) setting small, incremental learning goals just beyond the performer's ability; (d) engaging in repetitive behavioral rehearsal of specific skills; and (e) continuously assessing performance. Ericsson and his colleagues termed this process deliberate practice, a cyclical process that is illustrated in Figure 1.1.

FIGURE 1.1. Cycle of Deliberate Practice

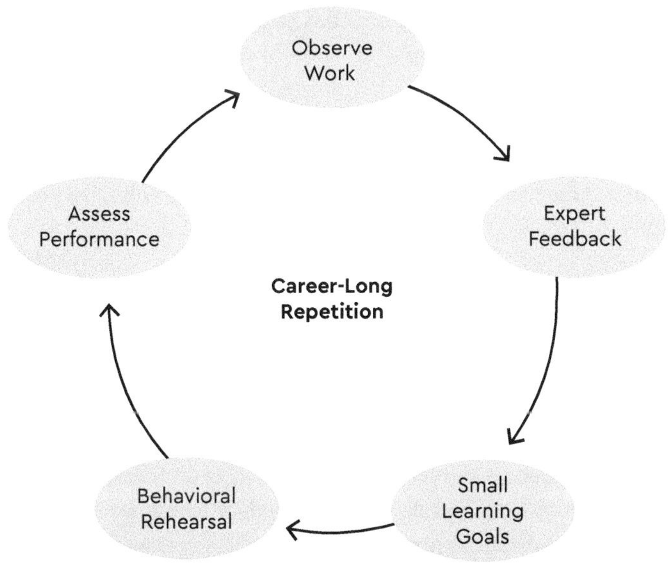

Note. From *Deliberate Practice in Emotion-Focused Therapy* (p. 7), by R. N. Goldman, A. Vaz, and T. Rousmaniere, 2021, American Psychological Association (https://doi.org/10.1037/0000227-000). Copyright 2021 by the American Psychological Association.

Research has shown that lengthy engagement in deliberate practice is associated with expert performance across a variety of professional fields, such as medicine, sports, music, chess, computer programming, and mathematics (Ericsson et al., 2018). People may associate deliberate practice with the widely known "10,000-hour rule" popularized by Malcolm Gladwell in his 2008 book *Outliers*, although the actual number of hours required for expertise varies by field and by individual (Ericsson & Pool, 2016). This, however, perpetuated two misunderstandings. First, that this is the number of deliberate practice hours that everyone needs to attain expertise, no matter the domain. In fact, there can be considerable variability in how many hours are required.

The second misunderstanding is that engagement in 10,000 hours of work performance will lead one to become an expert in that domain. This misunderstanding holds considerable significance for the field of psychotherapy, where hours of work experience with clients has traditionally been used as a measure of proficiency (Rousmaniere, 2016). Research suggests that the amount of experience alone does not predict therapist effectiveness (Goldberg et al., 2016). It may be that the quality of deliberate practice is a key factor.

Psychotherapy scholars, recognizing the value of deliberate practice in other fields, have recently called for deliberate practice to be incorporated into training for mental health professionals (e.g., Bailey & Ogles, 2019; Hill et al., 2020; Rousmaniere et al., 2017; Taylor & Neimeyer, 2017; Tracey et al., 2015). There are, however, good reasons to question analogies made between psychotherapy and other professional fields such as sports or music because by comparison, psychotherapy is so complex and free form. Sports have clearly defined goals, and classical music follows a written score. In contrast, the goals of psychotherapy shift with the unique presentation of each client at each session. Therapists do not have the luxury of following a score.

Instead, good psychotherapy is more like improvisational jazz (Noa Kageyama, as cited in Rousmaniere, 2016). In jazz improvisations, a complex mixture of group collaboration, creativity, and interaction are co-constructed among band members. Like psychotherapy, no two jazz improvisations are identical. However, improvisations are not a random collection of notes. They are grounded in a comprehensive theoretical understanding and technical proficiency that is only developed through continuous deliberate practice. For example, prominent jazz instructor Jerry Coker (1990) lists 18 skill areas that students must master, each of which has multiple discrete skills, including tone quality, intervals, chord arpeggios, scales, patterns, and licks. In this sense, more creative and artful improvisations are actually a reflection of a previous commitment to repetitive skill practice and acquisition. As legendary jazz musician Miles Davis put it, "You have to play a long time to be able to play like yourself" (Cook, 2005, p. 112).

The main idea that we would like to stress here is that we want deliberate practice to help EFCT therapists become themselves. The idea is to learn the skills so that you have them on hand when you want them. Practice the skills to make them your own. Incorporate those aspects that feel right for you. Ongoing and effortful deliberate practice should not be an impediment to flexibility and creativity. Ideally, it should enhance it. We recognize and celebrate that psychotherapy is an ever-shifting encounter and by no means want it to become or feel formulaic. Strong EFCT therapists mix an eloquent integration of previously acquired skills with properly attuned flexibility. The core EFCT responses provided are meant as templates or possibilities, rather than "answers." Please interpret and apply them as you see fit, in a way that makes sense to you. We encourage flexible and improvisational play!

Simulation-Based Mastery Learning

Deliberate practice uses simulation-based mastery learning (Ericsson, 2004; McGaghie et al., 2014). That is, the stimulus material for training consists of "contrived social situations that mimic problems, events, or conditions that arise in professional encounters" (McGaghie et al., 2014, p. 375). A key component of this approach is that the stimuli being used in training are sufficiently similar to the real-world experiences, so that they provoke similar reactions. This facilitates *state-dependent learning* in which professionals acquire skills in the same psychological environment where they will have to perform those skills (Fisher & Craik, 1977). For example, pilots train with flight simulators that present mechanical failures and dangerous weather conditions, and surgeons practice with surgical simulators that present medical complications. Training in simulations with challenging stimuli increases professionals' capacity to perform effectively under stress. For the psychotherapy training exercises in this book, the "simulators" are typical client statements that might actually be presented in the course of therapy sessions and call upon the use of the particular skill.

Declarative Versus Procedural Knowledge

Declarative knowledge is what a person can understand, write, or speak about. It often refers to factual information that can be consciously recalled through memory and often acquired relatively quickly. In contrast, procedural learning is implicit in memory and "usually requires *repetition of an activity*, and associated learning is demonstrated through *improved task performance*" (Koziol & Budding, 2012, p. 2694, emphasis added). Procedural knowledge is what a person can perform, especially under stress (Squire, 2004). There can be a wide difference between their declarative and procedural knowledge. For example, an "armchair quarterback" is a person who understands and talks about athletics well but would have trouble performing at a professional level. Likewise, most dance, music, or theater critics have a high ability to write about their subjects but would be flummoxed if asked to perform them.

The sweet spot for deliberate practice is the gap between declarative and procedural knowledge. In other words, effortful practice should target those skills that the trainee could write a good paper about but would have trouble actually performing with a real client. We start with declarative knowledge, learning skills theoretically and observing others perform them. Once learned, with the help of deliberate practice, we work toward the development of procedural learning, with the aim of therapists having "automatic" access to each of the skills that they can call on when necessary.

Now we turn to a little theoretical background on EFCT to help contextualize the skills of the book and how they fit into the greater training model.

Overview of Emotionally Focused Couple Therapy

EFCT was conceptualized by Leslie S. Greenberg and Susan M. Johnson in the early 1980s, culminating in a book on the topic in 1988. This version of EFCT was primarily a theoretical integration of two orientations—that of Rogers's (1961) intrapersonal, humanistic/experiential approach and that of Minuchin and Fishman's (1981) interpersonal, family systems approach. Johnson and Greenberg focused on the dancer and the dance and the system that held them together by simultaneously considering the intrapsychic experience (within the self) and the interpersonal experience (between the partners).

Emotion was privileged and seen as both the target and the agent of change. What resulted was an experiential, emotion-processing model to help distressed couples.

Johnson then expanded on the model by integrating John Bowlby's (1969, 1988) and Mary Ainsworth's (1962) attachment theory. She (Johnson, 2008) defined the core attachment question as "Are you there for me?" with each of the letters in the verb (ARE) standing for a different component of a secure bond: **a**ccessibility, **r**esponsiveness, and emotional **e**ngagement. "The approach became increasingly focused on strengthening a couple's bond" (Furrow et al., 2022, p. 5). The strategy for strengthening this bond is helping partners get in touch with their vulnerable (primary), attachment-based emotions; share their deep longings; and respond to their partners from a place of emotional vulnerability, ultimately building a safe and secure platform where various issues can be discussed and resolved. The approach was succinctly described by Wiebe and Johnson (2016):

> Couples are encouraged to explore here-and-now emotional experiencing, uncovering primary emotions that are often blocked from awareness by reactive surface emotions and responses, and share these with their partner in the session. Their partner will then be shown how to listen and respond in an emotionally attuned way. The new emotional music then elicits new responses and, gradually, changes the dance between partners. (p. 390)

Insecurely attached couples are wired, in moments of threat or danger, to fight, flee, freeze, or fawn, but they rarely reach for their partner in a vulnerable state to tell them that underlying their reactive (secondary) emotional response they feel hurt or afraid. Securely attached couples, by contrast, do reach for each other in moments of distress and talk openly about feeling sad, hurt, scared, or lonely. They have a more organized, coherent, and positive sense of self. They tend to view others as basically trustworthy, and their internal working model and view of self as lovable, competent, and worthy of care, comfort, and safety. Thus, when as therapists we can discover the implicit connection-seeking intent beneath the negative reactivity, change becomes possible. Many of the skills outlined in this book are designed to focus on the microskills to guide these couples to connectedness.

Today, EFCT has been modified so that it can be applied to individuals (Johnson, 2019; Johnson & Campbell, 2022) and families (EFFT; Furrow et al., 2019; Johnson, 2019). In this book, we focus on partners' bonding relationships.

Three Key Principles

EFCT is based on three core principles: attachment theory, emotion regulation, and a systemic approach.

Attachment Theory

EFCT draws heavily on attachment theory, which maintains that humans have an innate, hardwired need for emotional connection and security, especially when under threat. It emphasizes that the quality of the attachment formed in childhood influences adult relationships (Mikulincer & Shaver, 2017). We never outgrow our need for others. As Englishman Bowlby poetically stated, "Whilst especially evident during early childhood, attachment behaviour is held to characterise human beings from the cradle to the grave" (1969, p. 129). You might want to watch an 11-minute video that captures the essence of attachment behavior from the "cradle to grave" (Johnson, 2016).

Concurrent with the development of EFCT, the empirical, developmental, and theoretical literature on attachment theory exploded (Duschinsky et al., 2023). This increased information helped us understand that isolation, deprivation, loss, and rejection, as well as feelings of being intruded upon, pressured, and criticized by those we rely on in times of need, are inherently traumatizing. Burgeoning scientific work in the emerging specialization of the neurobiology of attachment (Coan, 2008; Cozolino, 2017; Siegel, 2020) has helped us understand how our nervous system is wired to recognize emotional disconnection from our loved ones as a threat signal to our security that in turn triggers pain, panic, fear, and disorientation. It is the attachment perspective that gives EFCT therapists a pragmatic way of seeing distress and conflict between partners as a means through which they are actually protesting their disconnection from each another. At the heart of EFCT lies the belief that emotions are the key drivers of human behavior and that a secure emotional bond is essential for a thriving relationship.

Johnson likes to say that emotions are like the music in the dance of intimates; the couple enters therapy dancing to the emotional music of their relationship. Unfortunately, they are often out of step with each another—mis-attuning and misinterpreting the signals their partner is sending them—and quick to say their own dance moves are the right ones. This dysfunctional dance unfortunately leaves both partners feeling threatened, which can manifest as withdrawal, anger, or both. What they perceive from their partner, and what they in turn send their partner, are danger cues or threat signals. By exploring and helping to change the dance steps (interactions) as well as the music driving the dance (emotional responsiveness), EFCT therapists can effectively improve the couple's intimacy, safety, and secure bonding. In keeping with the metaphor, it is not surprising that one of the roles the therapist plays is that of a choreographer, helping partners have more rewarding and intimate moves, enabling "conversations for a lifetime of love" (Johnson, 2008).

Accessing and Expressing Emotion

EFCT recognizes that emotions play a vital role in shaping thoughts, behaviors, and interactions. "It is seen as the essential transforming element in effective psychotherapy" (Furrow et al., 2022, p. 3). By helping couples identify, process, and express their emotions in a way their partner can hear, EFCT enables needs, fears, and desires to be recognized more effectively by themselves as well as their partners. Helping partners to identify and share their underlying, more vulnerable emotions fosters empathy, understanding, and compassion between them.

Systemic Approach

EFCT views the couple as a system, where the actions and emotions of one partner impact the emotions and actions of the other. It focuses on the dynamics and patterns within the individual and between the partners in the relationship, based on the understanding that negative cycles of interaction perpetuate distress. As outlined in the second edition of the workbook *Becoming an Emotionally Focused Therapist* (Furrow et al., 2022), EFCT is consistent with the basic tenets of systems theory: Causality is circular; behavior must be considered in context; couples' interactions are patterned and stable; all behavior is considered communication; and the major task of the therapist is to interrupt negative cycles of interaction. An important part of the initial stage of therapy is helping the couple identify their dysfunctional cycle and thereby realize that the enemy is the cycle, not their partner. By reshaping these cyclical patterns, EFCT aims to create positive cycles of connection and intimacy.

Thus, EFCT using an attachment frame, a systemic lens, and experiential interventions offers therapists a map of the couple's pain and stuck places, and what is needed to move them into health and well-being (Furrow et al., 2022; Johnson, 2019).

The EFCT Map: Three Stages, Nine Steps, and a Tango

The three stages of change comprise a series of nine recursive steps that are designed to restructure the attachment bond between couples. In the first stage, *de-escalation of the negative cycle*, the therapist helps the partners identify their interactional cycles and reframe this pattern as the problem, not each other. The EFCT therapist does this by carefully tracking the partners behaviors. In addition, the therapist validates the partners' protective behaviors while accessing the vulnerable emotions that underlie these defensive maneuvers. The second stage, *restructuring the interactional patterns* from insecure to secure, happens by helping each member of the couple reach for their partner and disclose to them in a vulnerable manner their attachment fears and longings. Process research on EFCT has consistently linked the clients' depth of emotional experiencing to positive therapeutic outcomes (Greenman & Johnson, 2013). The last stage, *consolidation*, focuses on appreciating the accomplishments in achieving a stronger bond and finding ways to foster continued success through attachment rituals. Throughout the therapy, the EFCT therapist maintains a stance of empathy, emotional presence, genuine attunement, and emotional responsiveness.

The most significant macroskill intervention that is used by EFCT therapists is a sequence of five key moves that, when combined, are commonly referred to as the *EFT tango*.[1] If you were to observe an EFCT therapist in action, you would notice them doing the same five moves in every session and in every step and stage of the model. In Move 1, the EFCT therapist focuses on the here-and-now inner emotional experience of each member of the couple as well as the experience between the partners. The therapist then focuses on each partner's triggers, meaning making and action tendencies, "assembling" their emotional experience in a coherent manner (Move 2), followed by choreographing an engaged encounter in which the partner vulnerably shares their heightened emotion with their partner (Move 3). The therapist then processes what it is like to share their feelings in this new, vulnerable way and what it is like for their partner to hear it (Move 4). The final move (Move 5) of the EFCT tango is a summary and an integration of this new way of engaging. Guiding partners to take new and often quite vulnerable emotional risks with each other is the primary way for EFCT therapists to promote corrective emotional experiences through healing interpersonal interactions.

The focus of this book is on learning EFCT skills that therapists can use to help clients more effectively access their underlying vulnerable emotions, communicate those in a vulnerable manner to a receptive partner, and engage in a series of positively cascading, interactive experiences.

Research on EFCT Practice and Training

Numerous studies have demonstrated the effectiveness of EFCT in improving relationship satisfaction, reducing distress, and promoting lasting change with a wide range of presenting problems (e.g., a partner facing end-stage cancer, infertility, posttraumatic stress disorder, attachment injuries requiring forgiveness; for reviews, see Furrow et al., 2022; Wiebe & Johnson, 2016). No other approach to couple therapy can claim the number of successful outcome studies (Sexton et al., 2011). A meta-analysis with a database

---

1. Sue Johnson became enamored with tango, the dance, while she was developing EFCT. She defines the tango, which originated in Argentina and Uruguay in the 1880s, as "a dance based on attunement and mutual resonance structured by emotional music. At first you have to learn the steps but then you dance it from muscle memory and can flexibly play with moves and music" (Johnson & Campbell, 2022, p. 72), which sounds a lot like the desired outcome from doing deliberate practice exercises.

of 20 studies and 332 couples provides support for EFCT as an evidence-based couple therapy approach, where 70% of couples are expected to be symptom free at the end of treatment, and 2-year follow-ups indicate maintenance of treatment gains (Spengler et al., 2024). Worthy of note is that the strongest moderator of outcome is EFCT treatment fidelity, indicating that the more one adheres to the EFCT model, the greater the therapeutic benefits to the couple. This finding of model specificity has particular relevance for the application of deliberate practice to EFCT skills training.

Regarding EFCT *efficacy* studies in naturalistic, clinical settings, significant improvements in relationship satisfaction have also been found. In addition, EFCT has been shown to increase attachment security in both anxious and avoidant partners, with this change maintained at follow-up (Burgess Moser et al., 2016; Wiebe et al., 2017). *Process-of-change* studies, linking therapeutic process and outcome in EFCT, have improved our understanding of how to create necessary conditions and procedures within the therapy and have added greatly to EFCT supervision and training specificity. For example, the therapist's ability to promote emotional depth and to direct enactments using heightened affect are related to successful outcomes (Bradley & Furrow, 2007; Burgess Moser et al., 2016; Greenman & Johnson, 2013). In addition, there are some excellent case studies (e.g., Mendelson, 2024a) and commentaries on the case studies (e.g., Kelly, 2024) and rejoinders (e.g., Mendelson, 2024b) that allow us to examine, in a more fine-grained manner, EFCT processes in light of the uniqueness of the individual case.

The research on the impact of EFCT training on therapist knowledge and competency is also robust. The usual pattern for formal learning in EFCT is to attend a 4-day externship training held by an International Centre for Excellence in Emotionally Focused Therapy (ICEEFT) certified trainer. The next step is to complete a core skills training, usually comprising four 2-day workshops led by an ICEEFT certified trainer or supervisor. The format for these trainings involves lecture, watching videos of clinical sessions with commentary, open-ended role-plays, and discussion. If one wishes to become a certified EFCT therapist, 8 hours of supervision by a certified EFCT supervisor is required.

Research using a self-report modification (Levenson et al., 2009) of the Emotionally Focused Therapy Therapist Fidelity Scale indicates that after externship training, therapists and trainees significantly increased their knowledge about and competency in EFCT (Montagno et al., 2011) and that much of the gains remained at follow-up. These findings have been replicated with therapists learning EFCT in Hungary (Koren et al., 2021) and six Spanish-speaking countries (Rodríguez-González et al., 2020, 2022). The Koren and colleagues (2021) study found that additional improvements in knowledge and competency also occurred after taking a course in core skills. In fact, most of the competency improvements were due to the core skills course, which makes sense because that course focuses on role-plays with individualized feedback, making another case for applying deliberate practice to EFCT.

The process of learning EFCT has also been studied in the United States (Sandberg & Knestel, 2011) and nine Spanish-speaking countries in Europe, Central America, and South America (Sandberg et al., 2020). In a questionnaire asking for their experiences learning EFCT, although the U.S. respondents mentioned many positive things (e.g., the EFCT framework and structure, improved personal relationships), the "results also show that the transition to EFT from another model can be taxing and requires time, support, and additional supervision/training to increase comfort level and competency with EFT" (Sandberg & Knestel, 2011, p. 393). The Spanish-speaking therapists, however, had a "heightened sense of appreciation for and resonance with the focus on core emotion in EFT and less frequent reports of difficulty learning and adapting to the model" (Sandberg et al., 2020, p. 256). The researchers concluded that these differences were in keeping with Latin American and Spanish cultural values and forms of emotional expression.

Concerning the Format of Skill Exercises: Diversity, Relationship Composition, and Pronouns

The pedagogical challenge of writing a deliberate practice workbook for EFCT skills has been to select critical skills, distill them into their component parts, and create straightforward exercises. As authors of this book, we have found that trying to do these tasks while holding people as complex, cultural beings has been a humbling experience. Although the attachment theory underpinnings of EFCT are considered universal, most of EFCT's formulation and intervention practices have been based on a Eurocentric, cis-gender, heterosexual, middle-class value system. Kelly (2024) has pointed out how all mainstream relationship therapy models are "assumed to be universally applicable despite being developed by, for, and with the dominant group" (p. 110). However, EFCT is ever-growing and becoming more inclusive, with an increasing number of papers and practice procedures highlighting diversity issues that need to be taken into consideration in the sessions (e.g., Allan et al., 2023; Franz et al., 2023; Greenman et al., 2009; Kelly, 2017; Kelly & Omar, 2017; Mendelson, 2024a, 2024b; Nightingale et al., 2019; Young et al., 2023). We certainly lack expertise with the many identities that readers will have. Nonetheless, we have intentionally set about to address three diversity-related matters in this book.

1. **Diversity:** In our skill exercises, we have included examples of individuals from diverse backgrounds (with regard to identities such as age, sexual orientation, culture), with a variety of issues (e.g., sexual dysfunction, life transitions, depression), and types of relationship distress cycles (e.g., pursue–withdraw, pursue–pursue, withdraw–withdraw). However, in the exercises, examples of individuals from explicitly named diverse backgrounds are limited. We found that including fully contextualized examples for every exercise was not possible without shifting the focus of this book and needing to add criteria and more exercises. Although we did not want our book to be devoid of multicultural references, we certainly did not want to provide just a token number in a performative manner either. In wrestling with this conflict, we consulted with a diverse group of EFCT certified therapists, supervisors, and trainers. There were clearly no simple answers. We eventually settled on a compromise solution of some inclusion but not primary focus. Hopefully, others (perhaps you?) will pick up where we left off and contribute further to creating skill-building exercises that can help EFCT therapists practice in culturally sensitive and informed ways.

2. **Relationship composition:** Although the title of this book contains the word *couple* (as does the approach itself!), we wish to acknowledge that there are many people involved in romantic and committed relationships who do not adhere to pair-bonded, monogamous partnerships. Our perspective is that whether the people seeking help are dyads or multiple members forming an attachment group or are in exclusive or explicitly open relationships (or some blended form of the two), the skills outlined in this book are applicable. However, additional EFCT training and even specialization are required to treat more complex relationship configurations successfully. This book does not presume advanced knowledge of EFCT; therefore, almost all the examples herein are based on two-person relationships.

3. **Personal pronouns:** In writing this book, we have tried to use pronouns for the therapist that are gender-neutral (e.g., they/them) so that all trainees will be able to move into the role of therapist more comfortably. In the exercises, we have written the client statements using a variety of personal pronouns (e.g., they/them, he/him, she/her). Trainees role-playing therapists responding to these client statements should try to use the pronouns that the clients prefer in referring to themselves and their partners. Attention to these aspects of the client's identity can be viewed as *microaffirmations* (Fischer et al., 2024).

The EFCT therapist needs to be accustomed to working skillfully with people who hold a variety of identities, with different cultural backgrounds and experiences in the world. Attending to the values of equity and inclusion in a diverse society allows for deeper and more authentic therapeutic relationships. It is critical that the therapist creates a safe enough space to bring topics of identity, power, culture, and difference into the session in the therapy process (PettyJohn et al., 2020). Under appropriate circumstances, conversations initiated by the therapist that attend to identity factors allow both the client and the therapist the opportunity to acknowledge their own positionality, intersectional identities, and points of privilege (Blow et al., 2023). When therapists develop the skills needed to engage sensitively and effectively with their clients, clients feel safe enough to speak openly about issues related to diversity and equity.

We direct readers to the book *Deliberate Practice in Multicultural Therapy* in which Harris and colleagues (2024) present a deliberate practice method for learning and developing the multicultural orientation (MCO) skills involved in manifesting *cultural humility* (open, curious, and oriented to clients' cultural identity), *cultural opportunities* (making use of moments in sessions to explore relevant cultural aspects), and *cultural comfort* (feeling at ease, open, and calm during culturally relevant conversations; Davis et al., 2018). These three pillars of MCO are associated with improvements in psychotherapy outcome and process (Davis et al., 2018; Owen et al., 2011). EFCT trainer Robert Allan has creatively integrated these "three pillars" into his EFCT teaching (personal communication, January, 2024), viewing them as similar to Sue Johnson's (2008) ARE acronym discussed earlier: He relates cultural humility to *accessible*; cultural opportunity to *responsive*; and cultural comfort to emotional *engagement*.

Another way to incorporate cultural aspects into the EFT frame is exemplified by the CARE model, which was an outgrowth of discussions among five prominent EFCT authors (Campbell et al., 2022). Here the letter C in the acronym stands for *context*, which includes

> various facets that shape identity and social location including identity (e.g., race, ethnicity, spirituality, religion, gender, sexuality), environment (e.g., socio-economic, work/organizational, neighbourhood), and related experiences (e.g., ableism, racism, sexism, and discrimination). Context is not a checklist of areas to cover but instead, a lens through which to listen and learn. (p. 1)

Similarly, Calamur and Seiff-Haron in their EFCT trainings include another culturally grounded perspective; theirs emphasizes action by including an S for *systemic change* in their CARES model. This added component highlights the need for actual systems change that might prevent harm to the individual(s) in the future.

We also recommend *Emotionally Focused Therapy With African American Couples: Love Heals* (Guillory, 2022) as another resource that can help EFCT therapists navigate diversity issues, especially when working with African American couples. Guillory (2022) wrote eloquently and with passion about how *race distress cues*, where the Black person's survival feels threatened, are similar to *attachment distress cues*. In a negative cycle, these two types of cues may interact. The sensitive EFCT clinician needs to be aware of how "racism—external or internalized—creates blocks to [the EFCT concepts of] accessibility, responsiveness, and emotional engagement" (Guillory, 2022, p. 201).

In EFCT, we try to see clients in all their diversity, including the beauty that makes their cultural experiences unique, the negative impact discrimination has on them, the growth and resilience they may have developed as a consequence, and the ways all these intersect to influence their inner working models and relationships. Talking about diversity can bring up difficult feelings and/or be used in ways that can cause unintentional pain by people who are still learning to become more culturally humble, aware, and responsible. To that end, when you role-play therapists working with clients who hold identities different from your own, you should try to do so in a culturally sensitive and informed manner without making stereotyped or limiting assumptions. In addition, when you role-play clients who hold an identity you do not share, (e.g., a male reading a female client's statement, a straight person reading a gay client's statement), please do not try to imagine how that person might act or sound. Instead, just follow the adjective descriptors (provided in brackets for every client statement) that suggest what emotional tone you should convey for that statement (e.g., sad, mad, glad).

We fervently hope that all the EFCT microskills presented in this book can be used to broach cultural and cross-cultural matters in ways that explore, expand, and deepen the clients' emotional experience. Although not every skill will function in that fashion for every person, we hope that they all can be useful in different ways for different people. The skills in this book should be practiced in a manner that sensitively considers the psychological and somatic impact of discrimination and immigration. An EFCT therapist needs to keep in mind that a client's attachment history, cultural stressors, trauma history, and unmet attachment needs all influence their internal working model (view of self and other) and that this in turn drives their behavioral reactivity associated with their presenting relationship problems. EFCT has been taught and conducted in many countries by therapists from many cultures, and helpful multicultural and diversity materials and relevant research papers can be found on the ICEEFT website (https://iceeft.com/).

The EFCT Skills Presented in Exercises 1–12

We have included 12 EFCT deliberate practice exercises in this text, each of which focuses on an individual skill. They represent foundational skills in emotionally focused therapy but are not an exhaustive list of all skills and techniques used by emotionally focused couple therapists. We have categorized the skills into three groups: beginner, intermediate, and advanced. The first five exercises represent fundamental EFCT skills, with the next seven skills being more complex (i.e., two intermediate and five advanced), combining and building on previous skills.

Beginner Skills

Each of the beginner skills reflects a key element of EFCT—evocative inquiry, evocative reflections, validating and tracking defensive behaviors, validating inner attachment fears, and deepening emotions—that must be understood before proceeding to other skills at the intermediate and advanced levels. Exercises 1 and 2 use the same set of client statements so that you can practice using a different skill with a different therapeutic intent prompted by the same client statement. Likewise, a new set of identical client statements is used in Exercises 3 through 5, which are designed to build on each other.

Skill 1: Evocative Inquiry

Evocative inquiry is a key technique to help clients become more aware of their feelings and bodily sensations as they speak and listen to their partners. It takes the form of the therapist's asking simple, open-ended questions, but is fundamental in focusing the clients on the importance of their emotions at a feeling and somatic level. In this exercise, the therapist will be speaking to both partners of a couple asking each of them what is going on inside as they say something to their partner, and what is going on inside as they listen to their partner.

Skill 2: Evocative Reflection

Whereas Skill 1 focuses partners on what they are aware of feeling, in this exercise the EFCT therapist tries to evoke a deeper, fuller emotional experience in each partner. Evocative reflection uses techniques such as vivid language, metaphor, and imagery to heighten emotions on the edge of awareness.

Skill 3: Validating Partners' Experiences and Tracking Dysfunctional Patterns

By validating each partner's self-protective (defensive) behaviors, you will strengthen the therapeutic alliance and create a safe space for clients to explore their emotions and experiences. You will help them come to understand the purpose of these self-protective behaviors by using the next skill.

Skill 4: Attachment-Reframed Validation

Using this skill you are not only validating the client's defensive behavioral reaction as understandable but also, more importantly, validating their inner attachment fears and longings that are driving the defense. Here the EFCT therapist begins to link the client's self-protective behavior to deep, vulnerable feelings of longing for connection. In this way, the therapist begins to seed the attachment needs of each partner for the other.

Skill 5: Deepening Emotions With RISSSSC

Finally, using the same client statement for the third time, you will get to practice going even deeper, using your voice to heighten the client's emotional experience of themselves or their partner. Depth of emotional experiencing has been shown to be related to outcome in EFCT. Thus, the capacity to use the prosody, tone, word phrasing, tempo, and timbre of one's voice is a critical EFCT skill. RISSSSC refers to the therapist's voice and phrasing—repeat (R), imagery (I), simple (S), slow (S), soft (S), specific (S), and using the client's words (C)—and is described in more detail later in this chapter. Exercise 5 focuses specifically on the simple, slow, and soft aspects of this skill.

Intermediate Skills

The intermediate skills involve becoming more aware of clients' inner experiences and offering couples a rationale for using EFCT.

Skill 6: Tracking the Therapist's Inner Experience

The format of practicing this skill is different from that of the other skills. Here the therapist does not practice what to say to clients; rather, the goal of this skill is to help therapists become more aware of their inner experiences, including feelings, thoughts, and bodily sensations, while they are listening to their clients. This awareness is known as self-reflection and has to do with what is referred to in EFCT as the *self-of-the-therapist*. By being aware of what they are thinking, feeling, and sensing in their bodies, therapists can better understand how their internal experiences might be at once informing them about their clients while also dynamically influencing their interactions with them. Such inner experiences are important to bring up in EFCT supervision sessions.

Skill 7: Providing a Rationale for EFCT

Often when people come into couple therapy, it is their first time. They probably do not know how couple therapy works—particularly an emotionally focused one. This exercise is designed to help trainees become more comfortable and verbally fluid with explaining EFCT concepts, theory, and interventions to couples. The therapist's being able to answer questions and concerns about EFCT in a matter-of-fact and straightforward manner can lessen the couple's anxiety, build hope, and promote their commitment to do the therapeutic work. It is an essential skill but one that is unfortunately often overlooked in training.

Advanced Skills

The following advanced skills are necessary to help a client make sense of relationship triggers and to distill reactive thoughts, sensations, meanings, and behaviors down to core vulnerable emotions such as sadness, fear, and loneliness. The EFT macrointervention, known as the EFT tango (described earlier), is an empirically supported collection of powerful intervention sequences that explore unmet attachment needs, longings, and fears and then harnesses them into courageous emotionally vulnerable revelations from one partner to another. Skills 8, 9, and 10 were written to be used in a sequence, similar to how the therapist would proceed in actual clinical sessions.

Skill 8: Gathering and Assembling Elements of Emotion

By using a series of questions in a specific order, the therapist helps the client understand in real time what is going on for them at bodily, cognitive, and behavioral levels when having an emotional reaction. In this way EFCT therapists help their clients to "assemble" their emotions to access their experience more clearly and fully with the goal of eventually being able to send a clearer and more vulnerable emotional signal to their partner aided by the therapist using the next skill.

Skill 9: Enactments

This skill focuses on inviting the client to turn to their partner (a choreographed enactment) and tell the partner what the client has learned about their own vulnerable emotional truths. However, sometimes the client refuses the therapist's invitation to do this because it feels too emotionally risky to be that vulnerable. Here the next skill comes to the rescue.

Skill 10: Slicing the Risk Thinner

When the client balks at revealing their vulnerable primary emotions to their partner, the therapist can invite them to express the reasons for their reluctance to share with their partner. This allows the client to communicate their emotions in a slightly less vulnerable ("more thinly sliced") way. With this skill, the therapist learns how to break down overwhelming or risky emotional experiences into smaller, more manageable parts, allowing clients to explore and process them in a safer way.

Skill 11: Catching a Bullet Early in Therapy

"Catching a bullet" is a metaphor used to describe the therapist's skill in intercepting and redirecting ("catching") negative or critical statements ("bullets") between partners during a therapy session. The so-called catching involves softening the emotional blow of a client's aggressive remark on their partner to avoid triggering the partner's reactive (self-protective) move of distancing or attacking back, thus fueling another negative interactional cycle. This skill also involves practicing how to set limits on what is acceptable in session behavior early on in therapy.

Skill 12: Catching a Bullet Later in Therapy

This skill focuses on another bullet-catching occasion later in therapy when the couple's cycle has been de-escalated. In this situation, one member of the couple says something from a place of vulnerability, and their partner mistrusts or minimizes or even denies what was just said and fires off a bullet as a form of attachment protest. To catch the bullet, the therapist must skillfully interrupt the speaking partner, validate any negative feelings engendered in the vulnerable partner, comment on the process, and ask the partner who fired the bullet what was happening for them. Sometimes the therapist can conjecture that the harmful words (the bullet) came from a place of disbelief that their partner could say something so vulnerable—especially if they had been longing to hear that very thing for so long.

A Note About Vocal Tone, Facial Expression, and Body Posture

As EFCT therapists, we are the agents of change. The skills you master will be rendered ineffective unless you bring your whole self into the work. For those doing in-person therapy, sitting close to your clients and leaning forward can signify caring and presence, consistent with attachment theory. Attunement and empathy demand that you use your voice and posture to signal that you are respectfully following or walking beside the couple, gently guiding and reflecting what you hear and see as they share their emotional experiences. Heightening is made possible with the use of a softer, simpler, slower, repetitive tone and, when needed, the use of self-involving, first-person grammar (e.g., "I"). EFCT is a humanistic, experiential, attachment-based therapy that privileges secure connection between therapist and client; therefore, the nonverbal and prosodic cues we use are the "pixie dust" that will make the other skills you are practicing much more meaningful, effective, and powerful. EFCT therapists keep the acronym RISSSSC in mind as it is a useful reminder of how to be with clients during a session. As noted earlier, the RISSSSC elements are as follows:

1. **R:** Repeat what the client is saying.
2. **I:** Use the client's imagery.
3. **S:** Use simple words.
4. **S:** Use a slow pace.
5. **S:** Use a soft voice.
6. **S:** Have a specific focus.
7. **C:** Use the client's words.

As pointed out by Feuerman (2018), therapists' use of RISSSSC is "the most potentiating element" (p. 30) of one's therapeutic presence in using EFCT skills. Practicing RISSSSC as a key EFCT skill (Exercise 5) is of critical importance because it is used liberally throughout the therapy to create emotional deepening. Research has indicated that therapists can modulate the quality of their voice to increase clients' emotional receptivity to approach their partners (Furrow et al., 2012). As EFCT therapists, we see ourselves as "amygdala whisperers." Similar to the parent–infant bond, where the parent can soothe a distressed infant's nervous system with a soft, soothing, and gentle way of speaking, so too can an EFCT therapist gently soothe their client's sympathetic nervous system. Reflections and insights are repeated numerous times as a way of aiding the client to resonate with the underlying emotional experience, attachment-reframed meaning, and views of self or other. As the therapist repeats the clients' words and uses the clients' own imagery, resistance and reactivity decrease, allowing for new, previously blocked information to come forth.

The Role of Deliberate Practice in EFCT Training

Training in EFCT takes place mainly through oversight provided by the ICEEFT based in Ottawa, Canada, and led by Johnson and the ICEEFT Board of Directors. Therapists interested in learning EFCT typically have earned or are in the process of obtaining graduate degrees in mental health treatment. They typically start their training in EFCT with a 4-day EFCT externship, led by certified EFCT trainers. This training offers a comprehensive introduction to the EFCT model, focusing on the science of attachment and the systematic approach to couple therapy.

The externship is usually followed by 24 to 48 hours of classes in core skills where students practice skills using traditional, spontaneous role-play exercises. There are also classes that go beyond core skills, as well as numerous master classes related to the treatment of trauma, addiction, attachment injuries, sexuality, and partner violence. Trainees interested in becoming certified as EFCT therapists by ICEEFT additionally participate in a minimum of 8 hours of clinical supervision, where they show recordings of their therapy sessions and get feedback from EFCT certified supervisors.

Because of EFCT's long-standing emphasis on experiential learning, deliberate practice exercises could easily be inserted at every stage of EFCT training. Especially during core skills, beyond core skills, and individual and group supervision, deliberate practice provides an ideal mechanism to teach and assess mastery.

For a full listing of training requirements and resources, see the ICEEFT website (https://iceeft.com/).

Overview of the Book's Structure

This book is organized into three parts. Part I contains this chapter and Chapter 2, which provides basic instructions on how to perform these exercises. We found through testing that providing too many instructions up front overwhelmed trainers and trainees, and as a result, they skipped past them. Therefore, we kept these instructions as brief and simple as possible to focus only on the most essential information that trainers and trainees will need to get started with the exercises. Further guidelines for getting the most about deliberate practice are provided in Chapter 3, and additional instructions for monitoring and adjusting the difficulty of the exercises are provided in Appendix A. **Do not skip the instructions in Chapter 2, and be sure to read the additional guidelines and instructions in Chapter 3 and Appendix A once you are comfortable with the basic instructions.**

Part II contains the 12 skill-focused exercises, which are divided into three categories based on their difficulty: beginner, intermediate, and advanced (see Table 1.1). Each exercise contains a brief overview of the exercise, example client–therapist interactions to help guide trainees, step-by-step instructions for conducting that exercise, and a list of criteria for mastering the relevant skill. The client statements and sample therapist responses are then presented, also organized by difficulty (beginner, intermediate, and advanced). The statements and responses are presented separately so that the trainee playing the therapist has more freedom to improvise responses without being influenced by the sample responses, which should only be turned to if the trainee has difficulty improvising their own responses. The last two exercises in Part II provide opportunities to practice the 12 skills within simulated psychotherapy sessions. Exercise 13 provides a sample psychotherapy session transcript in which the EFCT skills are used and clearly labeled, thereby demonstrating how they might flow together in an actual couple therapy session. EFCT trainees are invited to run through the sample transcript with one playing the therapist and two others playing the partners in the couple to get a feel for how a session might unfold. Exercise 14 provides suggestions for undertaking mock sessions, as well as couple profiles ordered by difficulty (beginner, intermediate, and advanced) that trainees can use for improvised role-plays.

Part III contains Chapter 3, which provides additional guidance for trainers and trainees. While Chapter 2 is more procedural, Chapter 3 covers big-picture issues. It highlights six key points for getting the most out of deliberate practice and describes the importance of appropriate responsiveness, attending to trainee well-being and respecting their privacy, and trainer self-evaluation, among other topics.

Three appendixes conclude this book. Appendix A provides instructions for monitoring and adjusting the difficulty of each exercise as needed. It provides a Deliberate Practice Reaction Form for the trainee playing the therapist to complete to indicate whether the exercise is too easy or too difficult. Appendix B includes a Deliberate Practice Diary Form that can be used during a training session's final evaluation to process the trainees' experiences, but its primary purpose is to provides trainees a format to explore and record their experiences while engaging in additional, between-session deliberate practice activities without the supervisor. Appendix C presents a sample syllabus demonstrating how the 12 deliberate practice exercises and other support material can be integrated into a wider EFCT training course. Instructors may choose to modify the syllabus or pick elements of it to integrate into their own courses.

Downloadable versions of this book's appendixes, including a color version of the Deliberate Practice Reaction Form, can be found in the "Resources" tab online (https://www.apa.org/pubs/books/deliberate-practice-emotionally-focused-couple-therapy).

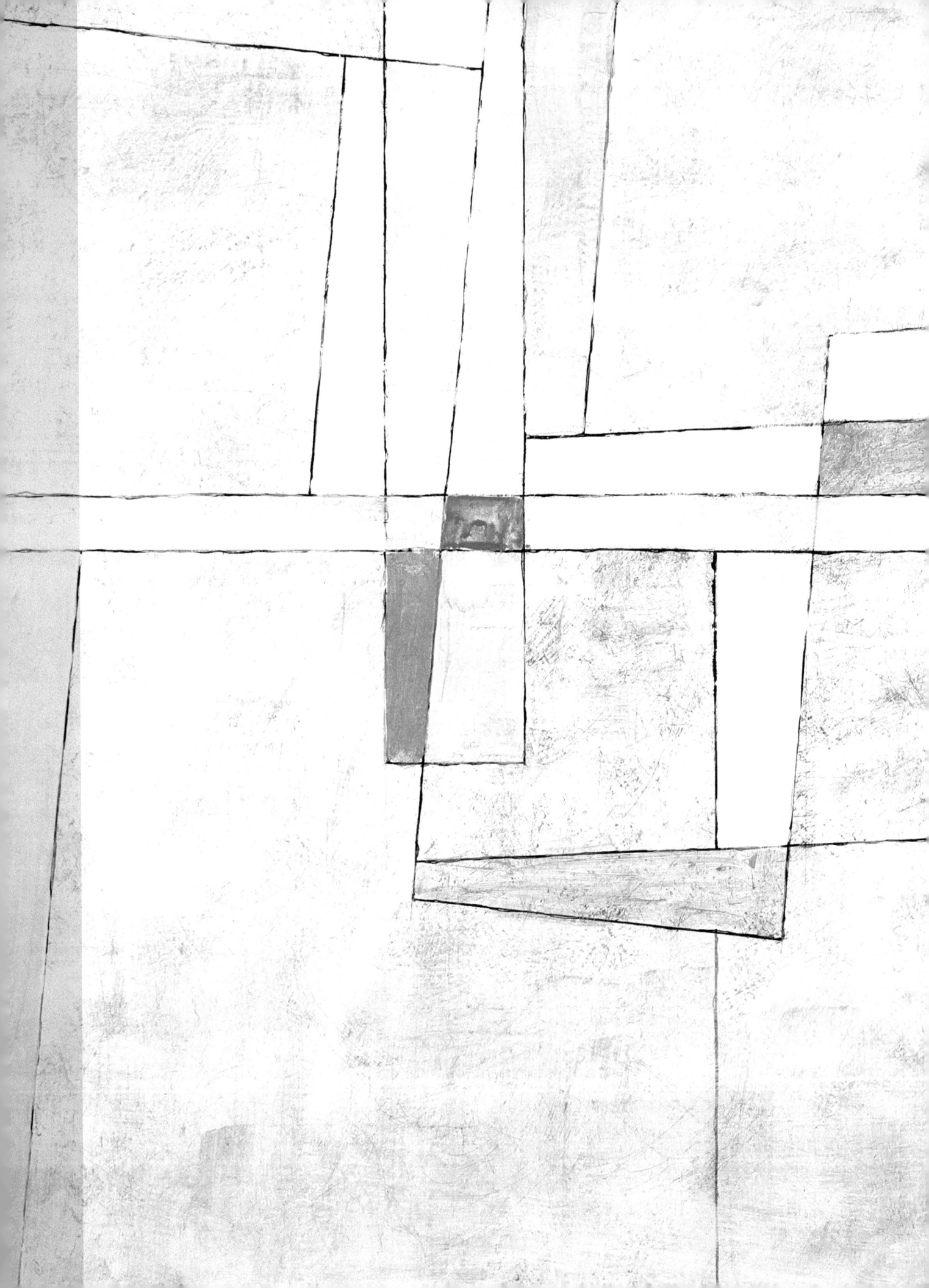

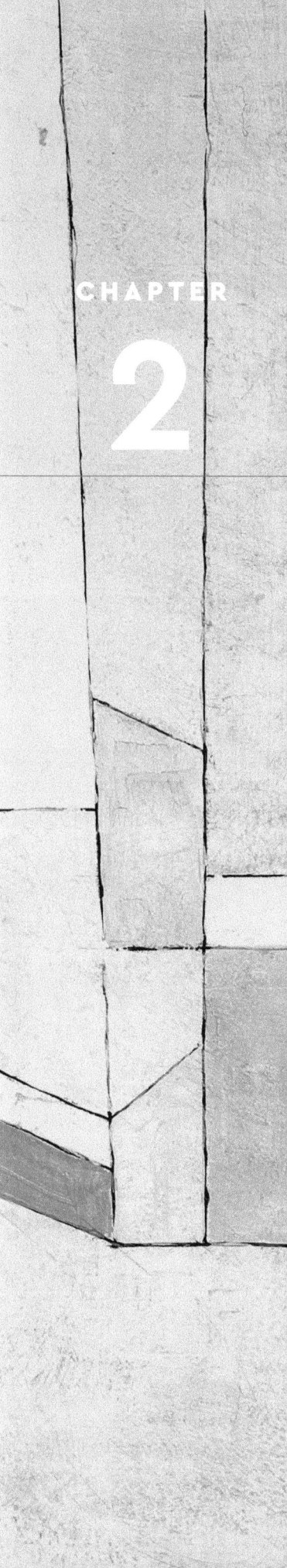

Instructions for the Emotionally Focused Couple Therapy Deliberate Practice Exercises

This chapter provides basic instructions that are common to all the exercises in this book. More specific instructions are provided in each exercise. Chapter 3 also provides important guidance for trainees and trainers that will help them get the most out of deliberate practice. Appendix A offers additional instructions for monitoring and adjusting the difficulty of the exercises as needed after getting through all the client statements in a single difficulty level, including a Deliberate Practice Reaction Form the trainee playing the therapist can complete to indicate whether they found the statements too easy or too difficult. **Difficulty assessment is an important part of the deliberate practice process and should not be skipped.**

Overview

The deliberate practice exercises in this book involve role-plays of hypothetical situations in therapy. The role-plays typically involve three people: One trainee role-plays the therapist, another trainee role-plays the client, and a trainer (professor/supervisor) observes and provides feedback. Alternatively, a peer can observe and provide feedback. For the last exercise, a third trainee role-plays the client's partner. Exercise 6 is unique in that two trainees act as fellow therapists with one expressing their inner experiences to the other.

This book provides a script for each role-play, each with a client statement and also with an example therapist response. The client statements are graded in difficulty from beginner to advanced, although these difficulty grades are only estimates. The actual perceived difficulty of client statements is very subjective and varies widely by trainee. For example, some trainees may experience a stimulus of a client being angry to be easy to respond to, whereas another trainee may experience it as very difficult. Thus, it is important for trainees to provide difficulty assessments and adjustments to ensure that they are practicing at the right difficulty level: neither too easy nor too hard.

https://doi.org/10.1037/0000436-002

Deliberate Practice in Emotionally Focused Couple Therapy, by H. Levenson, S. Jinich, A. Vaz, and T. Rousmaniere

Time Frame

We recommend a 90-minute time block for every exercise, structured roughly as follows:

- First 20 minutes: Orientation. The trainer explains the EFCT skill and demonstrates the exercise procedure with a volunteer trainee.

- Middle 50 minutes: Trainees perform the exercise in pairs. The trainer or a peer provides feedback throughout this process and monitors/adjusts the exercise's difficulty as needed after each set of statements (see Appendix A for more information about difficulty assessment).

- Final 20 minutes: Review, feedback, and discussion.

Preparation

1. Every trainee will need their own copy of this book.

2. Each exercise requires the trainer to fill out a Deliberate Practice Reaction Form after completing all the statements from a single difficulty level. The trainees should also complete a Deliberate Practice Diary Form during a training session's final evaluation and/or between sessions, particularly during additional deliberate practice activities. These forms are available online at https://www.apa.org/pubs/books/deliberate-practice-emotionally-focused-couple-therapy (see the "Resources" tab) and in Appendixes A and B, respectively.

3. Trainees are grouped into pairs for most exercises. One volunteers to role-play the therapist and one to role-play the client, except in Exercise 6 where the second trainee will play a colleague. The trainees will switch roles after 15 minutes of practice. In most exercises, the trainee playing the client will act as one partner in a couple with both they and the therapist imagining the other partner is there. In Exercises 8, 9, and 10, the trainee role-playing the client will alternate between playing both partners, although only one partner speaks at a time. Exercise 12 requires three trainees: one playing the therapist and two playing partners in a couple talking to each other. As noted previously, an observer who might be either the trainer or a fellow trainee will work with the trainees for every exercise.

The Role of the Trainer

The primary responsibilities of the trainer are to

1. provide corrective feedback, which includes both information about how well the trainees' response met expected criteria and any necessary guidance about how to improve the response, and

2. remind trainees to do difficulty assessments and adjustments after each level of client statements is completed (beginner, intermediate, and advanced).

How to Practice

Each exercise includes its own step-by-step instructions. Trainees should follow these instructions carefully because every step is important.

Skill Criteria

Each of the first 12 exercises focuses on one essential skill with skill criteria that describe the important components or principles for that skill.

The goal of the role-play is for trainees to practice improvising responses to the client statement in a manner that (a) is attuned to the client, (b) meets skill criteria as closely as possible, and (c) feels authentic for the trainee. Trainees are provided scripts with example therapist responses to give them a sense of how to incorporate the skill criteria into a response. **It is important, however, that trainees do not read the example responses verbatim in the role-plays!** Therapy is highly personal and improvisational; the goal of deliberate practice is to develop trainees' ability to improvise within a consistent framework. Memorizing scripted responses would be counterproductive for helping trainees learn to perform therapy that is responsive, authentic, and attuned to each individual client.

The authors (with input from other EFCT practitioners, supervisors, and trainers) wrote the scripted example responses. However, trainees' personal style of therapy may differ slightly or greatly from that in the example scripts. It is essential that, over time, trainees develop their own style and voice, while simultaneously being able to intervene according to the model's principles and strategies. To facilitate this, the exercises in this book were designed to maximize opportunities for improvisational responses informed by the skill criteria and ongoing feedback.

Review, Feedback, and Discussion

The review and feedback sequence after each role-play has these two elements:

- First, the trainee who played the client **briefly** shares how it felt to be on the receiving end of the therapist response. This can help assess how well trainees are attuning with the client.

- Second, the trainer provides **brief** feedback (less than 1 minute) based on the skill criteria for each exercise. Keep feedback specific, behavioral, and brief to preserve time for skill rehearsal. If one trainer is teaching multiple pairs of trainees, the trainer walks around the room, observing the pairs and offering brief feedback. When the trainer is not available, the trainee playing the client gives peer feedback to the therapist, based on the skill criteria and how it felt to be on the receiving end of the intervention. Alternately, a third trainee can observe and provide feedback.

Trainers (or peers) should remember to keep all feedback specific and brief and not to veer into discussions of theory. There are many other settings for extended discussion of EFCT theory and research. In deliberate practice, it is of utmost importance to maximize time for continuous behavioral rehearsal via role-plays.

Final Feedback

After both trainees have role-played the client and the therapist, the trainer provides some specific overall feedback followed by a short group discussion based on this feedback. This discussion can provide ideas for where to focus homework and future deliberate practice sessions. To this end, Appendix B presents a Deliberate Practice Diary Form, which can also be downloaded from the "Resources" tab online (https://www.apa.org/pubs/books/deliberate-practice-emotionally-focused-couple-therapy). This form can be used as part of the final feedback to help trainees process their experiences from that session with the supervisor. However, it is designed primarily to be used by trainees as a template for exploring and recording their thoughts and experiences between sessions, particularly when pursuing additional deliberate practice activities without the supervisor, such as rehearsing responses alone or if two trainees want to practice the exercises together, perhaps with a third trainee filling the supervisor's role. Then, if they want, the trainees can discuss these experiences with the supervisor at the beginning of the next training session.

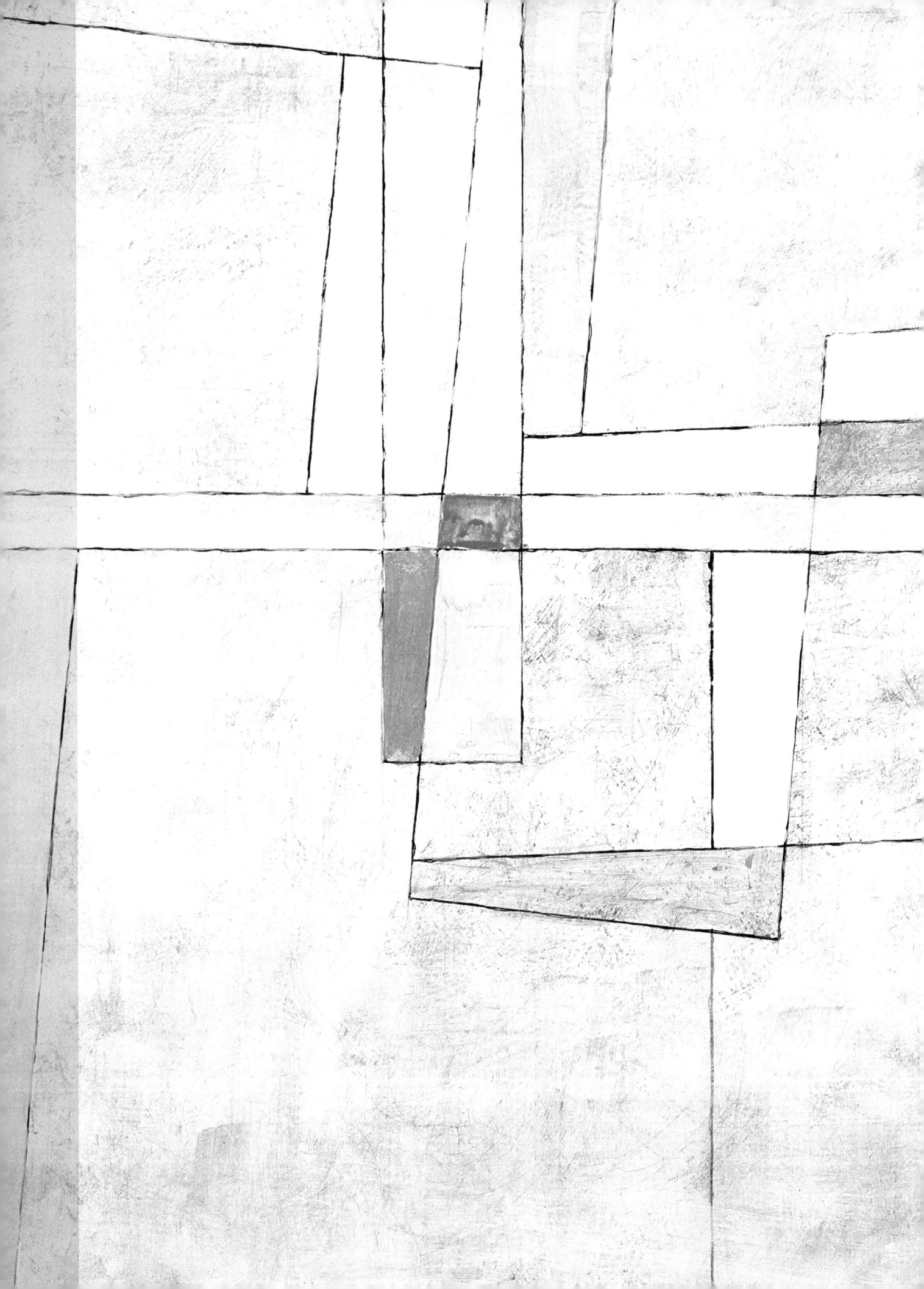

Deliberate Practice Exercises for Emotionally Focused Couple Therapy Skills

This part of the book presents 12 deliberate practice exercises for essential emotionally focused couple therapy (EFCT) skills. These exercises are divided into two groups—those that are more appropriate to someone just beginning EFCT training and those who have progressed to a more advanced level. Although we anticipate that most trainers would use these exercises in the order we have suggested, some trainers may find it more appropriate to their training circumstances to use a different order. We also provide two comprehensive exercises that bring together the EFCT skills using an annotated EFCT session transcript and mock EFCT sessions.

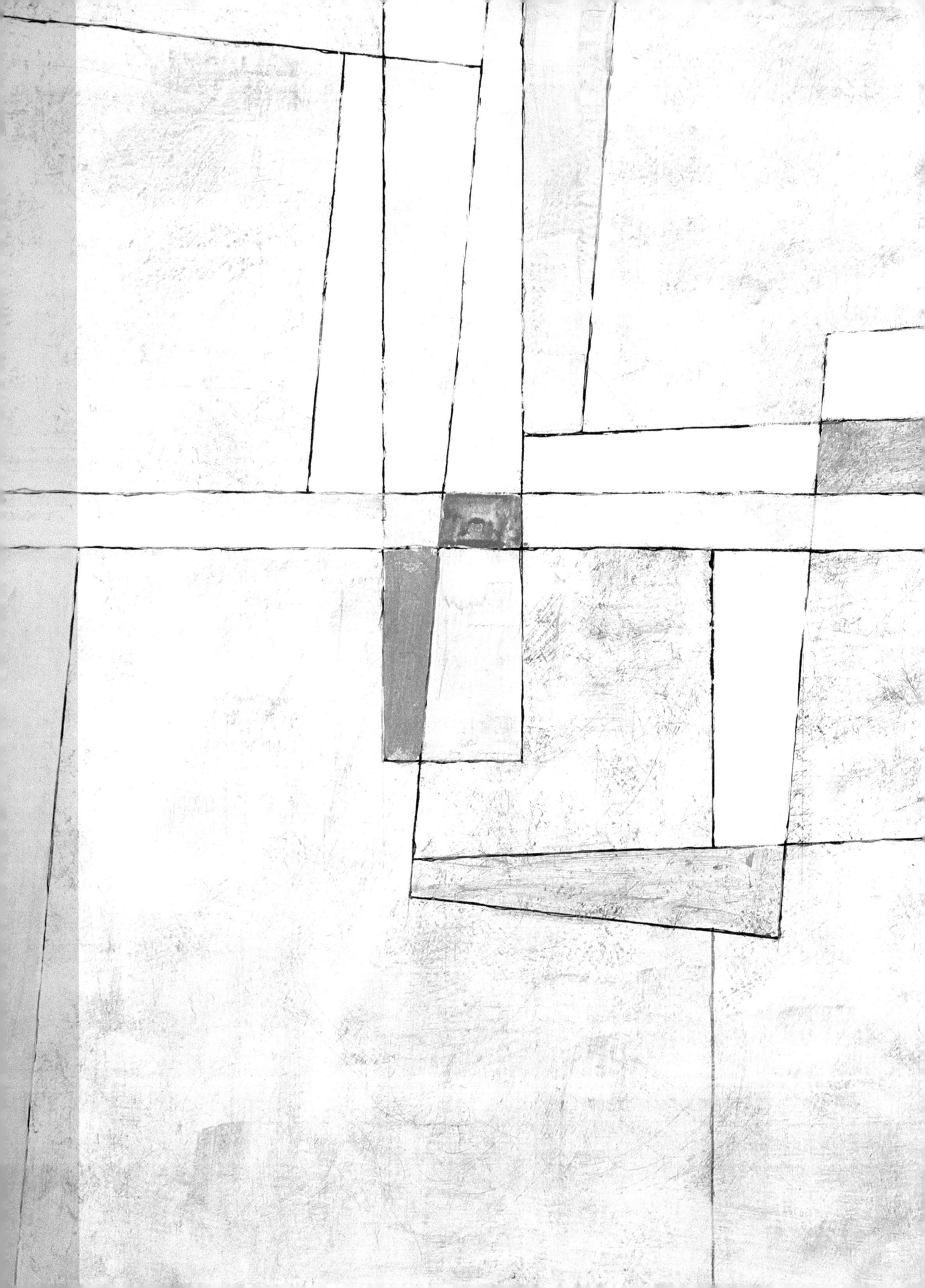

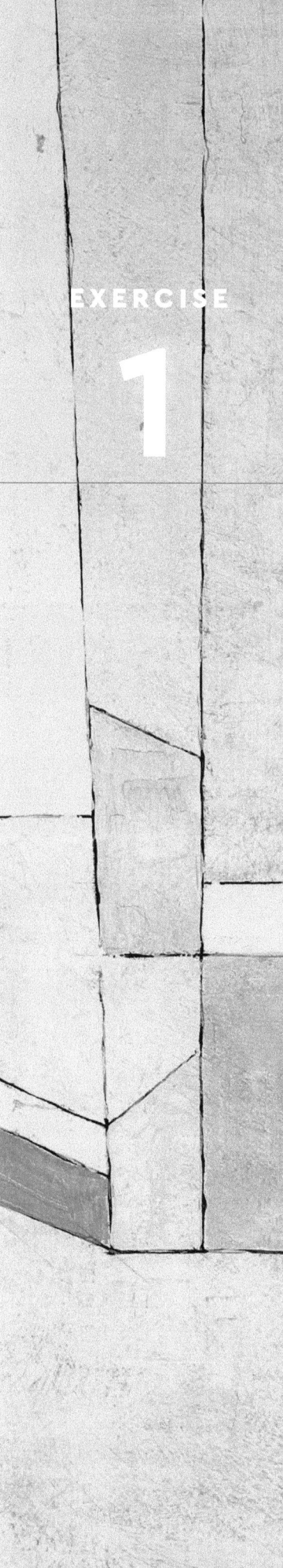

Evocative Inquiry: Identifying Patterns and Eliciting Attachment Fears and Needs

Preparations for Exercise 1

1. Read the instructions in Chapter 2.

2. Download the Deliberate Practice Reaction Form and the Deliberate Practice Diary Form at https://www.apa.org/pubs/books/deliberate-practice-emotionally-focused-couple-therapy (see the "Resources" tab; also available in Appendixes A and B, respectively).

Exercise Format

For this skill, you will need two trainees: one role-playing the therapist and one role-playing the client ("Partner 1"). The context for the skill is a couple therapy session where the therapist will be addressing both partners about only what "Partner 1" is saying.

Skill Description

Skill Difficulty Level: Beginner

Evocative inquiry is a key technique to help couples explore and understand their emotions and attachment needs. It involves the therapist asking open-ended questions and making empathetic statements to evoke and deepen emotional experiences further. It also helps partners have a better understanding of their unmet attachment longings and facilitates a safe and supportive environment where couples can explore their emotional experiences more deeply.

Evocative inquiry appears as simple, open-ended questions, but it quickly becomes a gateway for the therapist to reflect, expand, deepen, validate, empathize, and reframe

https://doi.org/10.1037/0000436-003

Deliberate Practice in Emotionally Focused Couple Therapy, by H. Levenson, S. Jinich, A. Vaz, and T. Rousmaniere

the client's experiences from an attachment perspective. The emotionally focused couple therapist is "evoking" emotional material that they then explore further. It is a tool for exploration rather than explanation, and it is not intended to put the client into an intellectually discursive or rationalizing mode; rather, it is designed to help individuals connect with their emotions and gain insight into their attachment patterns and needs.

The therapist's task is to improvise a response to each client statement following these skill criteria:

1. **Ask an open-ended question inviting Partner 1 to explore either (Option 1) their feelings or (Option 2) their bodily sensations about what they just said.** For example, for Option 1: "How do you feel listening to yourself talk about . . . ?" or for Option 2: "What's happening inside your body as you talk about . . . ?"

2. **Ask an open-ended question inviting Partner 2 to explore either (Option 1) their feelings or (Option 2) their bodily sensations about what Partner 1 just said.** For example, for Option 1: "How do you feel when your partner says . . . ?" or for Option 2: "What is happening inside your body as you listen to your partner talk about . . . ?"

Note: This exercise uses the same client statements as Exercise 2 so that trainees can get used to responding to the same prompts using different skills.

SKILL CRITERIA FOR EXERCISE 1

1. Ask an open-ended question inviting Partner 1 to explore one of the following options:
   - **Option 1: Their feelings.**
   - **Option 2: Their body sensations about what they just said.**
2. Ask an open-ended question inviting Partner 2 to explore one of the following options:
   - **Option 1:** Their **feelings.**
   - **Option 2:** Their **body** sensations about what Partner 1 just said.

Note: The descriptive words in bold here ("tags") and in the examples below are mnemonic devices to help you remember the criteria and their order.

HELPFUL HINTS FOR EXERCISE 1

1. For all the exercises, the therapist should respond using the pronouns used by the clients.
2. For this exercise, please assume that the therapist has a good relationship with the couple and has been working with them for a while.
3. Although no trainee will actually be playing Partner 2 in this exercise, the therapist should still address Partner 2 directly, as if they are also in the room.

Examples of Therapists Using Evocative Inquiry

Example 1

PARTNER 1: [*sad*] I really missed my partner. He traveled for a whole month, and I only got to see him once.

THERAPIST: [to Partner 1] What are you feeling right now as you talk about how much you missed your partner? (Criterion 1, Option 1—**Feelings**)

or

How is your body reacting as you talk about how much you missed your partner? (Criterion 1, Option 2—**Body**)

THERAPIST: [to Partner 2] What are you feeling as you hear that your partner missed you so much? (Criterion 2, Option 1—**Feelings**)

or

What's it like in your body for you to hear that your partner missed you so much? (Criterion 2, Option 2—**Body**)

Example 2

PARTNER 1: [*irritated*] Nothing I ever do is enough to make my partner satisfied.

THERAPIST: [to Partner 1] How are you feeling as you talk about how you can never satisfy your partner? (Criterion 1, Option 1—**Feelings**)

or

What is happening inside your body as you talk about how you can never satisfy your partner? (Criterion 1, Option 2—**Body**)

THERAPIST: [to Partner 2] How are you feeling listening to your partner saying no matter what they do, they can never satisfy you. (Criterion 2, Option 1—**Feelings**)

or

What is happening inside your body as you hear your partner talk about their frustration of never being able to satisfy you? (Criterion 2, Option 2—**Body**)

Example 3

PARTNER 1: [*angry*] You should have seen the pep in his step as he offered and helped our next-door neighbor carry her groceries into her house. I never see that kind of energy directed at what I need.

THERAPIST: [to Partner 1] How are you feeling as you talk about how you don't get from your partner what you see him give to others? (Criterion 1, Option 1—**Feelings**)

or

What happens in your body as you recall seeing your partner offer so much more of himself to the neighbor than he makes available to you? (Criterion 1, Option 2—**Body**)

THERAPIST: [to Partner 2] What do you feel when you hear your partner compare how much more enthusiastic you seem when offering your neighbor help, compared to when your own partner needs your help? (Criterion 2, Option 1—**Feelings**)

or

What do you feel in your body when you hear how much more enthusiastic you seem to be when helping your neighbor than your own partner? (Criterion 2, Option 2—**Body**)

INSTRUCTIONS FOR EXERCISE 1

Step 1: Role-Play and Feedback

- The client (Partner 1) says the first beginner client statement. The therapist **improvises** a response based on the skill criteria and delivers it to Partner 1 then improvises another response to Partner 2.
- The trainer (or, if not available, the client) provides **brief** feedback based on the skill criteria.
- The client then repeats the same statement, and the therapist again improvises a response. The trainer (or client) again provides brief feedback.

Step 2: Repeat

- Repeat Step 1 for all the statements **in the current difficulty level** (beginner, intermediate, or advanced).

Step 3: Assess and Adjust Difficulty

- The therapist completes the Deliberate Practice Reaction Form (see Appendix A) and decides whether to make the exercise easier or harder or to repeat the same difficulty level.

Step 4: Repeat for Approximately 15 Minutes

- Repeat Steps 1 through 3 for at least 15 minutes.
- The trainees then switch therapist/client roles and start over.

Now it's your turn! Follow Steps 1 and 2 from the instructions.

Remember: The goal of the role-play is for trainees to practice improvising responses to the client statements in a manner that (a) uses the skill criteria and (b) feels authentic for the trainee. **Example therapist responses for each client statement are provided at the end of this exercise. Trainees should attempt to improvise their own responses before reading the examples.**

BEGINNER-LEVEL CLIENT STATEMENTS FOR EXERCISE 1
Beginner Client Statement 1
[Sad] I really missed my partner. He traveled for a whole month, and I only got to see him once.
Beginner Client Statement 2
[Delighted] Yesterday, she looked at me with one of those warm, beautiful smiles I used to see years ago. I haven't seen one of those for a long time.
Beginner Client Statement 3
[Happy] And out of the blue, this week my partner told me they appreciated all I was doing to make our marriage better.
Beginner Client Statement 4
[Delighted] When I wasn't feeling well, he sent me several texts during the day with smiley faces and a message showing he was thinking of me.
Beginner Client Statement 5
[Smiling] On my birthday, she gave me a thoughtful gift and note apologizing for all the years she didn't remember.

Assess and adjust the difficulty before moving to the next difficulty level (see Step 3 in the exercise instructions).

INTERMEDIATE-LEVEL CLIENT STATEMENTS FOR EXERCISE 1
Intermediate Client Statement 1
[Frustrated] We don't speak all day, and we hardly connect at all during dinner, then at night in bed, he wants to get physically close. Why should I want to?
Intermediate Client Statement 2
[Frustrated] Every time I try to say something meaningful to her, she gets defensive or tunes me out. I'm tired of only being able to talk to my friends about things that are important to me.
Intermediate Client Statement 3
[Hurt] Even though I know that we both love each other very much, there is very little left between us. Maybe we are no longer supposed to be together. I don't know if he even remembers the last time we kissed!
Intermediate Client Statement 4
[Frustrated, to partner] I know I said I was leaving in 5 minutes, but something came up at the last minute that made me late. I don't know if she can trust that I have good intentions.
Intermediate Client Statement 5
[Sad] I hear his critical tone of voice, and I know we are going to have a fight. So I get defensive and then I shut down.

🛑 **Assess and adjust the difficulty before moving to the next difficulty level (see Step 3 in the exercise instructions).**

ADVANCED-LEVEL CLIENT STATEMENTS FOR EXERCISE 1
Advanced Client Statement 1
[Hurt, to partner] I don't really know how I am ever going to be able to trust you again. Everything seems different to me now.
Advanced Client Statement 2
[Frustrated] I would love to feel like I am enough just as I am. For years what I heard was how I didn't measure up.
Advanced Client Statement 3
[Sad] I feel excluded by my own family. I come home from work and it's like she and the kids have their little club that I don't belong to.
Advanced Client Statement 4
[Hurt] No matter how hard I try, or how loud I get, she says absolutely nothing. She just looks through me while I'm talking.
Advanced Client Statement 5
[Angry] He gives me the silent treatment and looks at me like I'm dangerous. I'm his life partner, not his enemy! I don't want this anymore.

Assess and adjust the difficulty here (see Step 3 in the exercise instructions). If appropriate, follow the instructions to make the exercise even more challenging (see Appendix A).

Example Therapist Responses: Evocative Inquiry

Remember: Trainees should attempt to improvise their own responses before reading the example responses. **Do not read the following responses verbatim unless you are having trouble coming up with your own responses!**

EXAMPLE RESPONSES TO BEGINNER-LEVEL CLIENT STATEMENTS FOR EXERCISE 1
Example Response to Beginner Client Statement 1
To Partner 1 • **Option 1:** What are you feeling right now as you talk about how much you missed your partner? • **Option 2:** How is your body reacting as you talk about how much you missed your partner? To Partner 2 • **Option 1:** What are you feeling as you hear that your partner missed you so much? • **Option 2:** What's it like in your body for you to hear that your partner missed you so much?
Example Response to Beginner Client Statement 2
To Partner 1 • **Option 1:** How do you feel when you recall the lovely way that she looked at you? • **Option 2:** What happens in your body right now as you recall the lovely way that she looked at you? To Partner 2 • **Option 1:** How does it feel to hear your partner delight in the way you looked at him and to hear him notice how long it's been since you looked at him this way? • **Option 2:** What happens in your body when you hear your partner delight in the way you looked at him or when he notices how long it's been since you looked at him this way?
Example Response to Beginner Client Statement 3
To Partner 1 • **Option 1:** How did you feel when you heard that from your partner? • **Option 2:** What did you sense in your body when you heard that from your partner? To Partner 2 • **Option 1:** What do you feel when you hear your partner tell me about your appreciation? • **Option 2:** What's it like in your body when you hear your partner tell me about your appreciation?

EXAMPLE RESPONSES TO BEGINNER-LEVEL CLIENT STATEMENTS FOR EXERCISE 1

Example Response to Beginner Client Statement 4

To Partner 1

- **Option 1:** How is that for you emotionally to be kept in mind and to receive that level of concern?

- **Option 2:** What is it like in your body as you recall how, when you weren't feeling well, he kept you in mind and wrote you several text messages showing he was thinking of you?

To Partner 2

- **Option 1:** How do you feel when he shares how attentive you were toward him?

- **Option 2:** What's it like in your body when you hear him talk about how attentive you were toward him?

Example Response to Beginner Client Statement 5

To Partner 1

- **Option 1:** How did it feel to have your day recognized in that way, especially with the acknowledgment of not remembering for all of those years?

- **Option 2:** What is it like in your body to have your day recognized in that way, especially with the acknowledgment of not remembering for all of those years?

To Partner 2

- **Option 1:** How did it feel just now to hear him acknowledging your thoughtfulness as well as your apology?

- **Option 2:** What happens in your body when he acknowledges your thoughtfulness and your apology?

EXAMPLE RESPONSES TO INTERMEDIATE-LEVEL CLIENT STATEMENTS FOR EXERCISE 1

Example Response to Intermediate Client Statement 1

To Partner 1

- **Option 1:** What are you feeling right now as you talk about this?

- **Option 2:** What is it like in your body as you talk about this?

To Partner 2

- **Option 1:** How are you feeling right now as you hear your partner talk about there being no connection between you all day and then you wanting to get physically close?

- **Option 2:** What happens in your body when your partner talks about there being no connection between you all day and then you wanting to get physically close?

Example Response to Intermediate Client Statement 2

To Partner 1

- **Option 1:** How do you feel as you talk about this?

- **Option 2:** What is happening right now in your body as you talk about this?

To Partner 2

- **Option 1:** What happens emotionally to you when you hear him complain that you react defensively or that you shut down when he tries to talk to you about something important?

- **Option 2:** What happens in your body when you hear him complain that you react defensively or that you shut down when he tries to talk to you about something important?

Example Response to Intermediate Client Statement 3

To Partner 1

- **Option 1:** What are you feeling right now as you wonder if the two of you are no longer supposed to be together?

- **Option 2:** What happens in your body when you wonder if you should be together?

To Partner 2

- **Option 1:** How do you feel as you hear "Maybe we are no longer supposed to be together"?

- **Option 2:** What happens in your body as you hear "Maybe we are no longer supposed to be together"?

Example Response to Intermediate Client Statement 4

To Partner 1

- **Option 1:** What are you feeling right now as you ask to be trusted?

- **Option 2:** What does it feel like in your body when your good intentions are not trusted?

To Partner 2

- **Option 1:** What do you feel when he says to you "trust me that I have good intentions"?

- **Option 2:** What happens in your body when you're asked to trust his good intentions?

EXAMPLE RESPONSES TO INTERMEDIATE-LEVEL CLIENT STATEMENTS FOR EXERCISE 1
Example Response to Intermediate Client Statement 5

To Partner 1

- **Option 1:** Tell me more about that. How do you feel when you hear his critical tone?

- **Option 2:** Tell me about that. Where do you feel it in your body when you hear his critical tone?

To Partner 2

- **Option 1:** How are you feeling right now as you hear her say that your critical tone is a cue that you will inevitably have a fight and that it leads her to get defensive and to shut down?

- **Option 2:** What happens on your side? What goes on in your body when you hear your partner talking about your critical tone and how it leads her to get defensive or shut down?

EXAMPLE RESPONSES TO ADVANCED-LEVEL CLIENT STATEMENTS FOR EXERCISE 1

Example Response to Advanced Client Statement 1

To Partner 1

- **Option 1:** How do you feel emotionally right now, as you say, "Everything seems different to me now"?
- **Option 2:** What happens in your body when you say you can never trust your partner again and that everything has changed?

To Partner 2

- **Option 1:** How do you feel when your partner tells you that they can never trust you again and that everything has changed?
- **Option 2:** Can you check in with your body right now? How does it react when you hear your partner say that you can never be trusted again and that everything has changed?

Example Response to Advanced Client Statement 2

To Partner 1

- **Option 1:** How do you feel right now, deep down, as you say, "I would love to hear that I am enough just as I am?"
- **Option 2:** Do you notice anything in your body right now as you say how much you long to hear that you are enough, just as you are?

To Partner 2

- **Option 1:** Can you tell me what you're feeling as you hear that your partner would love to hear that he is enough?
- **Option 2:** What do you notice in your body just now as you hear that your partner would love to hear from you that he is enough?

Example Response to Advanced Client Statement 3

To Partner 1

- **Option 1:** How does it feel not to belong?
- **Option 2:** What happens in your body as you relate your experience of being on the outside?

To Partner 2

- **Option 1:** How do you feel when he says he feels excluded, as if he isn't part of your club?
- **Option 2:** Can you tell me what happens in your body when he describes feeling excluded by you and the kids?

EXAMPLE RESPONSES TO ADVANCED-LEVEL CLIENT STATEMENTS FOR EXERCISE 1

Example Response to Advanced Client Statement 4

To Partner 1

- **Option 1:** What do you feel when she says absolutely nothing, or when she looks straight through you?

- **Option 2:** What are you experiencing in your body right now as you describe how she looks through you when you try to talk to her?

To Partner 2

- **Option 1:** How do you feel when he describes you as being so nonresponsive, no matter how hard he tries to get through to you?

- **Option 2:** When you hear him talk about your nonresponsiveness, can you tell me what happens in your body?

Example Response to Advanced Client Statement 5

To Partner 1

- **Option 1:** What were you feeling just now, as you said, "I don't want the silent treatment or the anger anymore"?

- **Option 2:** What is happening with your body as you let him know that you are not the enemy?

To Partner 2

- **Option 1:** Tell me how you feel emotionally right now as you hear her say, "I'm not the enemy. I'm not dangerous. I don't want this anymore"?

- **Option 2:** What happens in your body when she says that all she gets is the silent treatment and anger from you?

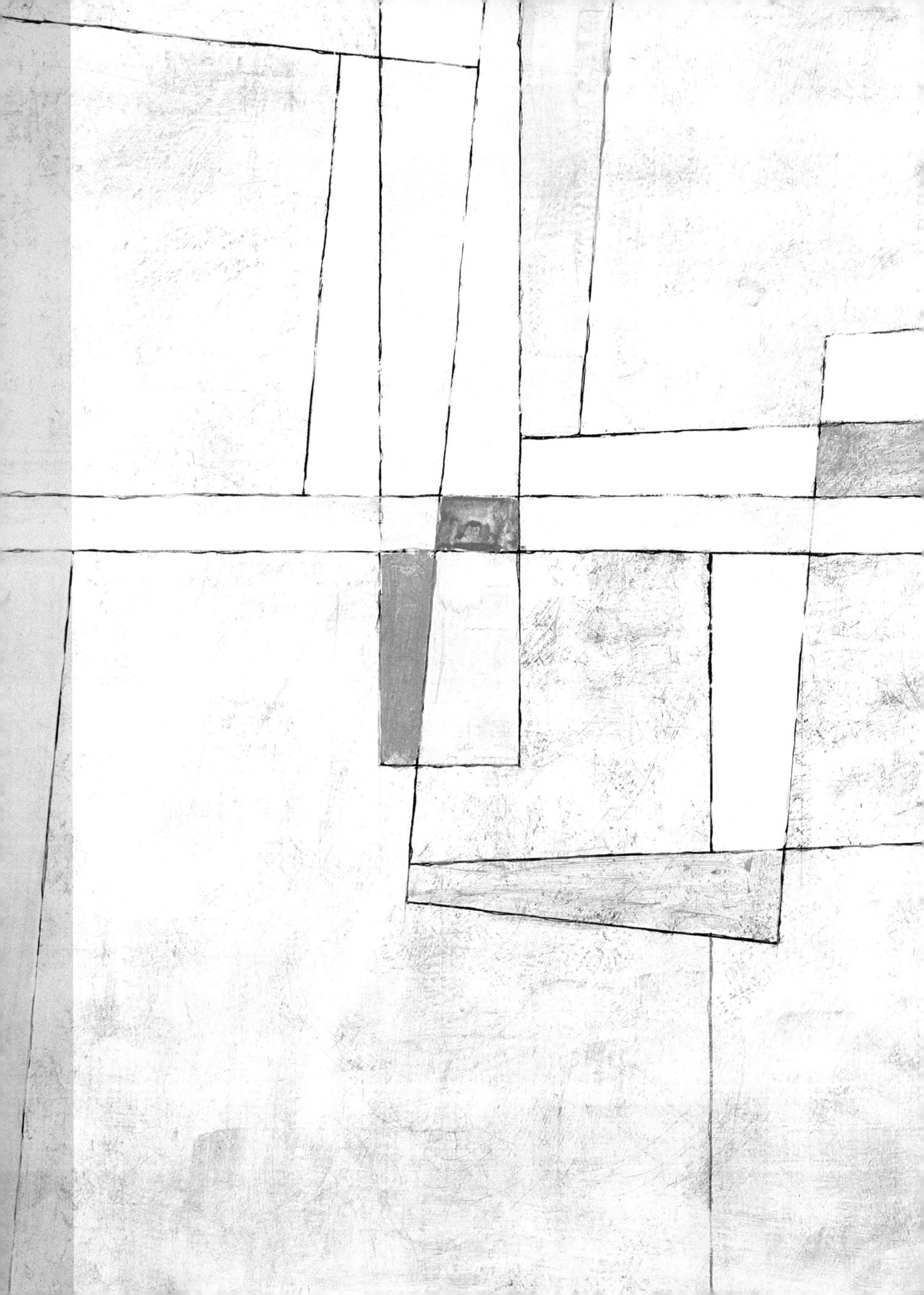

Evocative Reflection: Eliciting and Heightening Emotional Experience

Preparations for Exercise 2

1. Read the instructions in Chapter 2.

2. Download the Deliberate Practice Reaction Form and the Deliberate Practice Diary Form at https://www.apa.org/pubs/books/deliberate-practice-emotionally-focused-couple-therapy (see the "Resources" tab; also available in Appendixes A and B, respectively).

Exercise Format

For this skill, you will need two trainees: one role-playing the therapist and one role-playing the client. The context for the skill is a couple therapy session where you will imagine that both partners are present, but only one partner is speaking.

Skill Description

Skill Difficulty Level: Beginner

For this exercise you will practice two skills at the same time. The **first skill** comprises *"simple" reflections*, in which the therapist repeats back the client's words, or a close variant of the words. This skill is common to many therapeutic orientations and indicates that the therapist is interested and is listening carefully. In emotionally focused couple therapy (EFCT), these reflections have some additional benefits. For example, they slow down the pace of the session and give some extra time for the client to sit

https://doi.org/10.1037/0000436-004

Deliberate Practice in Emotionally Focused Couple Therapy, by H. Levenson, S. Jinich, A. Vaz, and T. Rousmaniere

with their words coming out of the therapist's mouth, often leading to a deepening of the experience of what is being reflected (Furrow et al., 2022). EFCT therapists use reflections to highlight particular emotional experiences that are likely to be significant clinically now or down the road. We are always looking for opportunities to deepen the affect between the couple and within the individual. These common types of reflections are important and are used liberally throughout the therapy, but especially in early sessions. Reflections, although seemingly simple, are potentially very powerful.

The **second skill** in this exercise is a specialized form of reflection: *evocative reflections*. This type of reflection is specifically designed to deepen the partners' experience by the therapist's saying what they are hearing on the edge of the client's awareness—to make what is implicit, explicit. Here the therapist must make inferences guided by attachment theory, the couple's unique background, and the therapist's empathic engagement in the client's experience. The goal is to capture the client's not yet fully formed emotional experience and increase the chances it will come forth. Using interventions that can heighten emotion such as vivid language, metaphor, and imagery are helpful in this regard.

Evocative reflections accomplish two things: (a) they give each partner more of a felt sense of what is going on at another, often more primary, emotional level within themselves and with their partners, and (b) they begin to seed attachment longings and fears, which will play a significant role in restructuring interactions later in the therapy.

The therapist uses their own "internal thesaurus" of affect-laden words, metaphors, and images in combination with their attunement to the implicit messages the client is sending to catalyze underlying primary feelings. For example, if a client were to say, "I often feel that my partner would rather be with his friends than with me," the therapist could evoke a more emotional experience by softly, slowly, and tentatively saying, "You feel excluded. Like you're not welcome, not invited. It's as if you're on the outside and they're on the inside. Something like that?" Now the client can hear back their own experience in a way that can affect them deeply and help them get in touch with the fullness of their experience. In this way, partners may eventually be able to get in contact with their attachment needs.

The therapist should improvise a response to each client statement following these skill criteria:

1. **Reflect back the most poignant part of what the client is saying or doing.** This is the simple reflection. It is key to pick the part of what the client is voicing that holds the most emotional charge or promise.

2. **Heighten this part by repeating it, using more vivid language, metaphor, or imagery.** This is this the evocative reflection. The therapist uses one of these interventions to evoke a fuller emotional experience. Therapists should pay careful attention to the client's words, phrasing, and nonverbals to discover clues as to what might be most evocative for the client.

3. **Check with the client to see if the evocative reflection fits.** Because the therapist is trying to convey something that may be on the edge of the client's awareness and makes inferences that may or may not be correct, it is critical to invite the client's response to what has been said to see if they agree.

Note: This exercise uses the same client statements as Exercise 1 so that trainees can get used to responding to the same prompts using different skills.

SKILL CRITERIA FOR EXERCISE 2

1. **Reflect** back the most poignant part of what the client is saying or doing.
2. **Heighten** this part by repeating it, using more vivid language, metaphor, or imagery.
3. Check with the client to see if the evocative reflection **fits**.

Examples of Therapists Using Evocative Reflections

Example 1

CLIENT: [*sad*] I really missed my partner. He traveled for a whole month, and I only got to see him once.

THERAPIST: You really missed your partner. (Criterion 1—**Reflect**) He was gone a very long time and your heart longed to see him. (Criterion 2—**Heighten**) Do I have that right? (Criterion 3—**Fit**)

Example 2

CLIENT: [*irritated*] Nothing I ever do is enough to make my partner satisfied.

THERAPIST: It seems nothing you do is ever enough for your partner. (Criterion 1—**Reflect**) You give, and you give, but it is like filling an empty hole. (Criterion 2—**Heighten**) Does that feel right? (Criterion 3—**Fit**)

Example 3

CLIENT: [*angry*] You should have seen the pep in his step as he offered and helped our next-door neighbor carry her groceries into her house. I never see that kind of energy directed at what I need.

THERAPIST: You don't experience your partner's enthusiasm to help you with what you need in the same way as he showed your neighbor. (Criterion 1—**Reflect**) It's as if he saves his best for others and then has nothing left for your needs. (Criterion 2—**Heighten**) Am I getting how it is for you when this happens? (Criterion 3—**Fit**)

INSTRUCTIONS FOR EXERCISE 2
Step 1: Role-Play and Feedback
<ul><li>The client says the first beginner client statement. The therapist **improvises** a response based on the skill criteria.</li><li>The trainer (or, if not available, the client) provides **brief** feedback based on the skill criteria.</li><li>The client then repeats the same statement, and the therapist again improvises a response. The trainer (or client) again provides brief feedback.</li></ul>
Step 2: Repeat
<ul><li>Repeat Step 1 for all the statements **in the current difficulty level** (beginner, intermediate, or advanced).</li></ul>
Step 3: Assess and Adjust Difficulty
<ul><li>The therapist completes the Deliberate Practice Reaction Form (see Appendix A) and decides whether to make the exercise easier or harder or to repeat the same difficulty level.</li></ul>
Step 4: Repeat for Approximately 15 Minutes
<ul><li>Repeat Steps 1 to 3 for at least 15 minutes.</li><li>The trainees then switch therapist and client roles and start over.</li></ul>

Now it's your turn! Follow Steps 1 and 2 from the instructions.

Remember: The goal of the role-play is for trainees to practice improvising responses to the client statements in a manner that (a) uses the skill criteria and (b) feels authentic for the trainee. **Example therapist responses for each client statement are provided at the end of this exercise. Trainees should attempt to improvise their own responses before reading the examples.**

BEGINNER-LEVEL CLIENT STATEMENTS FOR EXERCISE 2
Beginner Client Statement 1
[Sad] I really missed my partner. He traveled for a whole month, and I only got to see him once.
Beginner Client Statement 2
[Delighted] Yesterday, she looked at me with one of those warm, beautiful smiles I used to see years ago. I haven't seen one of those for a long time.
Beginner Client Statement 3
[Happy] And out of the blue, this week my partner told me they liked all that I was doing to try to make our marriage better.
Beginner Client Statement 4
[Delighted] When I wasn't feeling well, he sent me several texts during the day with smiley faces and a message showing he was thinking of me.
Beginner Client Statement 5
[Smiling] On my birthday, she gave me a thoughtful gift and a note apologizing for all the years she didn't remember.

 Assess and adjust the difficulty before moving to the next difficulty level (see Step 3 in the exercise instructions).

INTERMEDIATE-LEVEL CLIENT STATEMENTS FOR EXERCISE 2
Intermediate Client Statement 1
[Frustrated] We don't speak all day, and we hardly connect at all during dinner, then at night in bed, he wants to get physically close. Why should I want to?
Intermediate Client Statement 2
[Frustrated] Every time I try to say something meaningful to her, she either gets defensive or tunes me out. I'm tired of only being able to talk to my friends about things that are important to me.
Intermediate Client Statement 3
[Hurt] Even though I know that we both love each other very much, there is very little left between us. Maybe we are no longer supposed to be together. I don't know if he even remembers the last time we kissed!
Intermediate Client Statement 4
[Frustrated] I know I said I was leaving in 5 minutes, but something came up at the last minute that made me late. I don't know if she can trust that I have good intentions.
Intermediate Client Statement 5
[Sad] I hear his critical tone of voice, and I know we are going to have a fight. So I get defensive and then I shut down.

🛑 **Assess and adjust the difficulty before moving to the next difficulty level (see Step 3 in the exercise instructions).**

ADVANCED-LEVEL CLIENT STATEMENTS FOR EXERCISE 2
Advanced Client Statement 1
[Hurt] I don't really know how I am ever going to be able to trust her again. Everything seems different to me now.
Advanced Client Statement 2
[Frustrated] I would love to feel like I am enough just as I am. For years what I heard was how I didn't measure up.
Advanced Client Statement 3
[Sad] I feel excluded by my own family. I come home from work, and it's like she and the kids have their little club that I don't belong to.
Advanced Client Statement 4
[Hurt] No matter how hard I try or how loud I get, she says absolutely nothing. She just looks through me while I'm talking.
Advanced Client Statement 5
[Angry] He gives me the silent treatment and looks at me like I'm dangerous. I'm his life partner, not his enemy! I don't want this anymore.

Assess and adjust the difficulty here (see Step 3 in the exercise instructions). If appropriate, follow the instructions to make the exercise even more challenging (see Appendix A).

Example Therapist Responses: Evocative Reflections

Remember: Trainees should attempt to improvise their own responses before reading the example responses. **Do not read the following responses verbatim unless you are having trouble coming up with your own!**

EXAMPLE RESPONSES TO BEGINNER-LEVEL CLIENT STATEMENTS FOR EXERCISE 2
Example Response to Beginner Client Statement 1
You really missed your partner. (Criterion 1) A whole month felt like an eternity. (Criterion 2) Do I have that right? (Criterion 3)
Example Response to Beginner Client Statement 2
She flashed you a beautiful smile. (Criterion 1) It had been so long since you'd seen it that it really meant something to you. (Criterion 2) Does that feel right? (Criterion 3)
Example Response to Beginner Client Statement 3
They expressed liking all your efforts to improve the marriage. (Criterion 1) It was as if they could suddenly see you and appreciate all that you do for this marriage. (Criterion 2) Does that capture the feeling? (Criterion 3)
Example Response to Beginner Client Statement 4
He sent you reminders that he was thinking of you. (Criterion 1) It sounds like he was holding you in his heart and mind. (Criterion 2) Does that sound right? (Criterion 3)
Example Response to Beginner Client Statement 5
She apologized for not remembering your birthday all those years. (Criterion 1) Seems like remembering and apologizing for her past neglect was the best present. (Criterion 2) Does that ring true? (Criterion 3)

EXAMPLE RESPONSES TO INTERMEDIATE-LEVEL CLIENT STATEMENTS FOR EXERCISE 2
Example Response to Intermediate Client Statement 1
When he doesn't connect during the day, it's hard to connect physically at night. (Criterion 1) It's like he expects you to turn on at night, when you haven't been plugged in all day. (Criterion 2) Do I have that right? (Criterion 3)
Example Response to Intermediate Client Statement 2
You wish she was interested in hearing about things that are important to you. (Criterion 1) You get really tired of turning to your friends for meaningful conversation when she tunes you out. (Criterion 2) Is that right? (Criterion 3)
Example Response to Intermediate Client Statement 3
Even though you love each other, you are wondering if there is any hope for the two of you. (Criterion 1) It's like the spark has gone out and you are navigating in the dark. (Criterion 2) Is that how it seems to you? (Criterion 3)
Example Response to Intermediate Client Statement 4
You want her to believe that you had every intention of leaving when you said you would. (Criterion 1) You long to have her see that she can really trust you. (Criterion 2) Do I have that right? (Criterion 3)
Example Response to Intermediate Client Statement 5
When you feel a fight is inevitable, you shut down. (Criterion 1) It's as if the fight is going to be so painful or destructive that you need to go into a protective bunker just to survive. (Criterion 2) Is that an apt way of putting it for what goes on for you? (Criterion 3)

EXAMPLE RESPONSES TO ADVANCED-LEVEL CLIENT STATEMENTS FOR EXERCISE 2

Example Response to Advanced Client Statement 1

Now it seems like you'll never be able to trust her again. (Criterion 1) You are like a stranger in a strange land. The trust that was always there seems nowhere to be found. How disorienting! (Criterion 2) Is that how it feels? Please correct me if I have it wrong. (Criterion 3)

Example Response to Advanced Client Statement 2

For all this time you have felt like you didn't measure up in her eyes. (Criterion 1) You long to look into her eyes and see that you are enough just as you are. (Criterion 2) Is that how it feels? (Criterion 3)

Example Response to Advanced Client Statement 3

When you come home, you don't feel a part of your own family. (Criterion 1) It's as if you are on the outside with your nose pressed up to the window and they are cozy on the inside. (Criterion 2) Did I get that right? (Criterion 3)

Example Response to Advanced Client Statement 4

It seems no matter what you do, you can't get through to her. (Criterion 1) It's as if you are invisible to her; she doesn't see or hear you. (Criterion 2) Is that what it feels like? (Criterion 3)

Example Response to Advanced Client Statement 5

You seem desperate to convince him that you are his partner. (Criterion 1) It's as if no matter what you do to show him that you come in peace, he treats you like you are the enemy. (Criterion 2) Does this capture some of what you feel? Please correct me if I have it wrong. (Criterion 3)

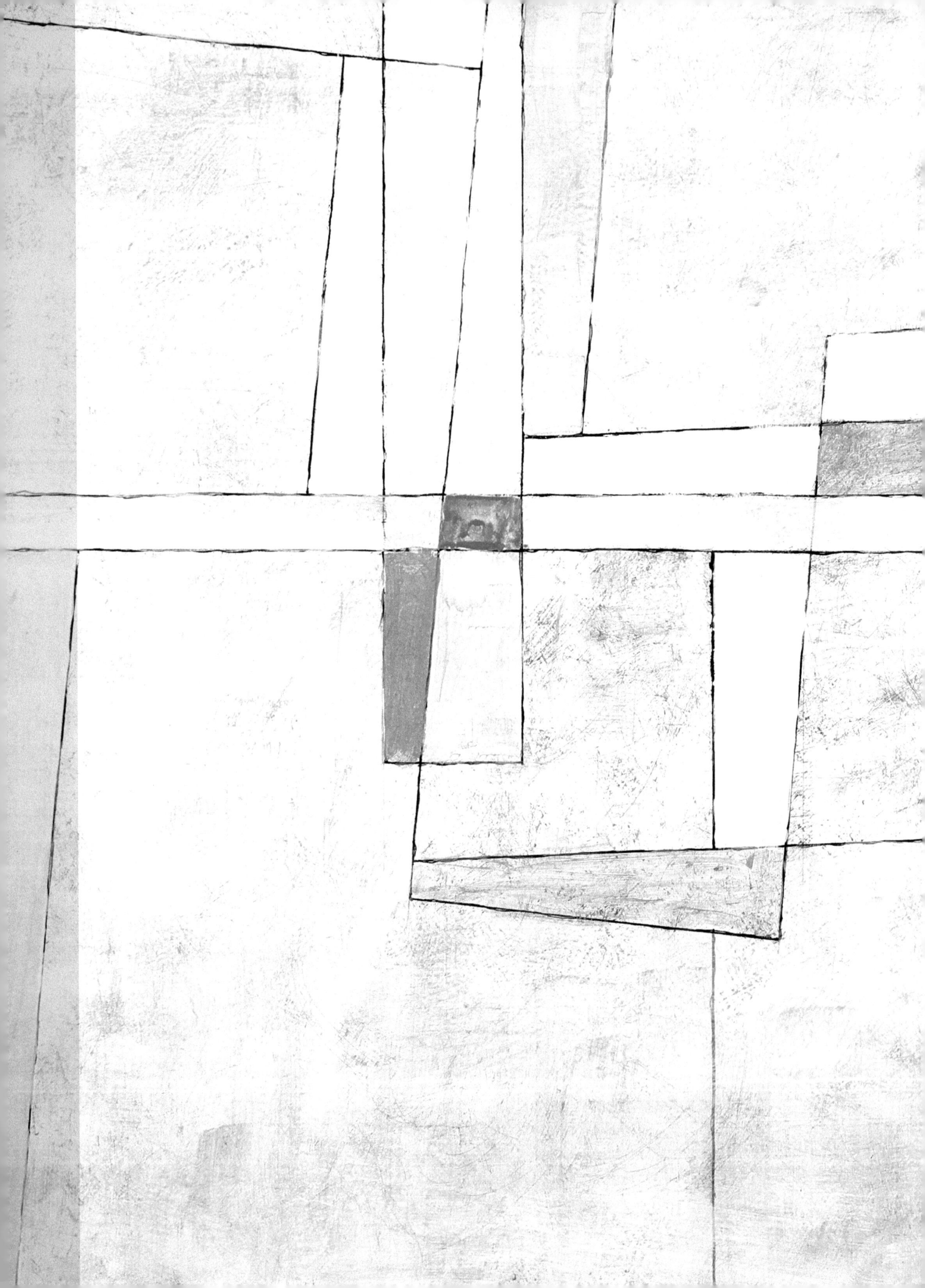

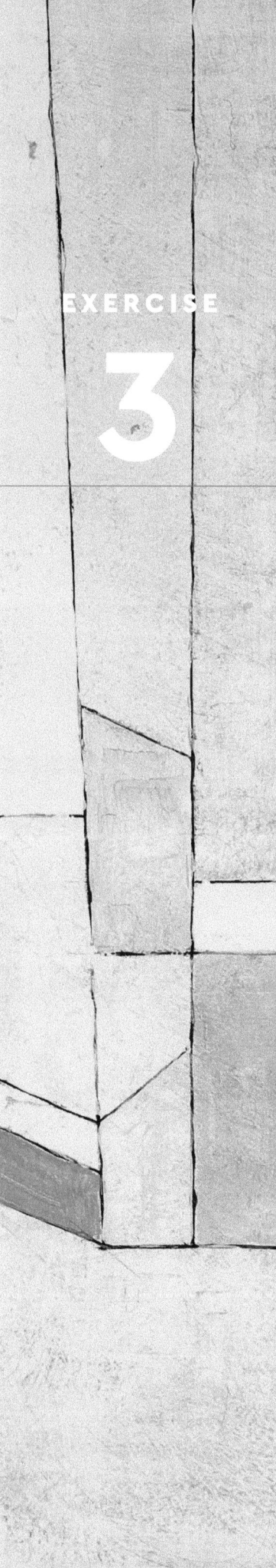

Validating Partners' Experiences and Tracking Dysfunctional Patterns

Preparations for Exercise 3

1. Read the instructions in Chapter 2.

2. Download the Deliberate Practice Reaction Form and the Deliberate Practice Diary Form at https://www.apa.org/pubs/books/deliberate-practice-emotionally-focused-couple-therapy (see the "Resources" tab; also available in Appendixes A and B, respectively).

Exercise Format

For this skill, you will need two trainees: one role-playing the therapist and one role-playing the client. The context for the skill is a couple therapy session where you will imagine both partners are present, but only one partner is speaking.

Skill Description

Skill Difficulty Level: Beginner

In this exercise, we are combining two skills: validation and tracking. Both are essential therapeutic skills in the therapist's toolbox.

Emotionally focused couple therapists validate what is happening in the present moment's experience by conveying, without judgment or criticism, that the person's thoughts, feelings, and reactions make sense. In emotionally focused couple therapy (EFCT), validation is particularly important because it helps individuals understand and feel understood in their emotional experiences. By validating clients' emotions, the therapist can help them feel safe and supported, which can facilitate emotional exploration

https://doi.org/10.1037/0000436-005

Deliberate Practice in Emotionally Focused Couple Therapy, by H. Levenson, S. Jinich, A. Vaz, and T. Rousmaniere

and healing. Additionally, validation helps to de-escalate conflicts and reduce negative interaction patterns. When individuals feel validated, they are more likely to be open to understanding their partners' perspective and engaging in healthier communication patterns.

Furthermore, validation can also help individuals develop a more secure attachment style by providing a corrective emotional perspective and fostering a sense of emotional safety within the therapeutic relationship. Validation creates a foundation for healing, growth, and the development of secure attachment bonds and therefore is an essential skill to master. Validation helps build and strengthen the therapeutic alliance by conveying to the couple that the therapist is understanding and accepting them, and it is essential in helping couples begin to see that their partner's behaviors or emotional reactions are understandable, given the context of their life experiences, past relationships, traumas, sensitivities, current situation, and unmet attachment needs. Importantly, validation is not meant to imply agreement, and it should never be used to convey that the therapist is taking sides by agreeing with one partner over the other.

The second skill of tracking is fundamental to the framework of EFCT. As the therapist tracks the triggers that lead to feelings and vice versa, relational patterns both within the individual and between individuals become more apparent. These cyclic patterns describe how Partner 1's behaviors stemming from their internal reactions trigger internal reactions in Partner 2, which in turn provoke their reciprocal behaviors, which then further affect Partner 1's internal emotional experience, and so on. By giving voice to tracking triggers and patterns, the therapist is seeding an awareness in the partners that allows them to begin to see how their reactions, expectations, and behaviors are part of the problem. They become aware of how the real issue is not their partner but the pattern of reciprocal defensive moves that has become chronic. The partners see that they are stuck in a repetitive dysfunctional pattern. In a nonpathologizing way, getting unstuck then becomes the goal of the EFCT.

In this exercise, the beginning elements of tracking will be practiced, focusing on linking Partner 1's reactive emotions to their interpretation of Partner 2's behavior.

The therapist should improvise a response to each client statement following these skill criteria:

1. **Match the client's vocal tone to convey attunement to their experience.** The EFCT therapist uses their voice to communicate to the clients just as much as their words do. The tone, intensity, and prosody of one's voice should match the client's current experience. For example, if the client is speaking loudly and forcefully, the therapist should match those qualities to indicate to the client that they are aligned with the client's affect. Saying words that validate the client's position is important; saying those words in a tone that resonates with the client's affect is equally important.

2. **Validate the client's feelings or thoughts.** If the client does not feel validated by the therapist, there is little likelihood that a good therapeutic alliance will be formed. Use validating phrases such as, "Yes, I can see how . . . ," "Yes, I hear what you are saying . . . ," and "What you are saying makes sense given that. . . ."

3. **Point out their partner's behavior that triggers those reactions.** Linking Partner 1's internal reactions to Partner 2's behavior is a first step toward framing the partners' interactions as part of a dysfunctional cycle. It is very important, however, that the partner's behavior is not portrayed as "bad" or purposely provocative, but nonetheless a trigger for Partner 1's internal reactions. Stick to simply pointing out the partner's behavior and don't attempt to clarify their intention or anything else under the

behavior. In Exercise 8 (Gathering and Assembling Elements of Emotion), you will have the opportunity to practice a fuller and more complex version of tracking.

Note: Exercises 3 through 5 use the same client statements so that trainees can get used to responding to the same prompts using different skills.

SKILL CRITERIA FOR EXERCISE 3

1. **Match** the client's vocal tone, intensity, and prosody to convey attunement to their current experience.
2. **Validate** the client's feelings or thoughts.
3. Point out their partner's behavior that **triggers** those reactions.

Examples of Therapists Validating Partners' Experiences and Tracking Dysfunctional Patterns

Example 1

CLIENT: [*devastated*] So now my partner wants to sleep in the guest room. That is the ultimate rejection of me. I feel so devastated and so alone.

THERAPIST: I can certainly understand why you feel completely devastated, (Criterion 2— **Validate**) given that your partner is thinking of sleeping in another room. (Criterion 3— **Trigger**)

Example 2

CLIENT: [*angry*] My partner seems to care more about her previous lover—the ex—than me. I hear so much about how wonderful the ex is, that I am thinking of ending this relationship. Then the two of them could be together forever.

THERAPIST: I can understand why it is so hard for you (Criterion 2—**Validate**) to constantly hear about how wonderful the ex is. (Criterion 3—**Trigger**)

Example 3

CLIENT: [*discouraged*] I feel so invisible in my marriage. Does my partner even know I exist? I cry myself to sleep every night, and I don't think they even notice.

THERAPIST: It makes sense how sad you get (Criterion 2—**Validate**) given that they don't even notice your tears. (Criterion 3—**Trigger**)

INSTRUCTIONS FOR EXERCISE 3
Step 1: Role-Play and Feedback
• The client says the first beginner client statement. The therapist **improvises** a response based on the skill criteria.   • The trainer (or, if not available, the client) provides **brief** feedback based on the skill criteria.   • The client then repeats the same statement, and the therapist again improvises a response. The trainer (or client) again provides brief feedback.
Step 2: Repeat
• Repeat Step 1 for all the statements **in the current difficulty level** (beginner, intermediate, or advanced).
Step 3: Assess and Adjust Difficulty
• The therapist completes the Deliberate Practice Reaction Form (see Appendix A) and decides whether to make the exercise easier or harder or to repeat the same difficulty level.
Step 4: Repeat for Approximately 15 Minutes
• Repeat Steps 1 to 3 for at least 15 minutes.   • The trainees then switch therapist and client roles and start over.

Now it's your turn! Follow Steps 1 and 2 from the instructions.

Remember: The goal of the role-play is for trainees to practice improvising responses to the client statements in a manner that (a) uses the skill criteria and (b) feels authentic for the trainee. **Example therapist responses for each client statement are provided at the end of this exercise. Trainees should attempt to improvise their own responses before reading the examples.**

BEGINNER-LEVEL CLIENT STATEMENTS FOR EXERCISE 3
Beginner Client Statement 1
[Frustrated] My partner is so insensitive to the things that are important to me, and when I try to point this out, she walks away and won't speak to me for hours. It's so frustrating! I haven't been happy in this marriage for years.
Beginner Client Statement 2
[Irritated] Well, my partner doesn't try to tell me how he feels; he just goes from zero to 100 within seconds, and there's nothing I can do to stop the onslaught of outrage and criticism. Eventually I just can't take it anymore, so I shut down and walk away.
Beginner Client Statement 3
[Discouraged] My partner turns away from me at the least little thing. There's nothing I can do to keep her engaged. I toss and turn trying to sleep every night, and I don't think she even notices.
Beginner Client Statement 4
[Sarcastic] Oh, I notice his tossing and turning. Each turning tells me I am a horrible person. In fact, the tossing and turning bothers me so much, I am thinking of sleeping in another room.
Beginner Client Statement 5
[Devastated] So now she wants to sleep in another room. That is the ultimate rejection of me. I feel so devastated and so alone.

 Assess and adjust the difficulty before moving to the next difficulty level (see Step 3 in the exercise instructions).

INTERMEDIATE-LEVEL CLIENT STATEMENTS FOR EXERCISE 3
Intermediate Client Statement 1
[Angry] My wife's family is always on my case just because I don't have a college degree. Instead of standing up for me, my wife ignores their subtle jabs. It's like they matter more than I do.
Intermediate Client Statement 2
[Hostile] My partner has always seen me as the problem in this relationship. He never talks about his lapses or mistakes. Instead, he goes on and on about what a big disappointment I've been in this relationship. I'm tired of always being blamed for everything.
Intermediate Client Statement 3
[Upset] So my partner just buys whatever he wants without consulting me. I just feel like I'm the bank funding whatever he wants. I'm tempted to cut up his credit cards and make him come to me for whatever he needs.
Intermediate Client Statement 4
[Hurt] Every time we sit down to a home-cooked meal, our teenager finds something to criticize me about. My husband just sits there and lets our child be so rude to me. I've told him I need his support and that I expect him to discipline our child, but nothing gets said and I'm all alone to set limits. Sometimes I feel completely ganged up on by the two of them.
Intermediate Client Statement 5
[Frustrated] No matter what I do, I can never get it right. Even last night after a full day of spring cleaning and shared projects, my partner had to go down the list of all the things I didn't have a chance to get to. It's just never good enough for them. I'm really frustrated.

🛑 **Assess and adjust the difficulty before moving to the next difficulty level (see Step 3 in the exercise instructions).**

ADVANCED-LEVEL CLIENT STATEMENTS FOR EXERCISE 3
Advanced Client Statement 1
[Irritated] Is there anything wrong with hanging out with my friends at a bar? But no, my partner has to call me every 10 minutes, screaming, "You need to come home!" It's makes me want to stay out even later.
Advanced Client Statement 2
[Discouraged] I feel so invisible in my marriage. Does my partner even know I exist? I cry myself to sleep every night, and I don't think they even notice.
Advanced Client Statement 3
[Indignant] He always puts pressure on me to move out for a few days when his parents come to town. It hurts me that he still hides his sexuality and our relationship. There's nothing wrong with the love that we feel for each other.
Advanced Client Statement 4
[Angry] My partner seems to care more about her previous lover—the ex—than me. She spends so much time talking about how wonderful the ex is and ignoring me, that I am thinking of ending this relationship. Then the two of them could be together forever.
Advanced Client Statement 5
[Angry] He is so cruel the way he just sits there with that smug look, saying nothing and just staring at the floor.

🛑 **Assess and adjust the difficulty here (see Step 3 in the exercise instructions). If appropriate, follow the instructions to make the exercise even more challenging (see Appendix A).**

Example Therapist Responses: Validating Partners' Experiences and Tracking Dysfunctional Patterns

Remember: Trainees should attempt to improvise their own responses before reading the examples. **Do not read the following responses verbatim unless you are having trouble coming up with your own!**

EXAMPLE RESPONSES TO BEGINNER-LEVEL CLIENT STATEMENTS FOR EXERCISE 3
Example Response to Beginner Client Statement 1
It makes so much sense that you're frustrated and have felt frustrated for so many years, (Criterion 2) given that when you try to tell her how ignored you feel, she withdraws and stops talking to you. (Criterion 3)
Example Response to Beginner Client Statement 2
Yes, I hear that you feel so helpless to stop his outrage, (Criterion 3) so it makes sense that you leave when you feel you just can't take it anymore. (Criterion 2)
Example Response to Beginner Client Statement 3
It makes sense how sad you get (Criterion 2) when your partner pulls away and doesn't even notice how you toss and turn every night. (Criterion 3)
Example Response to Beginner Client Statement 4
I can imagine it must feel terrible (Criterion 2) to hear your partner tossing and turning with each turn telling you how bad a partner you are. (Criterion 3) Of course, it makes you think about sleeping in another room. (Criterion 2)
Example Response to Beginner Client Statement 5
Of course you're devastated (Criterion 2) when your partner talks about sleeping in the other room. (Criterion 3)

EXAMPLE RESPONSES TO INTERMEDIATE-LEVEL CLIENT STATEMENTS FOR EXERCISE 3
Example Response to Intermediate Client Statement 1
It makes so much sense that you feel your wife's family matters more than you do, (Criterion 2) especially when she doesn't take your side against their criticism. (Criterion 3)
Example Response to Intermediate Client Statement 2
It sounds really hard (Criterion 2) to be blamed for everything and to be seen as the problem. (Criterion 3)
Example Response to Intermediate Client Statement 3
It makes sense that you feel like you're just a source of money to your partner (Criterion 2) when he spends freely and doesn't include you in the decision making. (Criterion 3) It makes sense that you would want to stop automatically funding his purchases and make him come to you. (Criterion 2)
Example Response to Intermediate Client Statement 4
Indeed, it must be very lonely for you (Criterion 2) to witness his passivity. (Criterion 3)
Example Response to Intermediate Client Statement 5
No matter what you do it's just never quite enough to satisfy your partner. (Criterion 3) It's frustrating. (Criterion 2)

EXAMPLE RESPONSES TO ADVANCED-LEVEL CLIENT STATEMENTS FOR EXERCISE 3
Example Response to Advanced Client Statement 1
So, when you are feeling controlled and told what to do, (Criterion 3) I can understand that you don't want to rush home. (Criterion 2)
Example Response to Advanced Client Statement 2
It makes sense how sad you get (Criterion 2) given that your partner doesn't even notice your tears. (Criterion 3)
Example Response to Advanced Client Statement 3
It makes a lot of sense that you feel hurt (Criterion 2) when he conceals your relationship and asks you to move out and pretend like you're just friends. (Criterion 3)
Example Response to Advanced Client Statement 4
Given how your partner praises the ex-partner while ignoring you, (Criterion 3) I can see how you get so hurt that thinking about leaving becomes an option. (Criterion 2)
Example Response to Advanced Client Statement 5
It seems so cruel to you when you're this upset for your partner to stare at the floor and not say anything. (Criteria 3) It's really hurtful, isn't it? That's understandable. (Criterion 2)

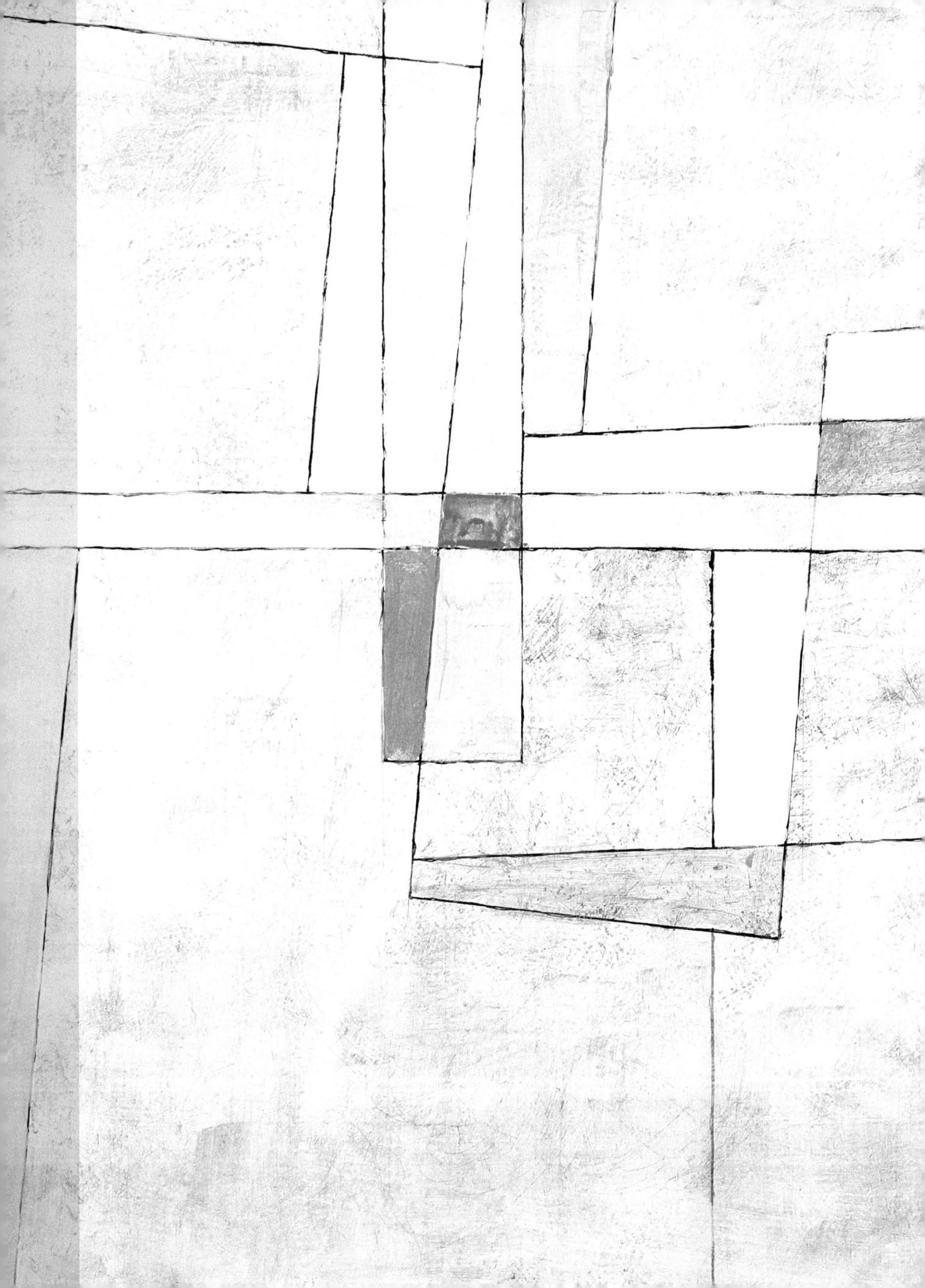

Attachment-Reframed Validation

Preparations for Exercise 4

1. Read the instructions in Chapter 2.

2. Download the Deliberate Practice Reaction Form and the Deliberate Practice Diary Form at https://www.apa.org/pubs/books/deliberate-practice-emotionally-focused-couple-therapy (see the "Resources" tab; also available in Appendixes A and B, respectively).

Exercise Format

For this skill, you will need two trainees: one role-playing the therapist and one role-playing the client. The context for the skill is a couple therapy session where you will imagine that both partners are present, but only one partner is speaking.

Skill Description

Skill Difficulty Level: Beginner

This exercise incorporates what you have just practiced in Exercise 3, validation of each couple's experience of their partner's triggering behavior. But this exercise goes one step further. In this exercise, you will begin seeding the importance of the partners' attachment fears and longings into the validation. One of the authors (SJ) calls this *attachment-reframed validation.*

From an emotionally focused couple therapy viewpoint, the reason a partner has such a strong reaction when the connection to their partner feels threatened is because that partner is so important to them. By focusing on how much their partner means to them

https://doi.org/10.1037/0000436-006

Deliberate Practice in Emotionally Focused Couple Therapy, by H. Levenson, S. Jinich, A. Vaz, and T. Rousmaniere

and their hope that this longing is reciprocated, the therapist begins to explore or conjecture about the vulnerable, primary emotions driving the partners attachment toward one another. Johnson (2019) underscored that strong attachment bonds are characterized by the perceived *accessibility*, *responsiveness*, and *emotional engagement* of the partners. These three elements are represented by the acronym A.R.E., which she uses as shorthand for the question predominant in each partner's mind—"Are you there for me?" (Johnson, 2019, p. 7). In this exercise, the feelings fueling this question are made explicit, rather than being implicitly hidden in the partners' blaming or withdrawing behavior. The therapist ends up validating the behavior of the partners because it is understandable given how they long to be attached and fear the loss of that attachment.

The therapist should improvise a response to each client statement following these skill criteria:

1. **Match the client's vocal tone, intensity, and prosody to convey attunement to their current experience.** For example, if the partner is speaking loudly and forcefully, you should match those qualities to indicate to the partner that you are aligned with their affect. If the partner is soft and hesitant, you can adjust your tone to be softer. Saying words that validate the partner's position is important; saying those words in a tone that resonates with their affect is equally important. In this exercise, your voice should be part of the validating intervention.

2. **Validate the client's feelings, behaviors, or thoughts.** This is more than reflecting back what you are hearing the client say. You want the client to feel that you see they are justified in what they are feeling, doing, and thinking having been triggered by their partner's behavior. You can use validating phrases such as, "Yes, I can see how . . . ," "Yes, I hear what you are saying," and "What you are saying makes sense given that. . . ."

3. **Point out their partner's behavior that triggers the client's reactions.** Linking the client's (Partner 1's) feelings, behaviors, or thoughts in reaction to their partner's (Partner 2's) behavior is a further step toward framing the partners' interactions as part of a dysfunctional cycle where one person's behavior triggers their partner's reactions and so on.

4. **Conjecture about the client's unmet attachment longings and/or fears.** Include in your validation an attachment-based rationale for seeing Partner 1's response as an understandable reaction to perceiving their partner as inaccessible, unresponsive, emotionally disengaged, uncaring, or even hostile. You are not only validating Partner 1's reactions (Criterion 3) as understandable, but also their hypothesized inner attachment fears and longings (Criterion 4). Here we begin to link the client's inner, vulnerable feelings of potential loss to what gets shown externally through their reactions.

Note: Exercises 3 through 5 use the same client statements so that trainees can get used to responding to the same prompts using different skills.

SKILL CRITERIA FOR EXERCISE 4

1. **Match** the client's vocal tone, intensity, and prosody to convey attunement to their current experience.
2. **Validate** the client's feelings, behaviors, or thoughts.
3. Point out their partner's behavior that **triggers** the client's reactions.
4. Conjecture about the client's unmet **attachment** longings and/or fears.

Examples of Therapists Using Attachment-Reframed Validation

Example 1

CLIENT: [*devastated*] So now my partner wants to sleep in the guest room. That is the ultimate rejection of me. I feel so devastated and so alone.

THERAPIST: I can certainly understand why you feel completely devastated, (Criterion 2—**Validate**) given that he is thinking of sleeping in another room. (Criterion 3—**Trigger**) Your partner is so important to you, that when he pulls away from you in this way, you feel so rejected. (Criterion 4—**Attachment**)

Example 2

CLIENT: [*angry*] My partner seems to care more about her previous lover—the ex—than me. I hear so much about how wonderful the ex is, that I am thinking of ending this relationship. Then the two of them could be together forever.

THERAPIST: I can understand why it's so hard for you (Criterion 2—**Validate**) to constantly hear about how wonderful the ex is, (Criterion 3—**Trigger**) when deep down what you want is to be the wonderful one in her eyes. (Criterion 4—**Attachment**)

Example 3

CLIENT: [*discouraged*] I feel so invisible in my marriage. Does my partner even know I exist? I cry myself to sleep every night, and I don't think they even notice.

THERAPIST: It makes sense how sad you get (Criterion 2—**Validate**) given that your partner doesn't even notice your tears. (Criterion 3—**Trigger**) Because they are so important to you, you want them to see your pain and feel it with you. (Criterion 4—**Attachment**)

INSTRUCTIONS FOR EXERCISE 4
Step 1: Role-Play and Feedback
• The client says the first beginner client statement. The therapist **improvises** a response based on the skill criteria.   • The trainer (or, if not available, the client) provides **brief** feedback based on the skill criteria.   • The client then repeats the same statement, and the therapist again improvises a response. The trainer (or client) again provides brief feedback.
Step 2: Repeat
• Repeat Step 1 for all the statements **in the current difficulty level** (beginner, intermediate, or advanced).
Step 3: Assess and Adjust Difficulty
• The therapist completes the Deliberate Practice Reaction Form (see Appendix A) and decides whether to make the exercise easier or harder or to repeat the same difficulty level.
Step 4: Repeat for Approximately 15 Minutes
• Repeat Steps 1 to 3 for at least 15 minutes.   • The trainees then switch therapist and client roles and start over.

Now it's your turn! Follow Steps 1 and 2 from the exercise instructions.

Remember: The goal of the role-play is for trainees to practice improvising responses to the client statements in a manner that (a) uses the skill criteria and (b) feels authentic for the trainee. **Example therapist responses for each client statement are provided at the end of this exercise. Trainees should attempt to improvise their own responses before reading the examples.**

BEGINNER-LEVEL CLIENT STATEMENTS FOR EXERCISE 4
Beginner Client Statement 1
[Frustrated] My partner is so insensitive to the things that are important to me, and when I try to point this out, she walks away and won't speak to me for hours. It's so frustrating! I haven't been happy in this marriage for years.
Beginner Client Statement 2
[Irritated] Well, my partner doesn't try to tell me how he feels; he just goes from zero to 100 within seconds, and there's nothing I can do to stop the onslaught of outrage and criticism. Finally, I just can't take it anymore, so I shut down and walk away.
Beginner Client Statement 3
[Discouraged] My partner turns away from me at the least little thing. There's nothing I can do to keep her engaged. I toss and turn trying to sleep every night, and I don't think she even notices.
Beginner Client Statement 4
[Sarcastic] Oh, I notice his tossing and turning. Each turning tells me I am a horrible person. In fact, the tossing and turning bothers me so much, I am thinking of sleeping in another room.
Beginner Client Statement 5
[Devastated] So now she wants to sleep in another room. That is the ultimate rejection of me. I feel so devastated and so alone.

 Assess and adjust the difficulty before moving to the next difficulty level (see Step 3 in the exercise instructions).

INTERMEDIATE-LEVEL CLIENT STATEMENTS FOR EXERCISE 4
Intermediate Client Statement 1
[Angry] My wife's family is always on my case just because I don't have a college degree. Instead of standing up for me, my wife ignores their subtle jabs. It's like they matter more than I do.
Intermediate Client Statement 2
[Hostile] My partner has always seen me as the problem in this relationship. He never talks about his lapses or mistakes. Instead, he goes on and on about what a big disappointment I've been in this relationship. I'm tired of always being blamed for everything.
Intermediate Client Statement 3
[Upset] So my partner just buys whatever he wants without consulting me. I just feel like I'm the bank funding whatever he wants. I'm tempted to cut up his credit cards and make him come to me for whatever he needs.
Intermediate Client Statement 4
[Hurt] Every time we sit down to a home-cooked meal, our teenager finds something to criticize me about. My husband just sits there and lets our child be so rude to me. I've told him I need his support and that I expect him to discipline our child, but nothing gets said and I'm all alone to set limits. Sometimes I feel completely ganged up on by the two of them.
Intermediate Client Statement 5
[Frustrated] No matter what I do, I can never get it right. Even last night after a full day of spring cleaning and shared projects, my partner had to go down the list of all the things I didn't have a chance to get to. It's just never good enough for them. I'm really frustrated.

🛑 **Assess and adjust the difficulty before moving to the next difficulty level (see Step 3 in the exercise instructions).**

ADVANCED-LEVEL CLIENT STATEMENTS FOR EXERCISE 4
Advanced Client Statement 1
[Irritated] Is there anything wrong with my hanging out with my friends at a bar? But no, my partner has to call me every 10 minutes, screaming, "You need to come home!" It's makes me want to stay out even later.
Advanced Client Statement 2
[Discouraged] I feel so invisible in my marriage. Does my partner even know I exist? I cry myself to sleep every night, and I don't think they even notice.
Advanced Client Statement 3
[Indignant] He always puts pressure on me to move out for a few days when his parents come to town. It hurts me that he still hides our relationship. There's nothing wrong with the love that we feel for each other.
Advanced Client Statement 4
[Angry] My partner seems to care more about her previous lover—the ex—than me. She spends so much time talking about how wonderful the ex is and ignoring me, that I am thinking of ending this relationship. Then the two of them could be together forever.
Advanced Client Statement 5
[Angry] He is so cruel the way he just sits there with that smug look, saying nothing and just staring at the floor.

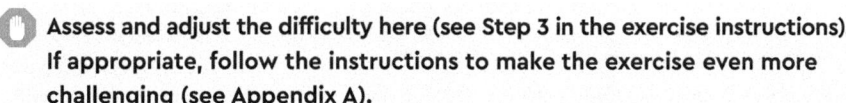 **Assess and adjust the difficulty here (see Step 3 in the exercise instructions). If appropriate, follow the instructions to make the exercise even more challenging (see Appendix A).**

Example Therapist Responses: Attachment-Reframed Validation

Remember: Trainees should attempt to improvise their own responses before consulting the examples. **Do not read the following responses verbatim unless you are having trouble coming up with your own!**

EXAMPLE RESPONSES TO BEGINNER-LEVEL CLIENT STATEMENTS FOR EXERCISE 4
Example Response to Beginner Client Statement 1
It makes so much sense that you're frustrated and have felt frustrated for so many years, (Criterion 2) given that when you try to tell her how ignored you feel, she withdraws and stops talking to you. (Criterion 3) It really matters to you to feel that what is important to you is also important to her. (Criterion 4)
Example Response to Beginner Client Statement 2
Yes, I hear that you feel so helpless to stop his outrage, (Criterion 3) and that when you feel you just can't take it anymore, you leave. (Criterion 2) It is especially hard when the person you care about so much acts in this uncaring and hostile way. (Criterion 4)
Example Response to Beginner Client Statement 3
It makes sense how sad you get (Criterion 2) when your partner turns away and doesn't even notice how you toss and turn every night. (Criterion 3) Deep down you need to know that you matter to her and that your sadness would grab her attention. (Criterion 4)
Example Response to Beginner Client Statement 4
I can imagine it must feel terrible (Criterion 2) to hear your partner tossing and turning with each turn telling you how bad a partner you are, (Criterion 3) especially when deep down you need him to acknowledge you as a good partner. (Criterion 4) I can understand why, it makes you think about sleeping in another room. (Criterion 2)
Example Response to Beginner Client Statement 5
Of course you're devastated (Criterion 2) when your partner talks about sleeping in the other room. (Criterion 3) She is so important to you, that when she pulls away from you in this way, you feel so alone. (Criterion 4)

EXAMPLE RESPONSES TO INTERMEDIATE-LEVEL CLIENT STATEMENTS FOR EXERCISE 4

Example Response to Intermediate Client Statement 1

It makes so much sense that you feel your wife's family matters more than you do, (Criterion 2) especially when she doesn't take your side against their criticism. (Criterion 3) You want to feel safe . . . and like you are the most important person [*pause*] in her life [*pause*] and that she would stand up to their jabs in a heartbeat for you. (Criterion 4)

Example Response to Intermediate Client Statement 2

It sounds really hard (Criterion 2) to be blamed for everything and to be seen as the problem. (Criterion 3) Your looking into his eyes and seeing disappointment is really hard for you, especially when he means the world to you. (Criterion 4)

Example Response to Intermediate Client Statement 3

It makes sense that if you feel like you are just a source of money to your partner, (Criterion 2) when he spends freely and doesn't include you in the decision-making, (Criterion 3) that you would want to stop automatically funding his purchases and make him come to you. (Criterion 2) This is especially hard when you really long to be included and considered by him. (Criterion 4)

Example Response to Intermediate Client Statement 4

Indeed, it must be very lonely for you (Criterion 2) to witness his passivity, (Criterion 3) especially since you long for him to be your support by setting clear limits with your child. (Criterion 4)

Example Response to Intermediate Client Statement 5

No matter what you do it's just never quite enough to satisfy your partner. (Criterion 3) It is frustrating (Criterion 2) never to be able to please the one person you most want to be appreciated by and seen in a positive light. (Criterion 4)

EXAMPLE RESPONSES TO ADVANCED-LEVEL CLIENT STATEMENTS FOR EXERCISE 4

Example Response to Advanced Client Statement 1

So, when you are feeling controlled and told what to do, (Criterion 3) I can understand that you don't want to rush home. (Criterion 2) You really long to feel trusted by your partner. (Criterion 4)

Example Response to Advanced Client Statement 2

It makes sense how sad you get (Criterion 2) given that your partner doesn't even notice your tears. (Criterion 3) Because they are so important to you, you want them to see your pain and feel for you. (Criterion 4)

Example Response to Advanced Client Statement 3

It makes a lot of sense that you feel hurt (Criterion 2) when he conceals this relationship and asks you to move out and pretend like you're just friends. (Criterion 3) You want him to be proud of you and your relationship because he means the world to you. (Criterion 4)

Example Response to Advanced Client Statement 4

Given how your partner praises the ex-partner while ignoring you, (Criterion 3) I can see how your hurt makes you think about leaving. (Criterion 2) If only she could show you how you are the most important person, then you would feel reassured and safe. (Criterion 4)

Example Response to Advanced Client Statement 5

It seems so cruel to you when you're this upset for your partner to stare at the floor and not say anything. (Criteria 3) It's really hurtful, isn't it? That's understandable. (Criterion 2) You desperately want him to hear your pleas and to show you that he cares about your pain. (Criterion 4)

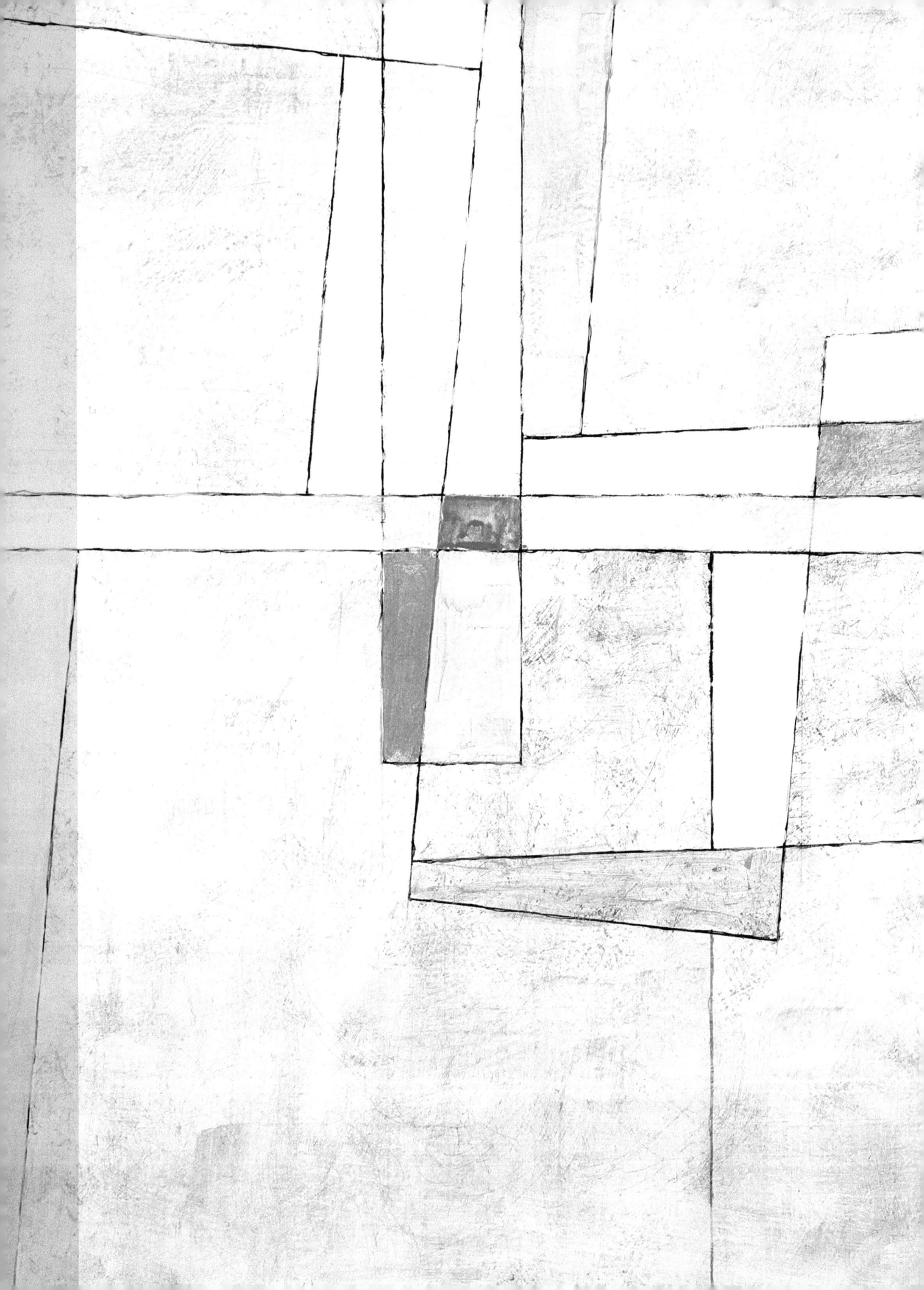

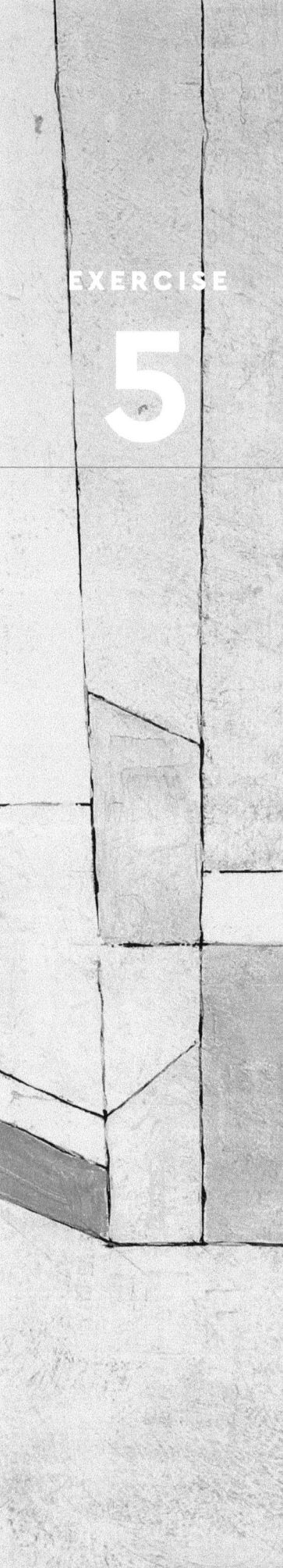

Deepening Emotions With RISSSSC: Speaking Simply, Slowly, and Softly

Preparations for Exercise 5

1. Read the instructions in Chapter 2.

2. Download the Deliberate Practice Reaction Form and the Deliberate Practice Diary Form at https://www.apa.org/pubs/books/deliberate-practice-emotionally-focused-couple-therapy (see the "Resources" tab; also available in Appendixes A and B, respectively).

Exercise Format

For this skill, you will need two trainees: one role-playing the therapist and one role-playing the client. The context for the skill is a couple therapy session where you will imagine that both partners are present, but only one partner is speaking.

Skill Description

Skill Difficulty Level: Beginner

In the previous two exercises, you learned to match the tone of your voice to that of the client. This is a way for the client to feel that you are attuning to them. There are other ways the emotionally focused couple therapist uses their voice. In this exercise you will learn how to use your voice to deepen the client's emotional experience of themselves and their partner. The intentionality of using one's prosody, tone, word phrasing, tempo, and timbre is a critical emotionally focused couple therapy (EFCT) skill. Deepening skills requires the EFCT therapist to attune to the client's affect and to use one's

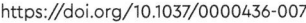

https://doi.org/10.1037/0000436-007

Deliberate Practice in Emotionally Focused Couple Therapy, by H. Levenson, S. Jinich, A. Vaz, and T. Rousmaniere

nonverbal and verbal presence to help the client to explore more vulnerable emotions. Once the therapist has identified something that they wish the client to grasp on an emotional level, they say it in a gentle caring manner using their voice, intonation, and word choice to help deepen the affect. The therapist has already discovered through exploration and discovery, areas that are difficult, painful, or just outside of awareness for the client. At these places, the therapist lingers longer. They slow down and focus on the more painful aspects of the experience that one partner is having with the other partner framed in attachment-based terms, so that the attachment fear or longing is emphasized. The assumption is that clients are not wanting to blame or alienate their partners (secondary emotions), but they end up using these defensive maneuvers when they are not in touch with their primary emotions.

Intonation, stress, rhythm, word phrasing, repetition, and use of key images can help clients feel their emotions more vividly. Also, it is important to realize that as you are speaking to one partner, you are also speaking to both of them. Partner 2 is listening to how you are reframing what Partner 1 cannot yet say to Partner 2 or might say in a confusing or triggering way. This can also have a profound effect on deepening Partner 2's emotions as they hear how much they mean to their partner.

EFCT uses the acronym RISSSSC to describe specific ways in which therapists use their voice and word phrasing: R standing for repeat, I for images, S for simple, S for slow, S for soft, S for specific, and C for client's words. For the purposes of this exercise, we will be focusing on three elements from this acronym:

- **Simple:** The therapist keeps words and phrases simple and concise.

- **Slow:** The therapist slows down the client enough to let their feelings catch up with their awareness. We have used "[*pause*]" in the example responses to help you establish a slower pace. For example, "You can hardly [*pause*] let yourself [*pause*] imagine [*pause*] that he still loves [*pause*] you." You will not read the word *pause* but rather take a pause at this place. Feel free to pause at different places that seem more natural for you. What is important is to pause at places you want the client to sink into and to have the opportunity to connect emotionally with what you are saying—especially those glimmering instances on the edge of awareness.

- **Soft:** A soft voice soothes and encourages deeper experiencing. It is reminiscent of a mother's soothing voice creating a safe and secure emotional cradle—rocking the child into a peaceful, emotionally regulated place—using the parent's nervous system to reregulate the child until maturity sets in.

The therapist should improvise a response to each client statement following these skill criteria:

1. **Conjecture the client's unmet attachment fear and/or longing.** You already did this in Exercise 2 as Criterion 4.
2. **As you point it out, say it simply, slowly, and softly.**

Note: This exercise uses the same client statements as the previous two exercises; however, the skill in this exercise focuses on the delivery of the response, not its content.

SKILL CRITERIA FOR EXERCISE 5
1. Conjecture the client's unmet **attachment** fear or longing.
2. As you point it out, say it simply, slowly, and softly (**SSS**).

Examples of Therapists Deepening Emotions With RISSSSC

Example 1

CLIENT: [*devastated*] So now my partner wants to sleep in the guest room. That is the ultimate rejection of me. I feel so devastated and so alone.

THERAPIST: [*softly*] Your partner [*pause*] is so important to you, [*pause*] that when they pull away from you in this way, [*pause*] you feel so rejected. (Criteria 1 and 2—**Attachment, SSS**)

Example 2

CLIENT: [*angry*] My partner seems to care more about her previous lover—the ex—than me. I hear so much about how wonderful the ex is, that I am thinking of ending this relationship. Then the two of them could be together forever.

THERAPIST: [*softly*] Deep down [*pause*] what you want [*pause*] is to be the wonderful one in her eyes. (Criteria 1 and 2—**Attachment, SSS**)

Example 3

CLIENT: [*discouraged*] I feel so invisible in my marriage. Does my partner even know I exist? I cry myself to sleep every night, and I don't think they even notice.

THERAPIST: [*softly*] Because they are so important to you, [*pause*] you want them to see your pain [*pause*] and feel for you. (Criteria 1 and 2—**Attachment, SSS**)

INSTRUCTIONS FOR EXERCISE 5

Step 1: Role-Play and Feedback

- The client says the first beginner client statement. The therapist **improvises** a response based on the skill criteria.
- The trainer (or, if not available, the client) provides **brief** feedback based on the skill criteria.
- The client then repeats the same statement, and the therapist again improvises a response. The trainer (or client) again provides brief feedback.

Step 2: Repeat

- Repeat Step 1 for all the statements **in the current difficulty level** (beginner, intermediate, or advanced).

Step 3: Assess and Adjust Difficulty

- The therapist completes the Deliberate Practice Reaction Form (see Appendix A) and decides whether to make the exercise easier or harder or to repeat the same difficulty level.

Step 4: Repeat for Approximately 15 Minutes

- Repeat Steps 1 to 3 for at least 15 minutes.
- The trainees then switch therapist and client roles and start over.

Now it's your turn! Follow Steps 1 and 2 from the exercise instructions.

Remember: The goal of the role-play is for trainees to practice improvising responses to the client statements in a manner that (a) uses the skill criteria and (b) feels authentic for the trainee. **Example therapist responses for each client statement are provided at the end of this exercise. Trainees should attempt to improvise their own responses before reading the examples.**

BEGINNER-LEVEL CLIENT STATEMENTS FOR EXERCISE 5
Beginner Client Statement 1
[Frustrated] My partner is so insensitive to the things that are important to me, and when I try to point this out, she walks away and won't speak to me for hours. It's so frustrating! I haven't been happy in this marriage for years.
Beginner Client Statement 2
[Irritated] Well, my partner doesn't try to tell me how he feels; he just goes from zero to 100 within seconds, and there's nothing I can do to stop the onslaught of outrage and criticism. Finally, I just can't take it anymore, so I shut down and walk away.
Beginner Client Statement 3
[Discouraged] My partner turns away from me at the least little thing. There's nothing I can do to keep her engaged. I toss and turn trying to sleep every night, and I don't think she even notices.
Beginner Client Statement 4
[Sarcastic] Oh, I notice his tossing and turning. Each turning tells me I am a horrible person. In fact, the tossing and turning bothers me so much, I am thinking of sleeping in another room.
Beginner Client Statement 5
[Devastated] So now she wants to sleep in another room. That is the ultimate rejection of me. I feel so devastated and so alone.

 Assess and adjust the difficulty before moving to the next difficulty level (see Step 3 in the exercise instructions).

INTERMEDIATE-LEVEL CLIENT STATEMENTS FOR EXERCISE 5

Intermediate Client Statement 1

[Angry] My wife's family is always on my case just because I don't have a college degree. Instead of standing up for me, my wife ignores their subtle jabs. It's like they matter more than I do.

Intermediate Client Statement 2

[Hostile] My partner has always seen me as the problem in this relationship. He never talks about his lapses or mistakes. Instead, he goes on and on about what a big disappointment I've been in this relationship. I'm tired of always being blamed for everything.

Intermediate Client Statement 3

[Upset] So my partner just buys whatever he wants without consulting me. I just feel like I'm the bank funding whatever he wants. I'm tempted to cut up his credit cards and make him come to me for whatever he needs.

Intermediate Client Statement 4

[Hurt] Every time we sit down to a home-cooked meal our teenager finds something to criticize me about. My husband just sits there and lets our child be so rude to me. I've told him I need his support and that I expect him to discipline our child but nothing gets said and I am all alone to set limits. Sometimes I feel completely ganged up on by the two of them.

Intermediate Client Statement 5

[Frustrated] No matter what I do, I can never get it right. Even last night after a full day of spring cleaning and shared projects, my partner had to go down the list of all the things I didn't have a chance to get to. It's just never good enough for them. I'm really frustrated.

 Assess and adjust the difficulty before moving to the next difficulty level (see Step 3 in the exercise instructions).

ADVANCED-LEVEL CLIENT STATEMENTS FOR EXERCISE 5
Advanced Client Statement 1
[Irritated] Is there anything wrong with my hanging out with my friends at a bar? But no, my partner has to call me every 10 minutes, screaming, "You need to come home." It's makes me want to stay out even later.
Advanced Client Statement 2
[Discouraged] I feel so invisible in my marriage. Does my partner even know I exist? I cry myself to sleep every night, and I don't think they even notice.
Advanced Client Statement 3
[Indignant] He always puts pressure on me to move out for a few days when his parents come to town. It hurts me that he still hides our relationship. There's nothing wrong with the love that we feel for each other.
Advanced Client Statement 4
[Angry] My partner seems to care more about her previous lover—the ex—than me. She spends so much time talking about how wonderful the ex is and ignoring me, that I am thinking of ending this relationship. Then the two of them could be together forever.
Advanced Client Statement 5
[Angry] He is so cruel the way he just sits there with that smug look, saying nothing and just staring at the floor.

Assess and adjust the difficulty here (see Step 3 in the exercise instructions). If appropriate, follow the instructions to make the exercise even more challenging (see Appendix A).

Example Therapist Responses: Deepening Emotions With RISSSSC

Remember: Trainees should attempt to improvise their own responses before consulting the examples. **Do not read the following responses verbatim unless you are having trouble coming up with your own!**

EXAMPLE RESPONSES TO BEGINNER-LEVEL CLIENT STATEMENTS FOR EXERCISE 5
Example Response to Beginner Client Statement 1
It especially matters to you [*pause*] to feel that what is important to you [*pause*] is also important to her. (Criteria 1 and 2)
Example Response to Beginner Client Statement 2
It is especially hard [*pause*] when the person you care about so much [*pause*] acts in this uncaring and hostile way. (Criteria 1 and 2)
Example Response to Beginner Client Statement 3
Deep down [*pause*] you need to know that you matter to her [*pause*] and that your sadness would grab her attention. (Criteria 1 and 2)
Example Response to Beginner Client Statement 4
Deep down [*pause*] you need him to acknowledge you as a good partner. (Criteria 1 and 2)
Example Response to Beginner Client Statement 5
She is so important to you [*pause*] that when she pulls away from you in this way [*pause*] you feel so alone. (Criteria 1 and 2)

EXAMPLE RESPONSES TO INTERMEDIATE-LEVEL CLIENT STATEMENTS FOR EXERCISE 5
Example Response to Intermediate Client Statement 1
You want to feel safe [*pause*] and like you are the most important person [*pause*] in her life [*pause*] and that she would stand up to her parents' criticism of you [*pause*] in a heartbeat. (Criteria 1 and 2)
Example Response to Intermediate Client Statement 2
You're looking into his eyes [*pause*] and seeing disappointment [*pause*]. It's really hard for you, especially when he means the world to you. (Criteria 1 and 2)
Example Response to Intermediate Client Statement 3
This is especially hard [*pause*] when you really long to be included and considered by him. (Criteria 1 and 2)
Example Response to Intermediate Client Statement 4
You long for him to be your support [*pause*] by setting clear limits with your child. (Criteria 1 and 2)
Example Response to Intermediate Client Statement 5
You long to please the one person [*pause*] who matters the most to you in your life. (Criteria 1 and 2)

EXAMPLE RESPONSES TO ADVANCED-LEVEL CLIENT STATEMENTS FOR EXERCISE 5
Example Response to Advanced Client Statement 1
You really long to feel trusted [*pause*] by your partner. (Criteria 1 and 2)
Example Response to Advanced Client Statement 2
They are so important to you. [*pause*] You want them to see your pain [*pause*] and feel for you. (Criteria 1 and 2)
Example Response to Advanced Client Statement 3
You want him to be proud of you [*pause*] and your relationship [*pause*] because he means the world to you. (Criteria 1 and 2)
Example Response to Advanced Client Statement 4
If only she [*pause*] could show you how you are the most important person, [*pause*] then you would feel reassured and safe. (Criteria 1 and 2)
Example Response to Advanced Client Statement 5
You desperately want him to hear your pleas [*pause*] and to show you that he cares about your pain. (Criteria 1 and 2)

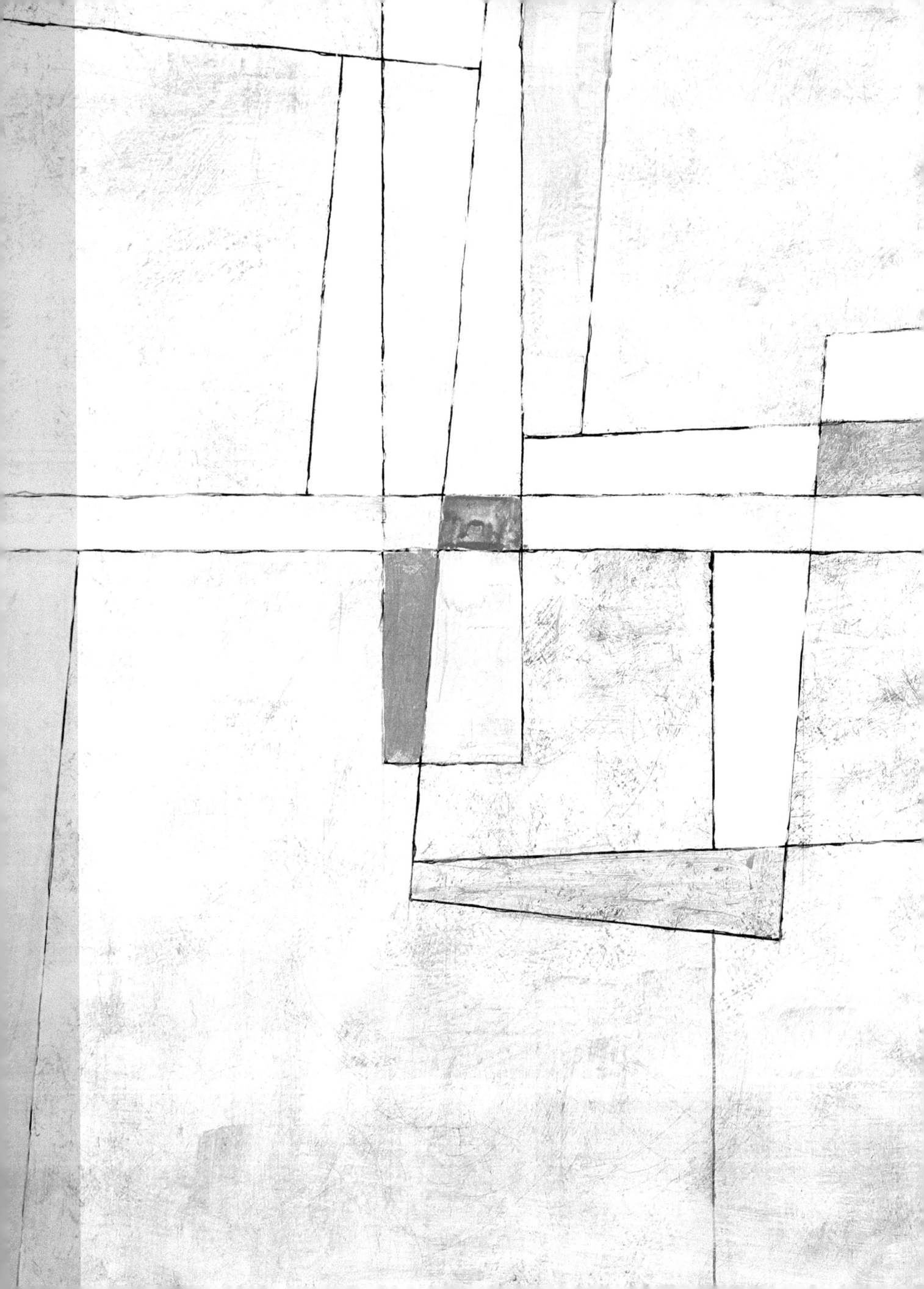

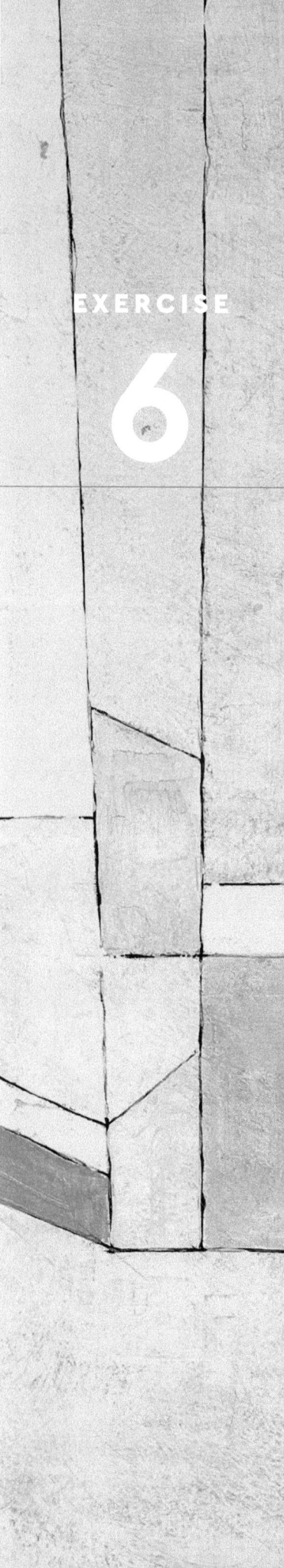

Tracking the Therapist's Inner Experience

Preparations for Exercise 6

1. Read the instructions in Chapter 2.

2. Download the Deliberate Practice Reaction Form and the Deliberate Practice Diary Form at https://www.apa.org/pubs/books/deliberate-practice-emotionally-focused-couple-therapy (see the "Resources" tab; also available in Appendixes A and B, respectively).

Exercise Format

For this skill, you will need two trainees: one role-playing the therapist and one reading a clinical situation. The therapist practices self-awareness by observing and speaking aloud their own internal reactions to the presented clinical situation. See the Exercise Instructions that follow.

Skill Description

Skill Difficulty Level: Intermediate

This exercise focuses on a very basic and essential underlying skill in emotionally focused couple therapy (EFCT)—being aware of how one is reacting internally while listening to and tracking the client.

When therapists track their own inner experience during a therapy session, it means that they pay attention to their own thoughts, feelings, somatic activation (bodily sensations), and visceral urges (gut-level directional responses) that arise within themselves while working with a client. This practice is often known as self-awareness or

https://doi.org/10.1037/0000436-008

Deliberate Practice in Emotionally Focused Couple Therapy, by H. Levenson, S. Jinich, A. Vaz, and T. Rousmaniere

self-reflection. The importance of therapists' tracking their own inner experience lies in the fact that therapy is a relational process, and the therapist's own internal state can directly influence their interventions and impact the couple and the therapeutic relationship. By being aware of what they are thinking, feeling, and sensing in their bodies, therapists can better understand how their internal experiences might be influencing their interactions with clients. This information also is excellent to bring up in supervision sessions.

Tracking inner experience allows therapists to gain insight into their own biases, countertransference (unconscious and conscious feelings and reactions toward the client), and personal triggers that may arise during therapy sessions. It helps them differentiate between their own issues and those of the client and can lessen their projecting their own unresolved emotions onto the client.

Self-compassion plays a crucial role in this process. *Self-compassion* refers to treating oneself with kindness, understanding, and acceptance, especially in moments of difficulty. Therapists need to cultivate self-compassion to avoid self-judgment or self-criticism when they encounter challenging emotions or thoughts during therapy sessions. By tracking and practicing self-compassion, therapists can create a safe and nonjudgmental space within themselves, allowing them to explore their own inner experiences without shutting down or becoming overwhelmed. A self-compassionate attitude helps therapists maintain their own well-being and prevent burnout as they learn to be gentle with themselves and acknowledge their own limitations. Moreover, self-compassion enables therapists to extend compassion and empathy toward their clients. When therapists are kind and accepting toward themselves, they can better understand and empathize with the struggles and vulnerabilities of their clients. This self-aware stance fosters a therapeutic environment that promotes healing and growth.

In summary, when therapists track their own inner experience during therapy sessions, it allows them to gain insight into their own biases, countertransference, and triggers. It is essential in the therapeutic process because it helps therapists create a nonjudgmental space within themselves and to maintain their well-being, and it also facilitates extending compassion toward their clients.

Exercise Instructions

This exercise involves tracking and reflecting on the therapist's own inner experience. This exercise is different from the others in this book because trainees are not practicing what to say out loud to couples in real therapy sessions. Instead, they practice self-awareness by observing and labeling their own internal reactions to a role-played, clinical situation, thus facilitating being aware of their inner voices when sitting with a real patient. To do this, trainees pair up as colleagues. One trainee will read the underlined text describing each clinical situation to provide context for their colleague who is listening as the therapist and then read the client statements for that scenario. The therapist monitors their own internal experience and reactions while listening to the material imagining they are in a session with the client, and then voices their reactions out loud to their colleague trainee. The therapist should not think about the *appropriate clinical interventions* or responses to the client but rather focus on their own internal reactions. Because each person's internal reactions are unique, this exercise does not include sample therapist responses.

The Deliberate Practice Reaction Form (Appendix A) provides lists of common internal responses, but you may notice your own responses that are not named on this form.

The therapist focuses on their own internal reactions following these skill criteria:

1. **The therapist observes and tracks their own internal experience (e.g., thoughts, feelings, somatic activation, visceral urges) in response to the clinical scenario and tries to stay self-compassionate to hear themselves better.** Sometimes the scenario might evoke deeply personal responses; sometimes it could evoke similar responses across a variety of therapists. What is important for this exercise is to be as aware as possible of one's own reactions.

2. **The therapist discloses what is going on internally (protecting their privacy and boundaries by not saying more than they want) to their colleague trainee.** Because this is a training session for educational purposes, the trainee should only say as much as they feel comfortable saying. There is no pressure intended in this exercise to be "completely open." It is imperative that trainees have the right not to reveal responses they wish to keep private. If the therapist has reactions to the clinical scenario in the "too hard" category on the Deliberate Practice Reaction Form, they should ask their colleague (or the trainer) to make the client's issues less provocative.

Reminder: The therapist is not practicing disclosing their inner reactions to the client. Rather, they are practicing self-awareness of their inner reactions by saying them aloud to a colleague.

SKILL CRITERIA FOR EXERCISE 6
1. The therapist observes and tracks their own internal experience (e.g., thoughts, feelings, somatic activation, visceral urges) in response to the clinical scenario and tries to stay self-compassionate to hear themselves better.
2. The therapist discloses what is going on internally (protecting their privacy and boundaries by not saying more than they want) to their colleague trainee.

Example of Therapists Tracking Their Inner Experience

Note: Underlined text is to be read aloud by the person playing the client to provide context.

At the beginning of the 11th session.

PARTNER 1: [*disappointed*] I'm sorry to say this, but I'm feeling a whole lot worse than when I started couples therapy with you.

THERAPIST: [Tracks their own internal experience to the scenario and shares what they are comfortable sharing with their colleague.]

INSTRUCTIONS FOR EXERCISE 6

Step 1: Role-Play and Feedback

- The colleague trainee reads aloud the <u>underlined text</u> before saying the first beginner client statement.
- The therapist describes their own experience out loud, sharing whatever thoughts, feelings, or bodily experiences they feel comfortable sharing.
- If you have reactions in the "too hard" category, ask the trainer (or your colleague) to make the role-play easier.

Step 2: Repeat

- Repeat Step 1 for all the scenarios **in the current difficulty level** (beginner, intermediate, or advanced).

Step 3: Assess and Adjust Difficulty

- The therapist completes the Deliberate Practice Reaction Form (see Appendix A) and decides whether to make the exercise easier or harder or to repeat the same difficulty level.

Step 4: Repeat for Approximately 15 Minutes

- Repeat Steps 1 to 3 for at least 15 minutes.
- The trainees then switch roles and start over.

Now it's your turn! Follow Steps 1 and 2 from the instructions.

Remember: We do not provide sample therapist responses to the statements because, unlike the other exercises, this one does not focus on developing the most appropriate response to the patient. **Instead, the main goal of this exercise is for trainees to explore and communicate their own genuine and uniquely personal internal reactions.**

   Note: Underlined text is to be read aloud by the person playing the client to provide context.

BEGINNER-LEVEL CLIENT STATEMENTS FOR EXERCISE 6
Beginner Client Statement 1
After 3 months of EFCT therapy, Partner 1 says to you:
[Delighted] You know, we have been to many therapists before you, and my husband could never open up. He always thought they didn't get him or weren't smart enough for him. He even ridiculed them on our way home after the sessions, and we would soon quit the therapy. I don't know what you're doing but keep doing it. I've never seen him so engaged. We joked last night that we want to name our first child after you.
Beginner Client Statement 2
Before initiating treatment with a couple and after meeting with them once together, you meet individually with each of the partners. When meeting with Partner 1, she says to you:
[Enthusiastic] I think you are really going to be able to help us. I've heard great things about you. None of the other couple therapists we've seen have done us any good, and one of them even did some harm.
Beginner Client Statement 3
Even though it has been 6 months since the couple began therapy, the couple continues to fight relentlessly. You've read papers on high-conflict couples and have tried everything to calm things down during the sessions. During the last session, you lost your temper and raised your voice. At the beginning of the next session, the husband says:
[Grateful] We left here last week feeling very embarrassed for how we have been behaving here. You're a great therapist and don't deserve to be stuck with us . . . and you're absolutely right, we really should stop fighting like 7-year-old children. Things have gone much better for us this week.
Beginner Client Statement 4
At the beginning of the 12th session, Partner 1 says:
[Cautiously] You know, we're doing somewhat better than when we started working with you, but frankly, it feels like you understand my partner much more than you understand me. When I come here, it sometimes feels like it's two against one trying to get me to say that I feel scared or something when I really don't.
Beginner Client Statement 5
At the end of a really difficult session with a couple, you were able to help Partner 1 put into words that it makes her feel sad when her partner takes care of everyone else before her. Partner 2 reacted really well to her revealing this and squeezed her hand. When you reflected on the power of her vulnerability, Partner 1 said:
[Challenging] But why do I have to be sad to have him show me a bit of attention and care?

 Assess and adjust the difficulty before moving to the next difficulty level (see Step 3 in the exercise instructions).

INTERMEDIATE-LEVEL CLIENT STATEMENTS FOR EXERCISE 6

Intermediate Client Statement 1

In an initial session one partner begins the session:

[Insistent] So I have a question for you. Are you married and do you have children? A simple yes or no will do.

Intermediate Client Statement 2

Partner 1 is having an individual session with you during a week when Partner 2 is out of town.

[Suggestive] I think it's obvious that you and I have feelings for each other. I see the way you look at me, the way you smile at me and get me like nobody else has understood me in my entire life. The other day when you leaned over to stop us from arguing, you lightly touched my knee, and it sent electricity up my spine. What should we do?

Intermediate Client Statement 3

At the beginning of a session early in the therapy, one partner starts the session by saying to his partner:

[Guilt-ridden] I have waited to bring this up and I just cannot hold it in anymore. I thought I had finally succeeded at controlling my impulses to spend money or doing stuff behind your back. I dipped into the college fund again. I thought it was a sure bet and that the investment would be a real winner, and it just kept dropping and I kept chasing it down. It's all gone. I didn't want you to find out because I knew you'd hate me.

Intermediate Client Statement 4

At the beginning of the sixth session, one partner says to you:

[Challenging] We clearly come from a different background than you do. Have you ever worked with clients like us? I mean, seriously, we often feel that you can't relate to us.

Intermediate Client Statement 5

One of the members of the couple you are treating is an EFCT trainee. In the second session, they say:

[Arrogant] I really think you could have gone deeper last week and then have me enact it. I have my couples deescalated way earlier than you are doing for us. If you can't do better, I really don't see how you'll be able to help us.

🛑 **Assess and adjust the difficulty before moving to the next difficulty level (see Step 3 in the exercise instructions).**

ADVANCED-LEVEL CLIENT STATEMENTS FOR EXERCISE 6
Advanced Client Statement 1
You have been working with a married couple for several months. The husband, who also is in individual therapy, begins the session.
[**Adamant**] My individual therapist really thinks that you need to get my wife into individual therapy. He thinks she is a borderline personality.
Advanced Client Statement 2
At the beginning of the 11th session, one partner says:
[**Angry**] Do you have a supervisor, or a boss, or something? I think they should know we are doing a whole lot worse since we started working with you.
Advanced Client Statement 3
In an individual session with a beginning couple, the girlfriend tells you that she is being physically and emotionally abused by her boyfriend. But she is very afraid of telling anyone.
[**Anxious**] My partner has told me that if I say anything, he will hurt me. What can I do?
Advanced Client Statement 4
You have been seeing this couple for almost a year. At the beginning of the last session, one partner says:
[**Distraught**] I just found out that the supposed love of my life has been having an affair and has been lying to me and to you this whole time.
Advanced Client Statement 5
In a first session with an elderly couple, one partner tells you that she has just been diagnosed with a rapidly progressive form of dementia and that she wants to end her life. Her wife desperately pleads with you:
[**Pleading**] I am here because I need your help. Please tell her that she can't abandon me and in this way.

⬢ **Assess and adjust the difficulty here (see Step 3 in the exercise instructions). If appropriate, follow the instructions to make the exercise even more challenging (see Appendix A).**

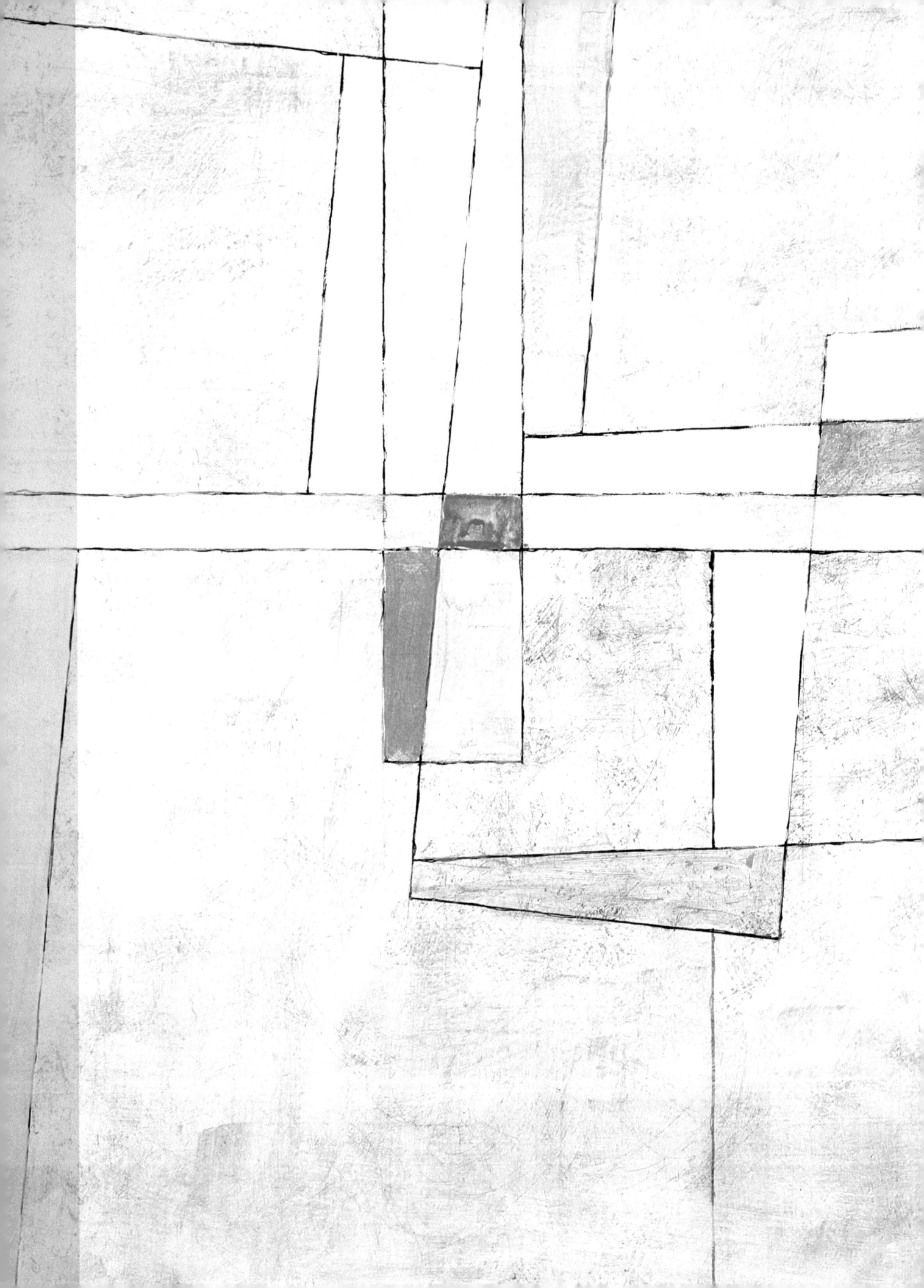

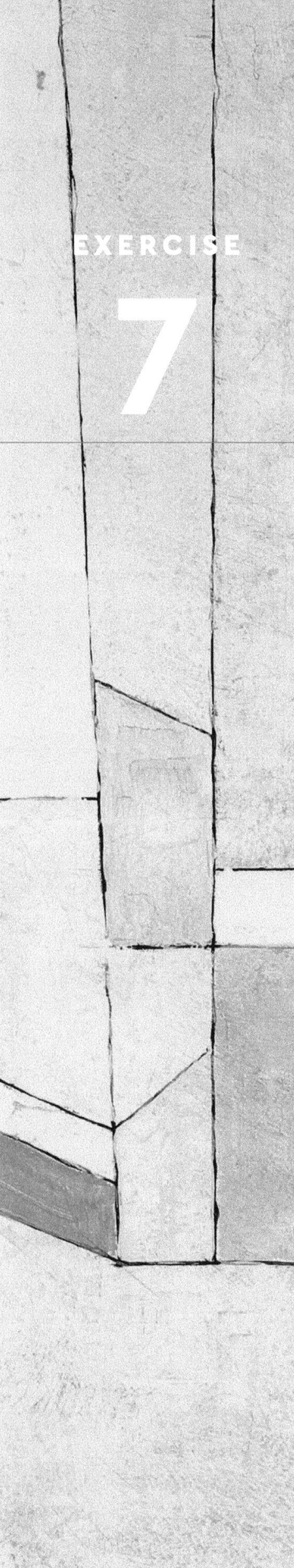

Providing a Rationale for Emotionally Focused Couple Therapy

Preparations for Exercise 7

1. Read the instructions in Chapter 2.

2. Download the Deliberate Practice Reaction Form and the Deliberate Practice Diary Form at https://www.apa.org/pubs/books/deliberate-practice-emotionally-focused-couple-therapy (see the "Resources" tab; also available in Appendixes A and B, respectively).

Exercise Format

For this skill, you will need two trainees: one role-playing the therapist and one role-playing a partner in a couple. The context for the skill is a couple therapy session where you imagine both partners are present, but only one partner is speaking.

Skill Description

Skill Difficulty Level: Intermediate

Often when people come into couple therapy, it is their first time. However, they may have seen portrayals of therapy (ridiculous ones or real-life examples) in the media. Sometimes they get the idea that therapy is about reducing conflict, learning to negotiate, or mastering communication skills. Sometimes they have the idea it is about not getting angry, having date nights, deciding how to raise their children, or even deciding who is right or wrong. It may be a way to end a relationship in the context of having "done everything possible" to save it. Whatever people's ideas, they will have questions about the particular approach of emotionally focused couple therapy (EFCT). If they don't have them at the outset, they will have them as the therapy evolves.

https://doi.org/10.1037/0000436-009

Deliberate Practice in Emotionally Focused Couple Therapy, by H. Levenson, S. Jinich, A. Vaz, and T. Rousmaniere

This exercise is to help therapists become more comfortable with explaining the rationale for EFCT in a verbally fluent manner (see Table E7.1).

The therapist's task is to improvise a response to each client statement following these skill criteria:

1. **Express appreciation for or validate the client's concern, question, or statement.** Expressing appreciation for the partner's concern or question about how EFCT works is an excellent opportunity to convey a respectful, transparent, and collaborative attitude—consistent with the therapeutic stance of the EFCT therapist. Especially at the beginning of the couple therapy, this stance will foster a working therapeutic alliance. In addition, throughout the therapy, answering questions about the therapist's actions and addressing concerns about the theory and approach of EFCT in a matter-of-fact and straightforward manner can lessen the couple's anxiety and promote their continued participation. When the partner's question is more reactive (coming from an interpersonally triggered place) than curious (see Example 2), it may require the therapist to validate the motive for the question rather than just appreciate that the partner asked the question. The therapist's intention would be that such validation could reduce the partner's reactivity.

2. **In response to the client's question, explain one or more relevant EFCT elements.** These responses will divide along two lines: (a) responses pertaining to the theory of EFCT, that is, the foundational pillars supporting the model, and (b) responses pertaining to what will happen in the sessions, especially the interventions the therapist will use in line with EFCT theory. Often people in couple therapy are surprised by the active, emotionally focused, and directive interventions of the therapist (e.g., telling partners what to say to each other, interrupting, focusing on what is driving the partners' behavior).

   Contextualizing the therapist's interventions as part of how EFCT works can make the process of the couple's work more understandable and less confusing. Similarly, learning about the empirical and scientific basis of EFCT can foster buy-in to the model and engender hope. Table E7.1 provides key EFCT elements that trainees can use to fulfill this criterion.

3. **Ask to confirm if your response(s) addressed the client's concern or question.** Asking if your answer was responsive to the question will provide useful information. It may open a fruitful dialogue about misunderstandings, differences in goals or strategies, and potential ruptures in the alliance. Your psychoeducational response may have

TABLE E7.1. Partner Concerns and Key Elements

Partner Concerns	Key Elements
Theory and approach of EFCT: What are the central elements of EFCT?	• Privilege emotion (e.g., gives us information about what we need/want; primary vs. secondary emotions) • Systems theory (reciprocal influences) • Foster safe and secure attachments (attachment theory)
Role of the therapist: What will happen in sessions?	• Process consultant (vs. content) • Choreographer (interrupt negative cycles, promote positive ones) • Follow a map of what needs to happen based on research (e.g., steps and stages)

Note. EFCT = emotionally focused couple therapy.

been objectively well-stated but ill-attuned to the actual needs of the person asking. Checking in with them gives you the opportunity to make necessary additions or corrections. The meta-message of this criterion is that you and the couple need to work as a team, making real-time, mid-course corrections as you go. You are dependent on their feedback to fine-tune your interventions.

SKILL CRITERIA FOR EXERCISE 7

1. Express appreciation for or **validate** the client's concern, question, or statement.
2. In response to the client's question, **explain** one or more relevant EFCT elements.
3. Ask to **confirm** if your response(s) addressed the client's concern or question.

Examples of Therapists Providing a Rationale for EFCT

Example 1

CLIENT: [*curious*] Our last couple therapist wasn't so active. I like when you are active, but what are you trying to do?

THERAPIST: What a perceptive question! (Criterion 1—**Validate**) My job is to help interrupt negative cycles of interaction and create opportunities for healthier patterns to take hold where people can see themselves and their partners in new and connecting ways. At the beginning of therapy, this requires me to be very active. (Criterion 2—**Explain**) Did what I said address the issue you raised? (Criterion 3—**Confirm**)

Example 2

CLIENT: [*indignant*] My partner can't see that I am right in this situation. You saw what happened. Can you tell them?

THERAPIST: Of course you would want me to weigh in here! It sounds really important to you that your partner sees that you are right. (Criterion 1—**Validate**) However, rather than trying to figure out who is right and who is wrong, what is important in this type of therapy is to identify dysfunctional dances that the two of you do—where one of you might get hurt and react defensively, triggering the other one to get defensive, for example. Before you know it, there are so many defensive walls going up that neither one of you can see one another anymore. (Criterion 2—**Explain**) Does that make sense? (Criterion 3—**Confirm**)

Example 3

CLIENT: [*curious*] So can you give me an overview of how the therapy will go? Is there a playbook? What can I expect?

THERAPIST: I'm glad you asked. (Criterion 1—**Validate**) Actually there is a playbook, constructed from years of research and clinical experience; this playbook has three phases. The first phase of our work together focuses on de-escalating negative interaction patterns. It can be the toughest part of our work as we identify how your self-protective behavior actually triggers your partner in unhelpful ways. In the second phase, we do the deeper work of seeing what each of you needs in the relationship and go about meeting those needs. Here I will be pretty active in structuring new interactions that help build more relationship satisfaction. The third stage is solidifying what you have learned. (Criterion 2—**Explain**) I know that's a pretty brief explanation, but does it give you some idea of how the therapy will go? (Criterion 3—**Confirm**)

INSTRUCTIONS FOR EXERCISE 7

Step 1: Role-Play and Feedback

- The client says the first beginner client statement (any <u>underlined text</u> before a statement should also be read aloud to provide context). The therapist **improvises** a response based on the skill criteria.
- The trainer (or, if not available, the client) provides **brief** feedback based on the skill criteria.
- The client then repeats the same statement, and the therapist again improvises a response. The trainer (or client) again provides brief feedback.

Step 2: Repeat

- Repeat Step 1 for all the statements **in the current difficulty level** (beginner, intermediate, or advanced).

Step 3: Assess and Adjust Difficulty

- The therapist completes the Deliberate Practice Reaction Form (see Appendix A) and decides whether to make the exercise easier or harder or to repeat the same difficulty level.

Step 4: Repeat for Approximately 15 Minutes

- Repeat Steps 1 to 3 for at least 15 minutes.
- The trainees then switch therapist and client roles and start over.

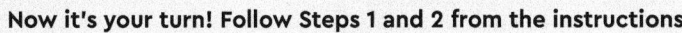 **Now it's your turn! Follow Steps 1 and 2 from the instructions.**

Remember: The goal of the role-play is for trainees to practice improvising responses to the client statements in a manner that (a) uses the skill criteria and (b) feels authentic for the trainee. **Example therapist responses for each client statement are provided at the end of this exercise. Trainees should attempt to improvise their own responses before reading the examples.**

BEGINNER-LEVEL CLIENT STATEMENTS FOR EXERCISE 7
Beginner Client Statement 1
[Curious] So can you give me an overview of how the therapy will go? Is there a playbook? What can we expect?
Beginner Client Statement 2
[Friendly] Our last couple therapist wasn't so active. I like when you are active, but what are you trying to do?
Beginner Client Statement 3
[Challenging] What's with all the slowing down stuff? You keep saying things like, "Let's slow down," and then you kind of repeat what I or my partner just said. Why all the slowing down? We don't have tons of time or money to do this.
Beginner Client Statement 4
[Anxious] It seems like you repeat everything I'm saying in here. It makes me wonder if you don't believe me the first time.
Beginner Client Statement 5
[Irritated] When I am talking with you, you sometimes have me turn to them and say the exact same thing again to them, when they are sitting right here and heard every word of our conversation already. What's with that?

🛑 **Assess and adjust the difficulty before moving to the next difficulty level (see Step 3 in the exercise instructions).**

INTERMEDIATE-LEVEL CLIENT STATEMENTS FOR EXERCISE 7
Intermediate Client Statement 1
[Forceful] So I travel a lot. When I am traveling, could you see my spouse alone?
Intermediate Client Statement 2
[Skeptical] I'm not sure getting into all our stuff is going to be helpful. Every time we start talking about our difficulties, it ends up in a big argument. Can you guarantee that if we come here, it won't go badly?
Intermediate Client Statement 3
[Fearful] Will you tell us if we should break up or stay together?
Intermediate Client Statement 4
[Engaged] Why is this approach called "emotionally focused"?
Intermediate Client Statement 5
[Dismayed] My partner and I are so different. I want to be close and loving but my partner is completely disinterested in being connected to me. I am at my wits end and thinking of getting divorced. Is there any hope for us?

🛑 **Assess and adjust the difficulty before moving to the next difficulty level (see Step 3 in the exercise instructions).**

ADVANCED-LEVEL CLIENT STATEMENTS FOR EXERCISE 7
Advanced Client Statement 1
[Reserved] I am thinking that our cultural background is different from most of your clients. Will the type of therapy you do be helpful to us?
Advanced Client Statement 2
[Irritated] You're always interrupting me!
Advanced Client Statement 3
[Frustrated] My partner can't see that I am right in this situation. You saw what happened. Can you tell them?
Advanced Client Statement 4
A prospective client asked the therapist a question over the phone.
[Hesitant] We are in a relationship made up of three partners, and we are struggling with some issues. Can EFCT work with polyamorous relationships?
Advanced Client Statement 5
[Resigned] We just don't have any passion. My partner always is demanding more sexual contact, and I just feel pressured. Eventually sex just became a turn off for me—another place where I didn't measure up. Is there any hope for us?

Assess and adjust the difficulty here (see Step 3 in the exercise instructions). If appropriate, follow the instructions to make the exercise even more challenging (see Appendix A).

Example Therapist Responses: Providing a Rationale for EFCT

Remember: Trainees should attempt to improvise their own responses before reading the examples. **Do not read the following responses verbatim unless you are having trouble coming up with your own!**

EXAMPLE RESPONSES TO BEGINNER-LEVEL CLIENT STATEMENTS FOR EXERCISE 7
Example Response to Beginner Client Statement 1
I'm glad you asked. (Criterion 1) Actually there is a playbook, constructed from years of research and clinical experience; the playbook has three phases. The first phase of our work together is called de-escalation, and it is the toughest stage as we identify how you trigger one another, and get that whole process to quiet down so you can really hear one another without setting one another off. In the second phase, we do the deeper work of seeing what each of you needs in the relationship and go about meeting those needs. The third stage is solidifying what you have learned so that the connection lasts. (Criterion 2) I know that's a pretty brief explanation, but does it give you some idea of how the therapy will go? (Criterion 3)
Example Response to Beginner Client Statement 2
What a perceptive question! (Criterion 1) My job is to help interrupt negative cycles of interaction and create opportunities for healthier patterns to take hold where people can see themselves and their partners in new and connecting ways. At the beginning of therapy that requires me to be very active. (Criterion 2) Did what I said address the issue you raised? (Criterion 3)
Example Response to Beginner Client Statement 3
Yeah, I'm glad you took notice of what I am doing there. You've got it just right. I do slow things down a lot. (Criterion 1) In this emotionally focused approach, we slow things down to make space for more than the fast, reactive emotions that often come up when we are triggered or emotionally dysregulated. Slowing down can help make space for the more vulnerable emotions to come through. And paradoxically, slowing down moment-by-moment really speeds up the work we can get done. (Criterion 2) In terms of what you've experienced in here when I do help slow things down, does this make sense? (Criterion 3)
Example Response to Beginner Client Statement 4
Yes, this is a good point you bring up about all the repeating I do. (Criterion 1) Repeating things back to you is my way of making sure that I am hearing you accurately and understanding you. I want you to know that your concerns are very important to me. I very much want you to correct me when I get it wrong. We need to work as a team in here, and your mid-course corrections will help me do a better job. (Criterion 2) Can we have an agreement that you will do that—let me know when something I've said doesn't represent how you really feel? (Criterion 3)

EXAMPLE RESPONSES TO BEGINNER-LEVEL
CLIENT STATEMENTS FOR EXERCISE 7

Example Response to Beginner Client Statement 5
Yes, I can see that this is confusing. They have clearly heard what you said to me, so why repeat the whole thing directly to them? (Criterion 1) Well, this repeating directly to our partners is a signature piece of this therapy. It's one thing for your partner to hear you talking to me about how you feel, but quite another when you look at them directly and tell them face to face about your feelings. When we look at our partners eye to eye, we *feel* what they are saying rather than just hearing it. It helps change the conversation from a more cognitive reactive one, into a more emotional receptive one. This is one of the key ways that we are trying to help you develop a more secure attachment with each other so you can take greater emotional risks and over time learn to do this on your own. (Criterion 2) Next time I ask you to do this, I will check out with both of you to see if it has made any emotional difference when you are talking face to face. OK? (Criterion 3)

EXAMPLE RESPONSES TO INTERMEDIATE-LEVEL CLIENT STATEMENTS FOR EXERCISE 7

Example Response to Intermediate Client Statement 1

Hmm. I'm so glad you brought this up because this is something we need to figure out. (Criterion 1) There may be some times when I would want to see each of you alone, but mainly I want to see the two of you together each session. The reason for that is I see my client as the couple—the two of you. The two of you make up a system of interactions that are characterized by certain patterns—patterns in the ways you influence each other. What I will be trying to do is influence those patterns, so instead of being distressing and dysfunctional, they can feel healthy and secure. It's sort of like I am a dance instructor helping you learn some smoother moves as you dance together, so to do that I need you in the same room together. (Criterion 2) How does what I am saying strike you? (Criterion 3)

Example Response to Intermediate Client Statement 2

I can really appreciate why you want to make sure that things won't get worse in your relationship if you start couple therapy. That's very understandable. (Criterion 1) The reason to come to therapy is to be able to explore your thoughts and feelings in some new ways you've probably never done before. My job is to keep things safe in here so that you can explore patterns of interacting that have been problematic and replace them with more positive patterns. The type of couple work that I do is empirically validated, and the process of change has been systemically studied and outlined. It's been used with many kinds of clients and problems. Of course I cannot make any promises about your specific outcome, but what I can guarantee is that this process will be respectful and collaborative. I will try to be transparent throughout. You should know in a few sessions if you feel that the work is going in a safe enough direction, and I invite your feedback every inch of the way. (Criterion 2) Is there more that you would like me to say at this point? (Criterion 3)

Example Response to Intermediate Client Statement 3

Wow! That's a really major question. I can see why you brought it up so directly. (Criterion 1) My job isn't to keep you together or conversely to tell you you shouldn't be together. My job is to keep the room from filling with smoke—the smoke of misperceptions built up over the years, convincing each of you that being with your partner is not safe. Often when people come to therapy it is because they fear they are not seen in the heart and mind of their partner. I would like to help you clear the smoke of defensiveness and repeated hurt, of recriminations of shame and guilt, so you can truly see each other again—or maybe for the first time—to help you get in touch with your authentic self and see your partner authentically. Then you will know what you want to do. (Criterion 2) Does that make sense? (Criterion 3)

Example Response to Intermediate Client Statement 4

That is a wonderful question! (Criterion 1) Sue Johnson, who cocreated EFCT, talks about emotions as being the dance music between couples. Research has shown that rather than help people solve content issues—for example, should we have children, where should we move, how do we share housework chores?—therapy works best when it helps couples develop comforting interactions and be able to stay emotionally engaged when they disagree. Emotion organizes our inner world and our relational world. So there is a lot of focus on emotion in the therapy I do. I'll be on the lookout for what is most emotionally relevant or painful for each of you. That will give us important information about what each of you is needing that you are not getting. (Criterion 2) Does that make sense? (Criterion 3)

**EXAMPLE RESPONSES TO INTERMEDIATE-LEVEL
CLIENT STATEMENTS FOR EXERCISE 7**

Example Response to Intermediate Client Statement 5

To answer your question, which is a critical one, (Criterion 1) let me have you imagine a porcupine and a tortoise. When threatened, they each do what is instinctual for them to do. They protect themselves. The porcupine's quills become rigid and dangerous, and they look angry, but really this is how they look when they are scared. Similarly, the tortoise defends itself by hiding within its hard shell. The tortoise may seem unaffected or impossible to reach, but in fact, it too is scared. To us humans, disconnection is threatening to our very survival. So, when we feel alone, some of us naturally defend by getting angry (the rigid quills), while others withdraw (into the shell). As we look at our partner, we see quills or a shell and wonder if they will really be there for us in our time of need. What we want to do in this therapy is to find out what is below these defensive strategies—what are your deeper, more vulnerable emotions which you are not sharing with each other in a way that can be heard. (Criterion 2) Does this story make sense to you? (Criterion 3)

EXAMPLE RESPONSES TO ADVANCED-LEVEL CLIENT STATEMENTS FOR EXERCISE 7

Example Response to Advanced Client Statement 1

You have raised a very important concern—will I be able to help you not only as a unique couple, but also given your cultural background? Of course I want to hear more about your concerns. They are very important for me to understand. (Criterion 1) Let me also say a word about how EFCT approaches therapy. EFCT is based on the science of attachment—that regardless of one's cultural background, we are all part of the human family and are therefore wired for connection—seeking safety and security in the bonds we form with one another. Consequently, couples from various cultures have been helped by EFCT. Having said that, however, your cultural background, as you suggest, is intricately intertwined with who you are—your view of self, your attachments, and your emotional life, and that makes you unique. In my collaborative work with you, I want to make sure that I understand how you see your culture impacting your relationship. Perhaps we can start there. (Criterion 2) I'm wondering how my answer to your concern has landed. Can you tell me? (Criterion 3)

Example Response to Advanced Client Statement 2

I am so sorry. I know that must be annoying and perhaps even feels disrespectful. I'm very glad you are letting me know. (Criterion 1) What I am trying to do is interrupt that negative cycle we've talked about. As the two of you trigger each other in your efforts to defend yourself and protest the behavior of the other, you are getting more and more disconnected from each other and more and more entrenched in that rut of despair. I wish to prevent your getting stuck in that rut and give you both the opportunity to see each other in a new light. (Criterion 2) Does that help explain where I am coming from when I interrupt? (Criterion 3)

Example Response to Advanced Client Statement 3

Of course you would want me to weigh in here! It is really important to you that your partner see that you are right. (Criterion 1) However, in this kind of therapy, it's not so simple to know who is right and who is wrong. I see it as a case where you both are getting caught up in a dysfunctional cycle—where one of you gets hurt and reacts defensively, triggering the other one to get defensive, and before you know it there are so many defensive maneuvers going on that neither one of you can see one another anymore. It's like the cycle is the enemy of your connectedness. (Criterion 2) Does that make sense? (Criterion 3)

Example Response to Advanced Client Statement 4

That's a very important question and I appreciate the way you framed it. (Criterion 1) Let me tell you the perspective of EFCT. EFCT sees human beings as capable of deeply loving more than one person. Think about how we can love more than one child or how we can love both parents. So having multiple adult others that we trust and can turn to in a moment of need is an amazing resource. EFCT therapists privilege one's wired-in need to be in secure relationships. We know how to process ruptures and how to explore what the underlying longings and fears are to help partners to learn to risk and to reach for each other. However, working with polyamorous partners is a unique skill set that I don't have. If you'd like, I could help you find such a qualified EFCT therapist to work with you and your partners. (Criterion 2) How does that sound? (Criterion 3)

Example Response to Advanced Client Statement 5

I can see that these sexual issues feel threating to your relationship. (Criterion 1) From an attachment perspective, when the emotional bonds between a couple feel tenuous and even broken, a couple's ability to resolve sexual issues is severely compromised. In EFCT, I would help you create emotional safety and connection with one another so that you could be open and responsive to what each other wants and needs regarding your intimacy. (Criterion 2) How does that sound? (Criterion 3)

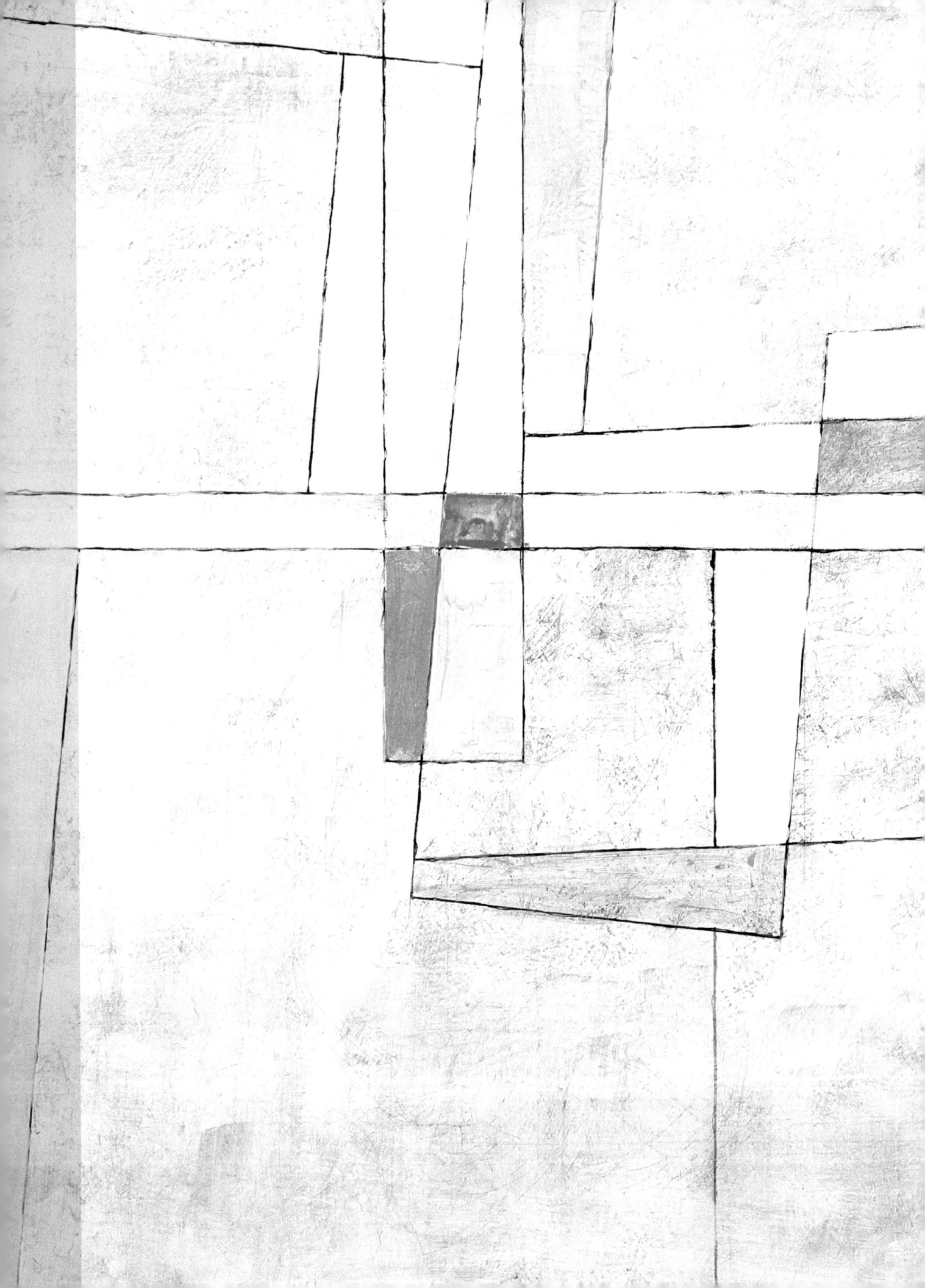

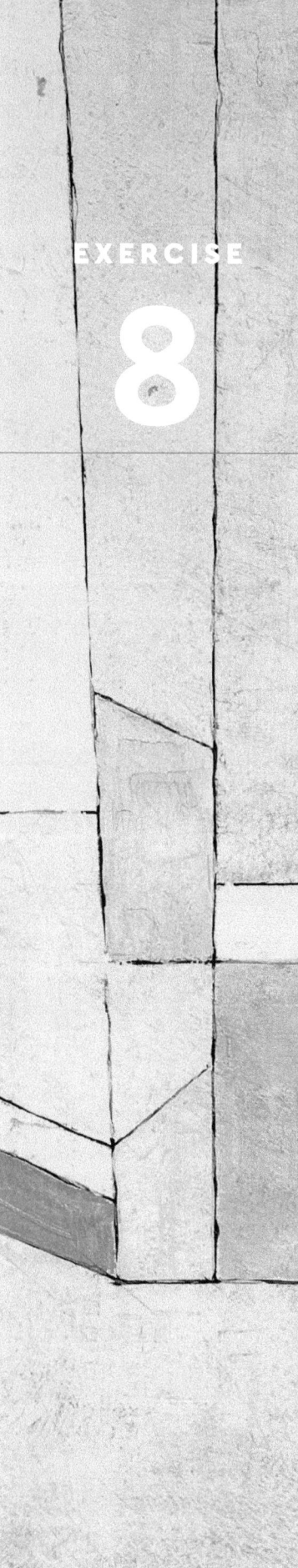

Gathering and Assembling Elements of Emotion

Preparations for Exercise 8

1. Read the instructions in Chapter 2.

2. Download the Deliberate Practice Reaction Form and the Deliberate Practice Diary Form at https://www.apa.org/pubs/books/deliberate-practice-emotionally-focused-couple-therapy (see the "Resources" tab; also available in Appendixes A and B, respectively).

Exercise Format

For this skill, you will need two trainees: one role-playing the therapist and one role-playing both partners in a couple, speaking as only one partner for each dialogue. The context for the skill is a couple therapy session where you will imagine that both partners are present, with only one partner speaking at a time.

Skill Description

Skill Difficulty Level: Advanced

This exercise represents the first step in a three-part process and is intended to be followed by deepening emotions and setting up enactments (Exercise 9) and inviting partners to say why they feel expressing their emotions directly is too challenging (referred to as "slicing the risk thinner"; Exercise 10). All three exercises follow the same five couples so that trainees can rehearse these skills sequentially with the same couple, as they would in actual practice. When a couple gets into one of their dysfunctional cycles, they need help organizing and understanding their emotional experience, so that eventually

https://doi.org/10.1037/0000436-010

Deliberate Practice in Emotionally Focused Couple Therapy, by H. Levenson, S. Jinich, A. Vaz, and T. Rousmaniere

they will be able to use that information to understand themselves (within) and to reconnect with their partner (between). The first step in assembling the elements of their emotional experience is to identify a *trigger* in the interpersonal communication—something their partner does that they perceive as a threat signal or danger cue. Couples are rarely able to slow down long enough to understand that deep down, the trigger feels scary. They don't turn to their partner and say that they feel afraid. Instead, what they typically do is react from a place of fear, resulting in defensive behavior.

Clients calm down and have greater access to more adaptive behavioral responses when they understand, in a more coherent and organized manner, the central elements of emotion (Johnson, 2019). According to Arnold (1960), a prominent psychologist known for her work on the study of emotions, emotions consist of three central elements: physiological changes, cognitive appraisal, and subjective feelings. Understanding and organizing these elements are crucial for developing adaptive behavioral responses.

Emotions are accompanied by physiological changes in the body, such as increased heart rate, sweating, or changes in facial expressions. These bodily responses are automatic and serve as signals to the individual and others about their emotional state. Recognizing and understanding these physiological changes can help individuals become more aware of their emotions and regulate them effectively. *Cognitive appraisal* refers to the evaluation and interpretation (*meaning making*) of a situation or event, that determines the emotional response. Different individuals may appraise the same situation differently, leading to varied emotional reactions. Understanding the cognitive appraisal process allows individuals to recognize their own thought patterns and beliefs that contribute to specific emotional responses. Subjective feelings refer to the conscious experience of emotions that individuals have. In sum, emotions are complex subjective experiences that involve cognitive processes, bodily sensations, and personal interpretations. They are influenced by an individual's thoughts, beliefs, and past experiences.

This exercise focuses on learning to help clients understand that triggers lead to physiological changes and cognitive appraisals, which in turn influence their action tendencies or behaviors. Organizing the central elements of emotions helps individuals regulate their emotional responses effectively. By recognizing the physiological changes and cognitive appraisals that trigger specific emotions, individuals can develop strategies to manage and control their emotional reactions. This ability to regulate emotions is crucial for adaptive behavior and maintaining healthy relationships.

Therapists who practice emotionally focused couple therapy help their clients to "assemble" their emotions to access their experience more clearly and fully with the goal of eventually being able to send a clearer and more vulnerable emotional signal to their partner. This in turn helps to create new bonding events between partners and, if done well, allows them to experience each other in a newer and safer manner. The skill of gathering and assembling the elements of emotion is a key building block toward developing secure attachment in couples.

Over the course of this exercise, the trainee playing the client will alternate between playing Partner 1 and Partner 2 within a couple. For instance, Partner 1 of a couple speaks in Beginner Dialogue 1, then Partner 2 of the same couple speaks in Beginner Dialogue 2. The therapist's task is to improvise a response to each client statement following these skill criteria:

1. **Ask the client who is speaking (Partner 1 or Partner 2) how their body feels when they are triggered by their partner's behavior.** Asking how the body feels (e.g., stomach tightening) is the first appraisal in assembling the elements of emotion. Getting the client in touch with their visceral reactions is a crucial first step.

2. **Ask the client what their triggered bodily response typically means to them.** Asking what the person thinks—what sense are they making of their sensations that occur in response to a trigger—is the second appraisal in this exercise. It involves meaning making.

3. **Ask the client about their typical action tendency in response to their triggered bodily response and the meaning it holds for them.** This is what the person customarily says or does—often as a protest to feeling abandoned or found inadequate—when experiencing the trigger, somatic reactions, and meaning.

4. **Organize all the elements into a summary, then check with the client for accuracy.** The assembling of the elements of emotion follows this format: "So, you get triggered when your partner does _____, and you experience the reaction in your body in this way _____. In making sense of your partner's behavior, you think they _____, and that causes you to say or do _____. Do I have that right?"

Because this exercise uses a dialogue format that is slightly different from most other skills in this book, please review the exercise instructions before initiating practice.

SKILL CRITERIA FOR EXERCISE 8

1. Ask the client (Partner 1 or Partner 2) how their **body** typically feels when they are triggered by their partner's behavior.
2. Ask client what their triggered bodily response typically **means** to them.
3. Ask client about their typical **action** tendency in response to their triggered bodily response and the meaning it holds for them.
4. Organize all the elements into a **summary**, then check with the client for accuracy.

Note: As a starting point, the triggers are identified in the text.

Example of a Therapist Gathering and Assembling Elements of Emotion

Note: Underlined text is to be read aloud by the person playing the client to provide context.

Example 1

This is Partner 1 of a couple that is stuck in a pursue–withdraw cycle.

PARTNER 1: [*irritated*] I beg my partner to clear off the dining room table of all his junk and stacks of paper, but he never does. It just keeps building up. (Trigger)

THERAPIST: And when you beg him to clear the dining table of all his papers and things, but he never does, are you aware of any reaction in your body? (Criterion 1—**Body**)

PARTNER 1: My stomach becomes one big, knotted mess.

THERAPIST: And when your stomach becomes a knotted mess, after he ignores your request to put his things away, what do you tell yourself about what is happening in those moments? (Criterion 2—**Means**)

PARTNER 1: [*irritated*] That what I want simply doesn't matter to him. He could care less what it is like for me to live this way. It's actually quite hurtful.

THERAPIST: When he doesn't do what you've asked and your stomach is in knots because what you want and need just doesn't seem to matter to him, what do you say or do? (Criterion 3—**Action**)

PARTNER 1: [*angry*] I raise my voice and I tell him, "I'm sick of living like this. It's a pigsty in here!" He can tell by my volume and tone that I'm angry and disappointed.

THERAPIST: So, you get triggered when your partner doesn't clear the dining table of all his papers and things, (Trigger) and you can feel your stomach becoming one big, knotted mess. (Criterion 1) In making sense of your partner's behavior, you think that what you want doesn't really matter to him, (Criterion 2) and that causes you to yell at him that you're sick of living like this. (Criterion 3) Do I have that right? (Criterion 4—**Summary**)

INSTRUCTIONS FOR EXERCISE 8

Step 1: Role-Play and Feedback

- The client says the first beginner statement and reads the therapist prompt for Criterion 1. The therapist **improvises** a response based on the skill criterion.
- The trainer (or, if not available, the partner) provides **brief** feedback based on the skill criterion. If the criterion is not met, the client repeats the same statement, and the therapist again improvises responses until it is easy to meet the skill criterion.
- The client reads the second beginner statement in the same dialogue, followed by the therapist prompt for Criterion 2. The therapist improvises a response.
- This continues until the dialogue has been completed.

Step 2: Repeat

- Repeat Step 1 for all the dialogues **in the current difficulty level** (beginner, intermediate, or advanced).

Step 3: Assess and Adjust Difficulty

- The therapist completes the Deliberate Practice Reaction Form (see Appendix A) and decides whether to make the exercise easier or harder or to repeat the same difficulty level.

Step 4: Repeat for Approximately 15 Minutes

- Repeat Steps 1 to 3 for at least 15 minutes.
- The trainees then switch therapist and client roles and start over.

Now it's your turn! Follow Steps 1 and 2 from the exercise instructions.

Remember: The goal of the role-play is for trainees to practice improvising responses to the client statements in a manner that (a) uses the skill criteria and (b) feels authentic for the trainee. **Example therapist responses for each client statement are provided at the end of this exercise. Trainees should attempt to improvise their own responses before reading the examples.**

BEGINNER-LEVEL DIALOGUE 1: COUPLE 1, PARTNER 1 (THIS IS PARTNER 1 OF A COUPLE THAT IS STUCK IN A PURSUE–WITHDRAW CYCLE.)
PARTNER 1: **[Irritated]** I beg my partner to clear off the dining room table of all their junk and stacks of paper, but they never do. It just keeps building up. (Trigger)
THERAPIST PROMPT (CRITERION 1): Ask Partner 1 how their body typically feels when they are triggered by their partner's behavior.
PARTNER 1: **[Matter-of-fact]** My stomach becomes one big, knotted mess.
THERAPIST PROMPT (CRITERION 2): Ask them what their triggered bodily response typically means to them.
PARTNER 1: **[Irritated]** That what I want simply doesn't matter to them. They could care less what it is like for me to live this way. It's actually quite hurtful.
THERAPIST PROMPT (CRITERION 3): Ask them about their typical action tendency in response to their triggered bodily response and the meaning it holds for them.
PARTNER 1: **[Angry]** I raise my voice and I tell them, "I'm sick of living like this. It's a pigsty in here!" They can tell by my volume and tone that I'm angry and disappointed.
THERAPIST PROMPT (CRITERION 4): Organize all the elements into a summary then check with Partner 1 for accuracy.

BEGINNER-LEVEL DIALOGUE 2:
COUPLE 1, PARTNER 2 (THIS IS PARTNER 2 OF THE SAME COUPLE STUCK IN A PURSUE–WITHDRAW CYCLE.)

PARTNER 2: [Frustrated] My partner is constantly on my case about being messy. I am criticized a lot. They never see what I do well. (Trigger)

THERAPIST PROMPT (CRITERION 1): Ask Partner 2 how their body typically feels when they are triggered by their partner's behavior.

PARTNER 2: [Worried] My heart races. I can feel my heart racing.

THERAPIST PROMPT (CRITERION 2): Ask them what their triggered bodily response typically means to them.

PARTNER 2: [Irritated] That I'll never catch a break. They will always make mountains out of mole hills, and everything will always be my fault. They'll never understand me or accept me.

THERAPIST PROMPT (CRITERION 3): Ask them about their typical action tendency in response to their triggered bodily response and the meaning it holds for them.

PARTNER 2: [Sad] I just shut down and say nothing. I walk away. I don't want any more criticism.

THERAPIST PROMPT (CRITERION 4): Organize all the elements into a summary, then check with Partner 2 for accuracy.

BEGINNER-LEVEL DIALOGUE 3:
COUPLE 2, PARTNER 1 (THIS IS PARTNER 1 IN A COUPLE WHO HAVE BEEN LIVING TOGETHER FOR 1 YEAR. THEY ARE SPEAKING ABOUT THEIR SEX LIFE.)

PARTNER 1: [Frustrated] My partner thinks he can ignore me all day and expect me to want to be sexually intimate at night. (Trigger)
THERAPIST PROMPT (CRITERION 1): Ask Partner 1 how her body typically feels when she is triggered by her partner's behavior.
PARTNER 1: [Upset] I feel myself get tearful, and I tense up.
THERAPIST PROMPT (CRITERION 2): Ask her what her triggered bodily response typically means to her.
PARTNER 1: [Worried] It's clear he doesn't get me or remember what I have said about needing more emotional connection before I can feel sexual desire.
THERAPIST PROMPT (CRITERION 3): Ask her about her typical action tendency in response to her triggered bodily response and the meaning it holds for her.
PARTNER 1: [Sad] I don't say anything. I just stay quiet while tears roll down my cheeks.
THERAPIST PROMPT (CRITERION 4): Organize all the elements into a summary, then check with Partner 1 for accuracy.

BEGINNER-LEVEL DIALOGUE 4: **COUPLE 2, PARTNER 2 (THIS IS PARTNER 2 OF THE SAME COUPLE** **SPEAKING ABOUT THEIR SEX LIFE.)**
PARTNER 2: [Matter-of fact] Anytime I want to talk about our sex life, she gets very quiet and tearful. (Trigger)
THERAPIST PROMPT (CRITERION 1): Ask Partner 2 how his body typically feels when he is triggered by his partner's behavior.
PARTNER 2: [Embarrassed] I feel really tense all over.
THERAPIST PROMPT (CRITERION 2): Ask him what his triggered bodily response typically means to him.
PARTNER 2: [Resigned] That my expressing my sexual needs hurts her. I think I will just have to accept feeling alone in this relationship.
THERAPIST PROMPT (CRITERION 3): Ask him about his typical action tendency in response to his triggered bodily response and the meaning it holds for him.
PARTNER 2: [Confused] I kind of freeze. I say things like, "Are you OK? Did I just upset you?" And then I won't bring up the topic for a couple of months.
THERAPIST PROMPT (CRITERION 4): Organize all the elements into a summary, then check with Partner 2 for accuracy.

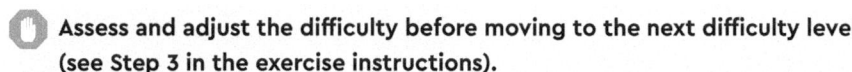 **Assess and adjust the difficulty before moving to the next difficulty level (see Step 3 in the exercise instructions).**

INTERMEDIATE-LEVEL DIALOGUE 1: COUPLE 3, PARTNER 1 (THIS IS THE HUSBAND OF A COUPLE WHO HAVE BEEN MARRIED FOR 4 YEARS. THEY ARE STUCK IN A PURSUE–WITHDRAW CYCLE.)
PARTNER 1: [Irritated] My wife always mumbles. (Trigger)
THERAPIST PROMPT (CRITERION 1): Ask Partner 1 how his body typically feels when he is triggered by his partner's behavior.
PARTNER 1: [Angry] My hands go into fists.
THERAPIST PROMPT (CRITERION 2): Ask him what his triggered bodily response typically means to him.
PARTNER 1: [Irritated] That I'm pissed off! It means my wife doesn't respect me enough to speak clearly.
THERAPIST PROMPT (CRITERION 3): Ask him about his typical action tendency in response to his triggered bodily response and the meaning it holds for him.
PARTNER 1: [Frustrated] I yell at her, "Speak clearly for a change!"
THERAPIST PROMPT (CRITERION 4): Organize all the elements into a summary, then check with Partner 1 for accuracy.

INTERMEDIATE-LEVEL DIALOGUE 2: COUPLE 3, PARTNER 2 (THIS IS THE WIFE OF THE SAME COUPLE STUCK IN A PURSUE–WITHDRAW CYCLE.)
PARTNER 2: [Angry] My husband accuses me of mumbling, and rather than asking me to please say it again, he immediately starts yelling at me for no good reason. (Trigger)
THERAPIST PROMPT (CRITERION 1): Ask Partner 2 how her body typically feels when she is triggered by her partner's behavior.
PARTNER 2: [Anxious] I start breaking out into a sweat.
THERAPIST PROMPT (CRITERION 2): Ask her what her triggered bodily response typically means to her.
PARTNER 2: [Anxious] He feels he can just go off on me for the least little thing. I feel like I am his emotional punching bag.
THERAPIST PROMPT (CRITERION 3): Ask her about her typical action tendency in response to her triggered bodily response and the meaning it holds for her.
PARTNER 2: [Ashamed] I just swallow my anger and get away from him to try to quiet myself down.
THERAPIST PROMPT (CRITERION 4): Organize all the elements into a summary, then check with Partner 2 for accuracy.

🛑 **Assess and adjust the difficulty before moving to the next difficulty level (see Step 3 in the exercise instructions).**

ADVANCED-LEVEL DIALOGUE 1: COUPLE 4, PARTNER 1 (THIS IS THE HUSBAND OF A POSTAFFAIR COUPLE WHO HAVE BEEN MARRIED FOR 42 YEARS.)
PARTNER 1: [Indignant] Every time I try to ask a simple question about my wife's past, her face gets really red. (Trigger)
THERAPIST PROMPT (CRITERION 1): Ask Partner 1 how his body typically feels when he is triggered by his partner's behavior.
PARTNER 1: [Irritated] How do you think I feel? Once again, I'm being punched in the stomach.
THERAPIST PROMPT (CRITERION 2): Ask him what his triggered bodily response typically means to him.
PARTNER 1: [Anxious] I think that she is cheating again and that I've caught her in another lie. I say to myself, "She's done it before; she'll do it again. You're a fool to trust her."
THERAPIST PROMPT (CRITERION 3): Ask him about his typical action tendency in response to his triggered bodily response and the meaning it holds for him.
PARTNER 1: [Furious] I demand to know the truth and I go after it. I turn and twist it every way I can, until I am sure that there is nothing I missed. I get so enraged that I won't let her leave the room until I get all the answers I need. I won't be tricked again!
THERAPIST PROMPT (CRITERION 4): Organize all the elements into a summary, then check with Partner 1 for accuracy.[1]

---

1. Expressions such as "I won't let her leave the room" may reflect an attitude rather than an actual physical infringement on a partner's freedom of movement. But even where there is physical infringement as in the case of "situational couple violence," such violence may be safely and successfully treated with emotionally focused couple therapy (EFCT). While Johnson (2004) originally held that partner violence was a contraindication for EFCT, she changed her mind, seeing that EFCT can be very helpful for such couples because the violence can be seen within the attachment frame as a product of escalating triggers and actions. In any case, trainees should seek close supervision for couples where violence may be present. For further information, see Slootmaeckers and Migerode (2020).

ADVANCED-LEVEL DIALOGUE 2: **COUPLE 4, PARTNER 2 (THIS IS THE WIFE OF A POSTAFFAIR COUPLE** **WHO HAVE BEEN MARRIED FOR 42 YEARS.)**
PARTNER 2: [Angry] My husband is constantly on my case, relentlessly demanding to know about everyone I've ever worked with. (Trigger)
THERAPIST PROMPT (CRITERION 1): Ask Partner 2 how her body typically feels when she is triggered by her partner's behavior.
PARTNER 2: [Upset] I feel my hands start shaking and my face reddens.
THERAPIST PROMPT (CRITERION 2): Ask her what her triggered bodily response typically means to her.
PARTNER 2: [Adamant] That I'm living in purgatory. I will never be forgiven even though I've apologized a million times.
THERAPIST PROMPT (CRITERION 3): Ask her about her typical action tendency in response to her triggered bodily response and the meaning it holds for her.
PARTNER 2: [Rebellious] I'm not proud of this, but I tell them it's no wonder that I had an affair.
THERAPIST PROMPT (CRITERION 4): Organize all the elements into a summary, then check with Partner 2 for accuracy.

ADVANCED-LEVEL DIALOGUE 3: COUPLE 5, PARTNER 1 (THIS IS PARTNER 1 OF A COUPLE WHO IS DEALING WITH THE AFTERMATH OF A TRAUMATIC INCIDENT.)
PARTNER 1: [Angry] Last week we talked about dancing at that straight club and how we weren't safe in that setting because we are gay. But after our session, I realized that I was still furious at my partner for blaming me when we were humiliated and pushed out of the club. OK, maybe we weren't so aware of our safety, but afterward I was so upset by my partner's blaming me. (Trigger)
THERAPIST PROMPT (CRITERION 1): Ask Partner 1 how his body typically feels when he is triggered by his partner's behavior.
PARTNER 1: [Embarrassed] I felt my hands start shaking, and my legs felt like they were turning into Jell-O.
THERAPIST PROMPT (CRITERION 2): Ask him what his triggered bodily response typically means to him.
PARTNER 1: [Angry] That I cannot count on him to be a team with me and I am basically all alone in this relationship.
THERAPIST PROMPT (CRITERION 3): Ask him about his typical action tendency in response to his triggered bodily response and the meaning it holds for him.
PARTNER 1: [Very angry] I get raging mad and yell insulting things to him and at times start breaking and throwing things. I feel desperate.
THERAPIST PROMPT (CRITERION 4): Organize all the elements into a summary, then check with Partner 1 for accuracy.

ADVANCED-LEVEL DIALOGUE 4:
COUPLE 5, PARTNER 2 (THIS IS PARTNER 2 OF THE COUPLE WHO IS DEALING WITH THE AFTERMATH OF A TRAUMATIC INCIDENT.)
PARTNER 2: [Frustrated] I am so tired of my partner being so out of control. He insults me and throws things. He is incapable of accepting responsibility for his behavior. (Trigger)
THERAPIST PROMPT (CRITERION 1): Ask Partner 2 how his body typically feels when he is triggered by his partner's behavior.
PARTNER 2: [Anxious] My throat is dry, and my stomach is very tight. I feel nauseous. I may have to excuse myself.
THERAPIST PROMPT (CRITERION 2): Ask about what this trigger and bodily response mean to him.
PARTNER 2: [Sad] That he'll never take responsibility for his behavior. He says he feels alone, but actually, I feel terribly alone and like maybe I deserve the insults. I really am frightened he will leave me.
THERAPIST PROMPT (CRITERION 3): Ask about his typical action tendency in response to his triggered bodily response and the meaning it holds for him.
PARTNER 2: [Scared] I shut down. I just don't know what else to do. I try not to break down, but inside I am destroyed and very scared.
THERAPIST PROMPT (CRITERION 4): Organize all the elements into a summary, then check with Partner 2 for accuracy.

⬡ **Assess and adjust the difficulty here (see Step 3 in the exercise instructions). If appropriate, follow the instructions to make the exercise even more challenging (see Appendix A).**

Example Therapist Responses: Gathering and Assembling Elements of Emotion

Remember: Trainees should attempt to improvise their own responses before reading the examples. **Do not read the following responses verbatim unless you are having trouble coming up with your own!**

EXAMPLE RESPONSES FOR BEGINNER-LEVEL DIALOGUE 1
PARTNER 1: [Irritated] I beg my partner to clear off the dining room table of all their junk and stacks of paper, but they never do. It just keeps building up. (Trigger)
THERAPIST: And when you beg them to clear the dining table of all their papers and things but they never do, are you aware of any reaction in your body?
PARTNER 1: [Matter-of-fact] My stomach becomes one big, knotted mess.
THERAPIST: And when your stomach becomes a knotted mess, after they ignore your request to put their things away, what do you tell yourself about what is happening in those moments?
PARTNER 1: [Irritated] That what I want simply doesn't matter to them. They could care less what it is like for me to live this way. It's actually quite hurtful.
THERAPIST: When they don't do what you've asked, and your stomach is in knots because what you want and need just doesn't seem to matter to them, what do you say or do?
PARTNER 1: [Angry] I raise my voice and I tell them, "I'm sick of living like this. It's a pigsty in here!" They can tell by my volume and tone that I'm angry and disappointed.
THERAPIST: So, you get triggered when your partner doesn't clear the dining table of all their papers and things, (Trigger) and you can feel your stomach becoming one big, knotted mess. (Criterion 1) In making sense of your partner's behavior, you think that what you want doesn't really matter to them, (Criterion 2) and that causes you to yell at them that you're sick of living like this. (Criterion 3) Do I have that right? (Criterion 4)

EXAMPLE RESPONSES FOR BEGINNER-LEVEL DIALOGUE 2
PARTNER 2: [Frustrated] My partner is constantly on my case about being messy. I am criticized a lot. They never see what I do well. (Trigger)
THERAPIST: When you experience your partner as critical of you, what do you typically feel in your body?
PARTNER 2: [Worried] My heart races. I can feel my heart racing.
THERAPIST: And when your partner criticizes you for being messy and your heart begins to race, what do you tell yourself in those moments?
PARTNER 2: [Irritated] That I'll never catch a break. They will always make mountains out of mole hills, and everything will always be my fault. They'll never understand me or accept me.
THERAPIST: When your partner criticizes you about the mess, your heart races, and it seems apparent that you'll never be understood or accepted, what do you typically do or say?
PARTNER 2: [Sad] I just shut down and say nothing. I walk away. I don't want any more criticism.
THERAPIST: So, you get triggered when your partner criticizes you for being messy, (Trigger) and you can feel your heart racing. (Criterion 1) In making sense of your partner's behavior, you conclude that you'll never be good enough for them, (Criterion 2) and that causes you to shut down and withdraw. (Criterion 3) Do I have that right? (Criterion 4)

EXAMPLE RESPONSES FOR BEGINNER-LEVEL DIALOGUE 3

PARTNER 1: [Frustrated] My partner thinks he can ignore me all day and expect me to want to be sexually intimate at night. (Trigger)

THERAPIST: When you've been ignored all day and then he suggests being sexually intimate, what happens in your body?

PARTNER 1: [Upset] I feel myself get tearful, and I tense up.

THERAPIST: When you're expected to be sexually intimate after being ignored all day, and you feel tearful and your body tenses up, what do you tell yourself about this?

PARTNER 1: [Worried] It's clear he doesn't get me or remember what I have said about needing more emotional connection before I can feel sexual desire.

THERAPIST: And what do you typically say or do when you are approached for sex after being ignored all day, and you get tense and tearful, realizing again that he doesn't remember how important emotional connection is for you to feel sexual?

PARTNER 1: [Sad] I don't say anything. I just stay quiet while tears roll down my cheeks.

THERAPIST: So, you get triggered when he wants to be sexually intimate after ignoring you all day, (Trigger) and you can feel your body tense up and you get tearful. (Criterion 1)
In making sense of his behavior, you think he doesn't understand you or your need for more emotional connection to feel sexual, (Criterion 2) and then you stay quiet and cry. (Criterion 3) Do I have that right? (Criterion 4)

EXAMPLE RESPONSES FOR BEGINNER-LEVEL DIALOGUE 4
PARTNER 2: [Matter-of-fact] Anytime I want to talk about our sex life, she gets very quiet and tearful. (Trigger)
THERAPIST: And when you want to talk and you see that even approaching the topic causes her to tear up and get quiet, what goes on with your body?
PARTNER 2: [Embarrassed] I feel really tense all over.
THERAPIST: What do you tell yourself when she gets quiet and tearful, and you find yourself tensing up?
PARTNER 2: [Resigned] That my expressing my sexual needs hurts her. I think I will just have to accept feeling alone in this relationship.
THERAPIST: When you want to talk to her about your sex life, and she becomes quiet and tearful and then you become tense and think that your needs are hurting her and you will have to resign yourself to feeling alone, what do you say or do?
PARTNER 2: [Confused] I kind of freeze. I say things like, "Are you OK? Did I just upset you?" And then I won't bring up the topic for a couple of months.
THERAPIST: So, you get triggered when you want to talk to her about your sex life and she gets very quiet and tearful, (Trigger) and you feel your body tense up. (Criterion 1) You believe that expressing your sexual needs is somehow hurting her, and you conclude that you just have to accept feeling alone in this relationship, (Criterion 2) which causes you to freeze and avoid the topic altogether for a couple of months. (Criterion 3) Do I have that right? (Criterion 4)

EXAMPLE RESPONSES FOR INTERMEDIATE-LEVEL DIALOGUE 1
PARTNER 1: [Irritated] My wife always mumbles. (Trigger)
THERAPIST: And when your wife mumbles, what is going on with your body?
PARTNER 1: [Angry] My hands go into fists.
THERAPIST: When your wife mumbles and your hands go into fists, what does that tell you?
PARTNER 1: [Irritated] That I'm pissed off! It means my wife doesn't respect me enough to speak clearly.
THERAPIST: So, when your wife mumbles, your hands go into fists, and you say to yourself "My wife doesn't respect me enough," what do you tend to say or do?
PARTNER 1: [Frustrated] I yell at her, "Speak clearly for a change!"
THERAPIST: So, when your wife is not speaking clearly to you, (Trigger) your body responds with closed fists. (Criterion 1) Because her mumbling means she doesn't respect you enough to speak clearly, (Criterion 2) you yell at her. (Criterion 3) Am I getting it? Is this what happens? (Criterion 4)

EXAMPLE RESPONSES FOR INTERMEDIATE-LEVEL DIALOGUE 2
PARTNER 2: [Angry] My husband accuses me of mumbling, and rather than asking me to please say it again, he immediately starts yelling at me for no good reason. (Trigger)
THERAPIST: And when your husband yells at you for no good reason, what happens inside your body?
PARTNER 2: [Anxious] I start breaking out into a sweat.
THERAPIST: So, when your husband yells at you for no good reason and you then break out into a sweat, what meaning do you make of it all?
PARTNER 2: [Anxious] He feels he can just go off on me for the least little thing. I feel like I am his emotional punching bag.
THERAPIST: When your husband yells at you and you break out into a sweat, and feel like you are being treated like an emotional punching bag, what do you end up doing or saying?
PARTNER 2: [Ashamed] I just swallow my anger and get away from him to try to quiet myself down.
THERAPIST: So, when your partner gets angry with you for no apparent reason, (Trigger) you get sweaty, (Criterion 1) and because you feel you are being used as an emotional punching bag, (Criterion 2) you swallow your anger and leave to quiet yourself down. (Criterion 3) Do I have that right? (Criterion 4)

EXAMPLE RESPONSES FOR ADVANCED-LEVEL DIALOGUE 1
PARTNER 1: [Indignant] Every time I try to ask a simple question about my wife's past, her face gets really red. (Trigger)
THERAPIST: When you ask her one of these questions and you notice your wife's face reddening, how does your body react?
PARTNER 1: [Irritated] How do you think I feel? Once again, I'm being punched in the stomach.
THERAPIST: And when you feel that pain in your stomach and you see your partner turning red, what do you make of it?
PARTNER 1: [Anxious] I think that she is cheating again, and that I've caught her in another lie. I say to myself, "She's done it before; she will do it again. You're a fool to trust her."
THERAPIST: What do you say or do in those moments when you're just asking a simple question and your partner's face gets red, and you feel like you've been punched in the stomach as you conclude that she's lying to you again?
PARTNER 1: [Furious] I demand to know the truth and I go after it. I turn and twist it every way I can, until I am sure that there is nothing I missed. I get so enraged that I won't let her leave the room until I get all the answers I need. I won't be tricked again!
THERAPIST: So, you get triggered when, in response to a simple question, your wife's face turns red, (Trigger) and it feels like you've been punched in the stomach. (Criterion 1) In making sense of her behavior, you believe you've caught her in a lie again. (Criterion 2) You become enraged, feeling you shouldn't trust her, and this causes you to interrogate her and prevent your wife from leaving the room until you've got your answers. You are making sure you aren't tricked again. (Criterion 3) Do I have that right? (Criterion 4)

EXAMPLE RESPONSES FOR ADVANCED-LEVEL DIALOGUE 2
PARTNER 2: [Angry] My partner is constantly on my case, relentlessly demanding to know about everyone I've ever worked with. (Trigger)
THERAPIST: What happens in your body when you're asked these kinds of questions?
PARTNER 2: [Upset] I feel my hands start shaking and my face redden.
THERAPIST: When your husband asks you about your work colleagues and you feel your hands shaking and your face turning red, what sense do you make of it?
PARTNER 2: [Adamant] That I'm living in purgatory. I will never be forgiven even though I've apologized a million times.
THERAPIST: When you are asked about the people you work with and your face turns red, and you get a sense that you are doomed to never be forgiven, what do you typically say or do?
PARTNER 2: [Rebellious] I'm not proud of this, but I tell them it's no wonder that I had an affair.
THERAPIST: So, you get triggered when your partner asks you questions about the people you work with or have worked with in the past, (Trigger) and you can feel your reaction in your body because your hands shake and your face turns red. (Criterion 1) You believe your husband will never forgive you for the affair even though you have apologized a lot. (Criterion 2) You are not proud of it, but you tell him that there was good cause for you to have that affair. (Criterion 3) Do I have that right? (Criterion 4)

EXAMPLE RESPONSES FOR ADVANCED-LEVEL DIALOGUE 3

PARTNER 1: [Angry] Last week we talked about dancing at that straight club and how we weren't safe in that setting because we are gay. But after our session, I realized that I was still furious at my partner for blaming me when we were humiliated and pushed out of the club. OK, we weren't so aware of our safety, but afterward I was so upset by my partner's blaming me. (Trigger)

THERAPIST: What happens in your body when your partner blamed you?

PARTNER 1: [Embarrassed] I felt my hands start shaking, and my legs felt like they were turning into Jell-O.

THERAPIST: When you remember your partner's blaming you and you feel your hands shaking and your legs turning into Jell-O, what sense do you make of it?

PARTNER 1: [Angry] That I cannot count on him to be a team with me and that I am basically all alone in this relationship.

THERAPIST: When you think about your partner's blaming you, and your hands starting to shake, and you get a sense that you are all alone in this relationship, what do you typically say or do?

PARTNER 1: [Very angry] I get raging mad and yell insulting things to him and at times start breaking and throwing things. I feel desperate.

THERAPIST: So, you get raging mad when you remember how your partner blamed you after the incident at the club, (Trigger) and you can feel your reaction in your body because your hands shake and your legs turn to Jell-O. (Criterion 1) You believe you don't have a partner—that you are all alone in this relationship. (Criterion 2) And then, out of desperation, you yell insulting things at your partner and even go so far as to break and throw things. (Criterion 3) Do I have that right? (Criterion 4)

EXAMPLE RESPONSES FOR ADVANCED-LEVEL DIALOGUE 4
PARTNER 2: [Frustrated] I am so tired of my partner being so out of control. He insults me and throws things. He is incapable of accepting responsibility for his behavior. (Trigger)
THERAPIST: What are you feeling in your body right now as you remember how your partner insulted you and threw things?
PARTNER 2: [Anxious] My throat is dry, and my stomach is very tight. I feel nauseous. I may have to excuse myself.
THERAPIST: When you remember your partner's insulting you and throwing things, and you feel your throat dry and your stomach so tight and this nausea, what meaning do you make of all of it?
PARTNER 2: [Sad] That he'll never take responsibility for his behavior. He says he feels alone, but actually, I feel terribly alone and like maybe I deserve the insults. I really am frightened he will leave me.
THERAPIST: When you think about your partner's insulting you and throwing things, your throat gets very dry, your stomach tightens and you feel sick, and you feel very alone. You get the sense that he will never take responsibility for what he does and at times you believe the negative things he says about you. And you are frightened he will leave. What do you typically say or do at those times?
PARTNER 2: [Scared] I shut down. I just don't know what else to do. I try not to break down, but inside I am destroyed and very scared.
THERAPIST RESPONSE: When you remember how your partner threw things and insulted you, (Trigger) you can feel your throat get dry and your stomach tighten. (Criterion 1) You believe he will never take responsibility for what he does. You also fear that maybe you sometimes deserve those insults, and you end up feeling very alone in this relationship and fearful he will leave you. (Criterion 2) And then you shut down and feel destroyed on the inside. (Criterion 3) Do I have that right? (Criterion 4)

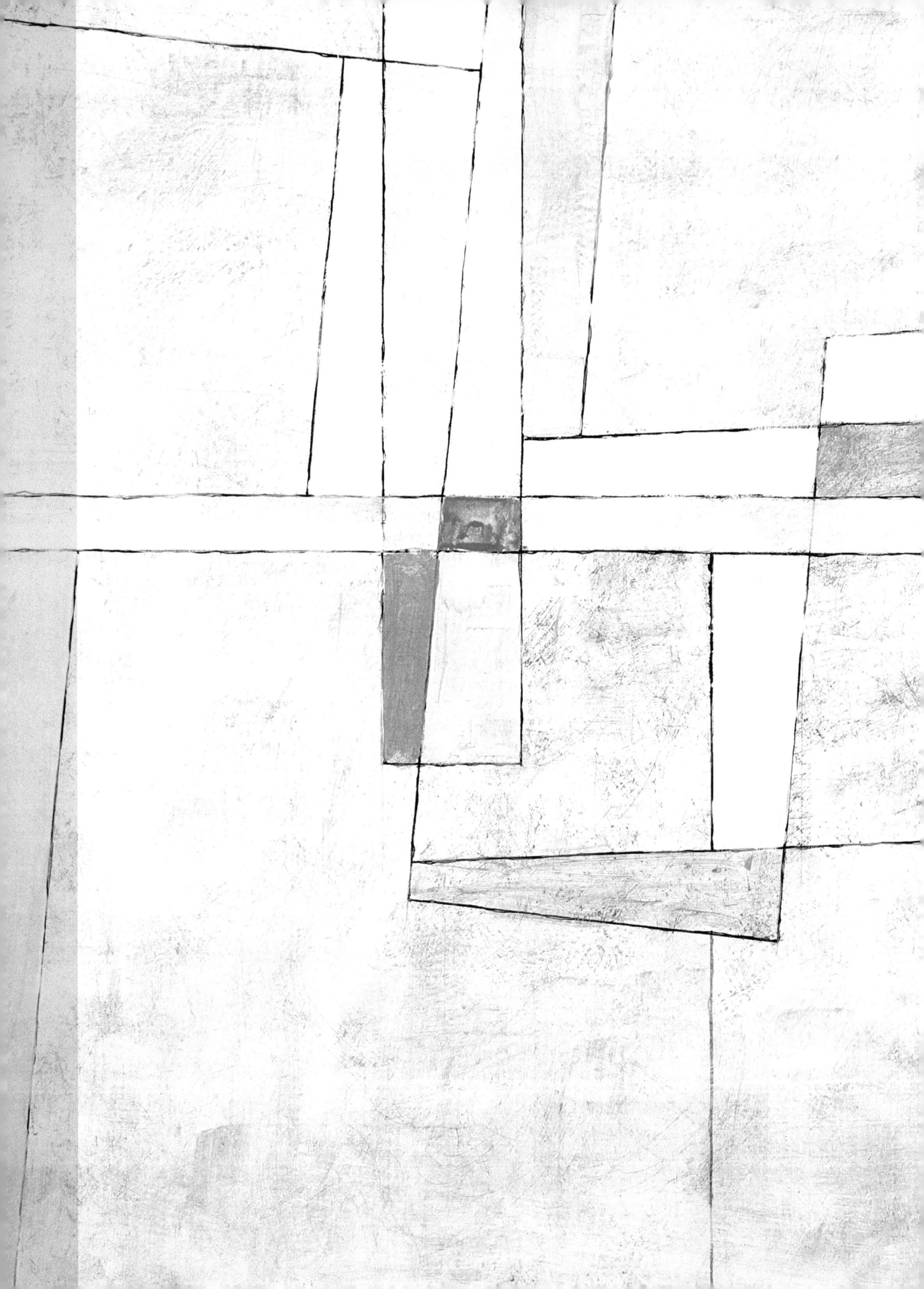

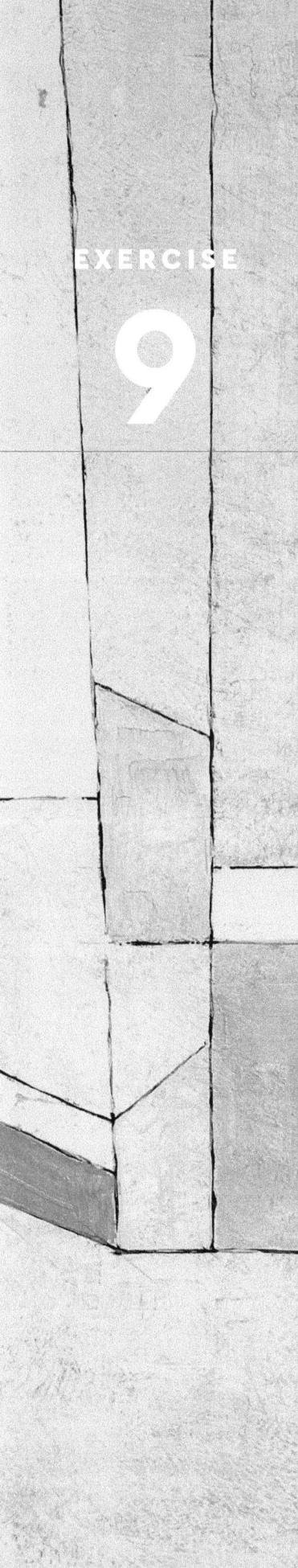

Enactments: Deepening Emotional Experience and Choreographing Engaged Encounters

Preparations for Exercise 9

1. Read the instructions in Chapter 2.

2. Download the Deliberate Practice Reaction Form and the Deliberate Practice Diary Form at https://www.apa.org/pubs/books/deliberate-practice-emotionally-focused-couple-therapy (see the "Resources" tab; also available in Appendixes A and B, respectively).

Exercise Format

For this skill, you will need two trainees: one role-playing the therapist and one role-playing both partners in a couple, speaking as only one partner for each dialogue. The context for the skill is a couple therapy session where you will imagine that both partners are present, with only one partner speaking at a time.

Skill Description

Skill Difficulty Level: Advanced

This exercise is second in the three-part process that begins with gathering and assembling emotion (Exercise 8) and ends with helping partners say why they feel expressing their emotions directly is too challenging (referred to as "slicing the risk thinner"; Exercise 10). As a reminder, the couples in this exercise are from the previous exercise and will appear again in Exercise 10 so that trainees can practice these skills sequentially with the same clients. The overarching goal of enactments is to create corrective emotional experiences within and between partners, eventually turning dysfunctional cycles into

https://doi.org/10.1037/0000436-011

Deliberate Practice in Emotionally Focused Couple Therapy, by H. Levenson, S. Jinich, A. Vaz, and T. Rousmaniere

lifetimes of safety and security. Enactments can be used at various times throughout the therapy. The particular shaping and depth of the encounter depends on what stage of therapy the couple is in.

The purpose of enactments is to restructure the couple's interactions so that the partners become more emotionally engaged. The role of the EFCT therapist as a choreographer comes to the fore, changing the emotional music and thereby changing the dance. When the therapist has sufficiently helped the couple move to a more emotionally receptive place and enabled one of the partners to identify their own attachment fears and longings, the therapist directs that partner to "turn and share" those vulnerable feelings with their partner. For example, "It's one thing to share these feelings with me, but telling your partner directly is the key."

We have constructed this exercise to follow Exercise 8, Gathering and Assembling Elements of Emotion, because it is important to identify the specific central and organizing elements that create distress before doing an enactment. In Exercise 8, the therapist has supported the partners to identify the vulnerable emotional experiences that would be most helpful to enact. In the current exercise, the EFCT therapist uses these vulnerable emotions to prime and change the interaction. In contrast to their customary negative interactions, couples are guided to share their softer, vulnerable feelings. Through the sharing of tender, primary emotions and attachment longings, the partners are naturally pulled toward each another. In sum, "the goal of an EFT enactment is to improve the security of the attachment bond through choreographing interactions that promote positive emotional engagement, enabling partners to build safety and security in their relationship" (Tilley & Palmer, 2013, p. 299).

This exercise begins with the therapist's reflecting the sharing partner's meaning making of the dysfunctional dance that they do with their partner. Then the therapist helps the sharing partner get in touch with their more primary emotions underlying that meaning. After deepening and setting the stage for the enactment, the therapist will invite Partner 1 to do an enactment—to turn to Partner 2 and to tell them in their own words about how their own defensive behavior is driven by their attachment longings and fears.

As with Exercise 8, the trainee playing the client will alternate between playing Partner 1 and Partner 2 within a couple. For instance, Partner 1 of a couple speaks in Beginner Dialogue 1, then Partner 2 of the same couple speaks in Beginner Dialogue 2. The therapist's task is to improvise a response to each client statement following these skill criteria:

1. **Reflect the client's meaning making back to them.** The purpose of summarizing the meaning Partner 1 makes of a triggering situation is to help heighten the vulnerable emotion behind the meaning. It is also a way of discovering the attachment theme embedded in the meaning. Meaning making is often a threat to Partner 1's attachment to their important other(s). It is in these moments that partners say to themselves, "No matter how hard I try, I'll never really be chosen. I will always feel excluded and 'second-class.'"

2. **Ask the client what vulnerable emotion they feel deep down as they hear you reflect their meaning making back to them.** One way to help the partner get in touch with their vulnerable emotion is by heightening the attachment valence of their meaning statement. "When you say to yourself, I will never really be special in their eyes, I will never be chosen or feel like I matter, what do you feel deep down? What do you feel right now as you hear me reflect this back to you?"

3. **Conjecture how the client's reactive behavior is linked to their vulnerable emotion.** The therapist's conjecture gives an in-depth understanding to the partner as to the function of their reactive behavior to protect their vulnerability. Just as important, this statement serves as critical information for Partner 2 to better understand their partner's vulnerability. "When you raise your voice and demand to know what your partner is thinking and feeling, it sounds like there is a lot of fear deep down that doesn't get expressed."

4. **Invite the client to turn to their partner and tell them, in their own words, about their own vulnerable feelings and how it drives their reactive behavior.** "Please turn to your partner and in your own words tell them about your feeling: [pause] (e.g., fear, sadness, hopelessness, feelings of inadequacy, etc.) [pause] and how it leads you to: [pause] (e.g., become critical, get loud, get angry, shut down, withdraw, etc.)." When the therapist can choreograph encounters between partners that focus on vulnerability, the couple can have new and powerful affective experiences that offer opportunities for deeper emotional connection. As with most EFCT skills, the therapist's vocal tone and demeanor is vital to the deepening process. (See Exercise 5 on Deepening Emotions With RISSSSC.)

SKILL CRITERIA FOR EXERCISE 9

Note: All of the following actions should be done in a soft, simple, slow manner.

1. Reflect the client's **meaning** making back to them.
2. Ask the client what vulnerable **emotion** they feel deep down as they hear you reflect their meaning making back to them.
3. Conjecture how the client's reactive **behavior** is linked to their vulnerable emotion.
4. Invite the client to **turn** to their partner and tell them, in their own words, about their own vulnerable feelings and how it drives their reactive behavior.

Example of Therapist Using Enactments

Note: Underlined text is to be read aloud by the person playing the client to provide context. Pauses are indicated in brackets, but the therapist should pause in places that seem natural for them.

This is a couple who has been living together for 1 year. They are speaking about their sex life.

PARTNER 1: When my partner wants to be sexually intimate after ignoring me all day, I get mad, and I become quiet and tearful. It confirms to me that my partner doesn't remember what I've said about needing more emotional connection for me to want to get physically close.

THERAPIST: [*softly*] So you're left thinking to yourself, [*pause*] "He doesn't remember me or my emotional needs." (Criterion 1—**Meaning**)

PARTNER 1: Yes.

THERAPIST: [*softly*] What do you feel just now as I say this to you? (Criterion 2—**Emotion**)

PARTNER 1: I feel really sad about this, and I feel very alone.

THERAPIST: [*softly*] So when this happens [*pause*] deep down inside [*pause*] you feel sad [*pause*] and very alone, and then you get quiet and tearful. (Criterion 3—**Behavior**)

PARTNER 1: Yes. Exactly.

THERAPIST: [*softly*] Please turn to him and tell him. Tell him about the sadness and the loneliness you feel. Help him understand what is going on when he sees you being quiet and tearful. (Criterion 4—**Turn**)

INSTRUCTIONS FOR EXERCISE 9

Step 1: Role-Play and Feedback

- The client says the first beginner client statement and reads the therapist prompt for Criterion 1. The therapist **improvises** a response based on the skill criterion.

- The trainer (or, if not available, the partner) provides **brief** feedback based on the skill criterion. If the criterion is not met, the client then repeats the same statement, and the therapist again improvises responses until it is too easy to meet the skill criterion.

- The client reads the second beginner client statement in the same dialogue, followed by the therapist prompt for Criterion 2. The therapist improvises a response.

- This continues until the dialogue has been completed.

Step 2: Repeat

- Repeat Step 1 for all the dialogues **in the current difficulty level** (beginner, intermediate, or advanced).

Step 3: Assess and Adjust Difficulty

- The therapist completes the Deliberate Practice Reaction Form (see Appendix A) and decides whether to make the exercise easier or harder or to repeat the same difficulty level.

Step 4: Repeat for Approximately 15 Minutes

- Repeat Steps 1 to 3 for at least 15 minutes.
- The trainees then switch therapist and client roles and start over.

Now it's your turn! Follow Steps 1 and 2 from the exercise instructions.

Remember: The goal of the role-play is for trainees to practice improvising responses to the client statements in a manner that (a) uses the skill criteria and (b) feels authentic for the trainee. **Example therapist responses for each client statement are provided at the end of this exercise. Trainees should attempt to improvise their own responses before reading the examples.**

BEGINNER-LEVEL DIALOGUE 1: COUPLE 1, PARTNER 1 (THIS IS PARTNER 1 OF A COUPLE WHO IS STUCK IN A PURSUE–WITHDRAW CYCLE.)
PARTNER 1: [Angry] When my partner doesn't clear the dining room table, I feel it in my body—my stomach tenses. It's then that I realize that what I want really doesn't matter to them. I get so mad that I yell, "I can't live like this anymore!"
THERAPIST PROMPT (CRITERION 1): Reflect Partner 1's meaning making back to them.
PARTNER 1: [Pause and soft] Right.
THERAPIST PROMPT (CRITERION 2): Ask Partner 1 what vulnerable emotion they feel deep down as they hear you reflect their meaning back to them.
PARTNER 1: [Sad] I feel quite sad.
THERAPIST PROMPT (CRITERION 3): Conjecture how their reactive behavior is linked to their vulnerable emotion.
PARTNER 1: [Soft] Yes. Exactly.
THERAPIST PROMPT (CRITERION 4): Invite Partner 1 to turn to Partner 2 and tell them, in their own words, about their own vulnerable feelings and how it drives their reactive behavior.

BEGINNER-LEVEL DIALOGUE 2: COUPLE 1, PARTNER 2 (THIS IS PARTNER 2 OF THE SAME COUPLE STUCK IN A PURSUE–WITHDRAW CYCLE.)
PARTNER 2: [Anxious] I get triggered when my partner criticizes me for being messy; my heart races, and there's a pounding in my chest. I often say to myself that my partner will never accept me for who I am, and that's when I shut down and withdraw.
THERAPIST PROMPT (CRITERION 1): Reflect Partner 2's meaning making back to them.
PARTNER 2: [Soft] Uh-hum.
THERAPIST PROMPT (CRITERION 2): Ask Partner 2 what vulnerable emotion they feel deep down as they hear you reflect their meaning back to them.
PARTNER 2: [Sad] Worthless and sad. [*pause*] I am a big disappointment.
THERAPIST PROMPT (CRITERION 3): Conjecture how their reactive behavior is linked to their vulnerable emotion.
PARTNER 2: [Embarrassed] That's true.
THERAPIST PROMPT (CRITERION 4): Invite Partner 2 to turn to Partner 1 and tell them, in their own words, about their own vulnerable feelings and how it drives their reactive behavior.

BEGINNER-LEVEL DIALOGUE 3: **COUPLE 2, PARTNER 1 (THIS IS A COUPLE WHO HAS BEEN LIVING TOGETHER** **FOR 1 YEAR. THEY ARE SPEAKING ABOUT THEIR SEX LIFE.)**
PARTNER 1: [Soft] When my partner wants to be sexually intimate after ignoring me all day, I get mad, and I become quiet and tearful. It confirms to me that my partner doesn't remember what I've said about needing more emotional connection for me to want to get physically close.
THERAPIST PROMPT (CRITERION 1): Reflect Partner 1's meaning making back to her.
PARTNER 1: [Sad] Yes.
THERAPIST PROMPT (CRITERION 2): Ask Partner 1 what vulnerable emotion she feels deep down as she hears you reflect her meaning back to her.
PARTNER 1: [Sad] I feel really sad about this, and I feel very alone.
THERAPIST PROMPT (CRITERION 3): Conjecture how her reactive behavior is linked to her vulnerable emotion.
PARTNER 1: [Soft] Yes. Exactly.
THERAPIST PROMPT (CRITERION 4): Invite Partner 1 to turn to Partner 2 and tell him, in her own words, about her own vulnerable feelings and how it drives her reactive behavior.

BEGINNER-LEVEL DIALOGUE 4:
COUPLE 2, PARTNER 2 (THIS IS PARTNER 2 OF THE SAME COUPLE.)

PARTNER 2: [Resigned] It's really hard for me when I want to talk to my partner about our sex life, and she gets very quiet and tearful. That's when I think my needs are somehow hurting her, and so I tell myself that perhaps it's better to just accept feeling alone in this relationship, and then I avoid the topic altogether for a couple of months until I can't.

THERAPIST PROMPT (CRITERION 1): Reflect Partner 2's meaning making back to him.

PARTNER 2: [Sad] That's right.

THERAPIST PROMPT (CRITERION 2): Ask Partner 2 what vulnerable emotion he feels deep down as he hears you reflect his meaning back to him.

PARTNER 2: [Sad] I don't know. I just feel guilty. I don't want to hurt her. I feel so alone.

THERAPIST PROMPT (CRITERION 3): Conjecture how his reactive behavior is linked to his vulnerable emotion.

PARTNER 2: [Head hung in shame] Yes. Exactly.

THERAPIST PROMPT (CRITERION 4): Invite Partner 2 to turn to Partner 1 and tell her, in his own words, about his own vulnerable feelings and how it drives his reactive behavior.

🛑 **Assess and adjust the difficulty before moving to the next difficulty level (see Step 3 in the exercise instructions).**

INTERMEDIATE-LEVEL DIALOGUE 1: **COUPLE 3, PARTNER 1 (HUSBAND, COUPLE MARRIED 4 YEARS,** **STUCK IN A PURSUE–WITHDRAW CYCLE.)**
PARTNER 1: **[Irritated]** My wife always mumbles. It's clear she doesn't respect me when she does this. It makes me so angry that she doesn't respect me, so I yell at her and tell her to stop mumbling.
THERAPIST PROMPT (CRITERION 1): Reflect Partner 1's meaning making back to him.
PARTNER 1: **[Confused, then sad]** Hmm. Right.
THERAPIST PROMPT (CRITERION 2): Ask Partner 1 what vulnerable emotion he feels deep down as he hears you reflect his meaning back to him.
PARTNER 1: **[Confused then sad]** It's strange. As I hear you say it, I feel really empty and sad.
THERAPIST PROMPT (CRITERION 3): Conjecture how his reactive behavior is linked to his vulnerable emotion.
PARTNER 1: **[Soft]** Yes. Exactly.
THERAPIST PROMPT (CRITERION 4): Invite Partner 1 to turn to Partner 2 and tell her, in his own words, about his own vulnerable feelings and how it drives his reactive behavior.

INTERMEDIATE-LEVEL DIALOGUE 2: **COUPLE 3, PARTNER 2 (WIFE, COUPLE MARRIED 4 YEARS,** **STUCK IN A PURSUE–WITHDRAW CYCLE.)**
PARTNER 2: [Angry] When my husband accuses me of mumbling and starts yelling at me for no good reason, I usually break out into a sweat. He acts like he just doesn't love me. He just goes off on me for the least little thing. I get angry inside, and I usually walk away and quiet myself down.
THERAPIST PROMPT (CRITERION 1): Reflect Partner 2's meaning making back to her.
PARTNER 2: [Sad] Right.
THERAPIST PROMPT (CRITERION 2): Ask Partner 2 what vulnerable emotion she feels deep down as she hears you reflect her meaning back to her.
PARTNER 2: [Anxious] It makes me very scared, actually, to think that he doesn't love me. Maybe he'll leave me, and I really love him.
THERAPIST PROMPT (CRITERION 3): Conjecture how her reactive behavior is linked to her vulnerable emotion.
PARTNER 2: [Confused] Probably that's true.
THERAPIST PROMPT (CRITERION 4): Invite Partner 2 to turn to Partner 1 and tell him, in her own words, about her own vulnerable feelings and how it drives her reactive behavior.

🛑 **Assess and adjust the difficulty before moving to the next difficulty level (see Step 3 in the exercise instructions).**

ADVANCED-LEVEL DIALOGUE 1: COUPLE 4, PARTNER 1 (PARTNER 1 IS THE HUSBAND OF A MARRIED, POSTAFFAIR COUPLE.)
PARTNER 1: **[Suspicious]** Even when I ask a simple question, my wife's face becomes red, and that's all it takes for me to feel like I've been punched in the stomach. I feel like I've caught her in a lie again and that I shouldn't trust her. I become an interrogator and prevent her from leaving the room until I've got my answers. I will not be tricked again.
THERAPIST PROMPT (CRITERION 1): Reflect Partner 1's meaning making back to him.
PARTNER 1: **[Indignant]** Yes!
THERAPIST PROMPT (CRITERION 2): Ask Partner 1 what vulnerable emotion he feels deep down as he hears you reflect his meaning back to him.
PARTNER 1: **[Anxious]** I am scared. It was the worst pain I have ever experienced.
THERAPIST PROMPT (CRITERION 3): Conjecture how his reactive behavior is linked to his vulnerable emotion.
PARTNER 1: **[Downcast]** Yes.
THERAPIST PROMPT (CRITERION 4): Invite Partner 1 to turn to Partner 2 and tell her, in his own words, about his own vulnerable feelings and how it drives his reactive behavior.

ADVANCED-LEVEL DIALOGUE 2: COUPLE 4, PARTNER 2 (THIS IS THE WIFE OF THE SAME POSTAFFAIR COUPLE DEALING WITH THE AFTERMATH OF THE ATTACHMENT INJURY.)
PARTNER 2: [Irritated] Yeah, it's really hard for me when my husband drills me with questions about the people I work with or have worked with in the past. I can feel my hands shaking, and my face feels hot and I'm sure it gets very red. I'll never be believed or forgiven for the affair no matter how many times I have cried and apologized for it. I'm not proud of what happens to me, but in desperation, I end up yelling at him that there was good cause for me to have that affair.
THERAPIST PROMPT (CRITERION 1): Reflect Partner 2's meaning making back to her.
PARTNER 2: [Resigned] Exactly. I am condemned for life. Nothing will ever be the same again.
THERAPIST PROMPT (CRITERION 2): Ask Partner 2 what vulnerable emotion she feels deep down as she hears you reflect her meaning back to her.
PARTNER 2: [Ashamed] I feel so hopeless and so worn out. I mostly feel gut-wrenching sadness for doing this to the person I love most in the world.
THERAPIST PROMPT (CRITERION 3): Conjecture how her reactive behavior is linked to her vulnerable emotion.
PARTNER 2: [Very sad] I do.
THERAPIST PROMPT (CRITERION 4): Invite Partner 2 to turn to Partner 1 and tell him, in her own words, about her own vulnerable feelings and how it drives her reactive behavior.

ADVANCED-LEVEL DIALOGUE 3:
COUPLE 5, PARTNER 1 (PARTNER 1 OF A COUPLE WHO IS DEALING WITH THE AFTERMATH OF A TRAUMATIC INCIDENT.)

PARTNER 1: [Upset] When my partner blames me, I cannot count on him to be a team with me. I yell insulting things and even go so far as to break and throw things. I feel I am basically all alone in this relationship.

THERAPIST PROMPT (CRITERION 1): Reflect Partner 1's meaning making back to him.

PARTNER 1: [Softly] Right.

THERAPIST PROMPT (CRITERION 2): Ask Partner 1 what vulnerable emotion he feels deep down as he hears you reflect his meaning back to him.

PARTNER 1: [Sad] [*pause*] I feel overwhelmed with sadness.

THERAPIST PROMPT (CRITERION 3): Conjecture how his reactive behavior is linked to his vulnerable emotion.

PARTNER 1: [Softly] I guess so.

THERAPIST PROMPT (CRITERION 4): Invite Partner 1 to turn to Partner 2 and tell him, in his own words, about his own vulnerable feelings and how it drives his reactive behavior.

ADVANCED-LEVEL DIALOGUE 4: COUPLE 5, PARTNER 2 (PARTNER 2 OF A COUPLE WHO IS DEALING WITH THE AFTERMATH OF A TRAUMATIC INCIDENT.)
PARTNER 2: [Upset] When I remember how my partner throws things and insults me, I just end up feeling so very alone in this relationship. I tend to shut down and feel destroyed on the inside. He never takes responsibility for what he does. I am so frightened he will leave me.
THERAPIST PROMPT (CRITERION 1): Reflect Partner 2's meaning making back to him.
PARTNER 2: [Sad, nodding] Right.
THERAPIST PROMPT (CRITERION 2): Ask Partner 2 what vulnerable emotion he feels deep down as he hears you reflect his meaning back to him.
PARTNER 2: [Sad] [*pause*] I feel sad and really anxious about him leaving me.
THERAPIST PROMPT (CRITERION 3): Conjecture how his reactive behavior is linked to his vulnerable emotion.
PARTNER 2: [Head hung] Umm-hmm. Yeah.
THERAPIST PROMPT (CRITERION 4): Invite Partner 2 to turn to Partner 1 and tell him, in his own words, about his own vulnerable feelings and how it drives his reactive behavior.

🛑 **Assess and adjust the difficulty here (see Step 3 in the exercise instructions). If appropriate, follow the instructions to make the exercise even more challenging (see Appendix A).**

Example Therapist Responses: Enactments

Remember: Trainees should attempt to improvise their own responses before reading the examples. **Do not read the following responses verbatim unless you are having trouble coming up with your own!**

EXAMPLE RESPONSES TO BEGINNER-LEVEL DIALOGUE 1
PARTNER 1: [Angry] When my partner doesn't clear the dining room table, I feel it in my body—my stomach tenses. It's then that I realize that what I want really doesn't matter to them. I get so mad that I yell, "I can't live like this anymore!"
THERAPIST: [Softly] You [*pause*] don't matter to them. (Criterion 1)
PARTNER 1: [Pause and soft] Right.
THERAPIST: [Softly] What do you feel [*pause*] deep down [*pause*] when you say to yourself [*pause*] "I don't matter"? (Criterion 2)
PARTNER 1: [Sad] I feel quite sad.
THERAPIST: [Softly] So it seems there is really a lot of sadness deep down, when you raise your voice [*pause*] and you yell at them you can't tolerate living like this? (Criterion 3)
PARTNER 1: [Soft] Yes. Exactly.
THERAPIST: [Softly] I'd like to ask you [*pause*] to please turn to your partner [*pause*] and in your own words, tell them about this sadness. [*pause*] Tell them how it's easier to show anger rather than the deep-down sadness. (Criterion 4)

EXAMPLE RESPONSES TO BEGINNER-LEVEL DIALOGUE 2
PARTNER 2: [Anxious] I get triggered when my partner criticizes me for being messy; my heart races, and there is a pounding in my chest. I often say to myself that my partner will never accept me for who I am, and that's when I shut down and withdraw.
THERAPIST: [Softly] It's as if [*pause*] you will never be good enough for them. (Criterion 1)
PARTNER 2: [Resigned] Uh-hum.
THERAPIST: [Softly] I wonder, what vulnerable emotion are you feeling deep down right now [*pause*] as I reflect this back to you? (Criterion 2)
PARTNER 2: [Sad] Worthless and sad. [*pause*] I am a big disappointment.
THERAPIST: [Softly] On the inside, you are very sad, [*pause*] you feel worthless and like you are a disappointment, [*pause*] and yet on the outside [*pause*] what your partner sees is that you shut down, withdraw, and distance? (Criterion 3)
PARTNER 2: [Embarrassed] That's true.
THERAPIST: [Softly] I'd like you to tell your partner about that. Can you turn to them [*pause*] and let them in a bit? Help them understand [*pause*] how when they see you shut down and withdraw, [*pause*] deep down [*pause*] you are really filled with sadness and fear that you are a disappointment to them. Tell them about this part. (Criterion 4)

EXAMPLE RESPONSES TO BEGINNER-LEVEL DIALOGUE 3
PARTNER 1: [Soft] When my partner wants to be sexually intimate after ignoring me all day, I get mad, and I become quiet and tearful. It confirms to me that my partner doesn't remember what I've said about needing more emotional connection for me to want to get physically close.
THERAPIST: [Softly] So you're left thinking to yourself, "He doesn't remember me or my emotional needs." (Criterion 1)
PARTNER 1: [Sad] Yes.
THERAPIST: [Softly] What do you feel just now as I say this to you? (Criterion 2)
PARTNER 1: [Sad] I feel really sad about this, and I feel very alone.
THERAPIST: [Softly] So when this happens [*pause*] deep down inside [*pause*] you feel sad [*pause*] and very alone, and then you get quiet and tearful. (Criterion 3)
PARTNER 1: [Soft] Yes. Exactly.
THERAPIST: [Softly] Please turn to him and tell him. Tell him about the sadness and the loneliness you feel. Help him to understand what is going on when he sees you being quiet and tearful. (Criterion 4)

EXAMPLE RESPONSES TO BEGINNER-LEVEL DIALOGUE 4
PARTNER 2: [Resigned] It's really hard for me when I want to talk to my partner about our sex life, and she gets very quiet and tearful. That's when I think my needs are somehow hurting her, and so I tell myself that perhaps it's better to just accept feeling alone in this relationship, and then I avoid the topic altogether for a couple of months until I can't.
THERAPIST: [Softly] So what you tell yourself in these moments [*pause*] when you want to get close to your partner [*pause*] and you see her being quiet and tearful [*pause*] is that [*pause*] your needs are hurting her and that you just have to accept things as they are [*pause*] such as feeling alone in this relationship. (Criterion 1)
PARTNER 2: [Sad] That's right.
THERAPIST: [Softly] How are you feeling right now deep down as I reflect this back to you? (Criterion 2)
PARTNER 2: [Sad] I don't know. I just feel guilty. I don't want to hurt her. I feel so alone.
THERAPIST: [Softly] So you feel guilty [*pause*] and so alone. But you don't show this part, right? You withdraw [*pause*] and don't bring up your needs for her until the loneliness gets overwhelming. Hmm? (Criterion 3)
PARTNER 2: [Head hung in shame] Yes. Exactly.
THERAPIST: [Softly] I would like for you to turn toward your partner now [*pause*] and tell her how [*pause*] even when you seem so distant [*pause*] when you don't approach her for intimacy or talk about what you need, [*pause*] you're feeling so alone [*pause*] and guilty for hurting her. (Criterion 4)

EXAMPLE RESPONSES TO INTERMEDIATE-LEVEL DIALOGUE 1
PARTNER 1: [Irritated] My wife always mumbles. It's clear she doesn't respect me when she does this. It makes me so angry that she doesn't respect me, so I yell at her and tell her to stop mumbling.
THERAPIST: [Softly] So [*pause*] she doesn't respect you. (Criterion 1)
PARTNER 1: [Confused, then sad] Hmm. Right.
THERAPIST: [Softly] What do you feel deep down [*pause*] when you hear yourself say, "My partner doesn't respect me"? (Criterion 2)
PARTNER 1: [Confused, then sad] It's strange. As I hear you say it, I feel really empty and sad.
THERAPIST: [Softly] So you feel quite empty [*pause*] and sad [*pause*] down deep [*pause*] when you yell at her about her mumbling? (Criterion 3)
PARTNER 1: [Soft] Yes. Exactly.
THERAPIST: [Softly] I'd like you [*pause*] to please turn to your wife [*pause*] and tell her about this emptiness [*pause*] and sadness [*pause*] that you feel. Please tell her in your own words how these softer feelings sometimes get expressed as criticism and yelling. (Criterion 4)

EXAMPLE RESPONSES TO INTERMEDIATE-LEVEL DIALOGUE 2
PARTNER 2: [Angry] When my husband accuses me of mumbling and starts yelling at me for no good reason, I usually break out into a sweat. He acts like he just doesn't love me. He just goes off on me for the least little thing. I get angry inside, and I usually walk away and quiet myself down.
THERAPIST: [Softly] So your partner goes off on you [*pause*] for no good reason [*pause*] and you wonder if he just doesn't love you. So then you go off to quiet yourself down. (Criterion 1)
PARTNER 2: [Sad] Right.
THERAPIST: [Softly] What do you feel deep down when you say to yourself, "He acts as if he doesn't love me"? (Criterion 2)
PARTNER 2: [Anxious] It makes me very scared, actually, to think that he doesn't love me. Maybe he'll leave me, and I really love him.
THERAPIST: [Softly] So when you go off to quiet yourself down, [*pause*] you are actually feeling quite scared [*pause*] that perhaps he will leave you. (Criterion 3)
PARTNER 2: [Confused] Probably that's true.
THERAPIST: [Softly] I would like to ask you to turn to him and to say this directly to him. Tell him [*pause*] about this fear [*pause*] and about how scary it is [*pause*] that he could decide [*pause*] to leave you. (Criterion 4)

EXAMPLE RESPONSES TO ADVANCED-LEVEL DIALOGUE 1

PARTNER 1: [Suspicious] Even when I ask a simple question, my wife's face becomes red, and that's all it takes for me to feel like I've been punched in the stomach. I feel like I've caught her in a lie again, and that I shouldn't trust her. I become an interrogator and prevent her from leaving the room until I've got my answers. I will not be tricked again.

THERAPIST: [Softly] It's in these moments [*pause*] when you most need some kind of reassurance, that you tell yourself [*pause*] something is going on, [*pause*] don't trust her again, [*pause*] don't be made a fool again. [*pause*] (Criterion 1)

PARTNER 1: [Indignant] Yes!

THERAPIST: [Softly] What are you feeling right now [*pause*] as I reflect this back to you? (Criterion 2)

PARTNER 1: [Anxious] I am scared. It was the worst pain I have ever experienced.

THERAPIST: [Softly] Of course, and so [*pause*] when you feel such deep fear that you could be tricked again, that you could once again be kept in the dark [*pause*] and once again experience such terrible pain, [*pause*] you become hyperfocused, and you go after the truth. You block your wife's exit, [*pause*] you interrogate her, [*pause*] but deep down [*pause*] you are feeling so [*pause*] much [*pause*] fear. [*pause*] This really hurt you deeply. [*pause*] (Criterion 3)

PARTNER 1: [Downcast] Yes.

THERAPIST: [Softly] I'd like to ask you to tell your wife about your fear of being hurt again. Turn to her and let her know how behind your actions of a detective following clues. [*pause*] For you it's all about calming your own fears [*pause*] so you never have to experience that kind of awful pain again. Can you tell her this, in your own words? (Criterion 4)

EXAMPLE RESPONSES TO ADVANCED-LEVEL DIALOGUE 2

PARTNER 2: [Irritated] Yeah, it's really hard for me when my husband drills me with questions about the people I work with or have worked with in the past. I can feel my hands shaking, and my face feels hot and I'm sure it gets very red. I'll never be believed or forgiven for the affair no matter how many times I have cried and apologized for it. I'm not proud of what happens to me, but in desperation, I end up yelling at him that there was good cause for me to have that affair.

THERAPIST: [Softly] It's as if no matter what you say or do, you will never be seen differently, [*pause*] you will never be forgiven, [*pause*] it will always be like this, [*pause*] frozen in time. (Criterion 1)

PARTNER 2: [Resigned] Exactly. I am condemned for life. Nothing will ever be the same again.

THERAPIST: [Softly] What do you feel deep down when you say to yourself, "I will never be forgiven. It doesn't matter how much regret I feel and express, [*pause*] I will always be guilty and under suspicion forever"? (Criterion 2)

PARTNER 2: [Ashamed] I feel so hopeless and so worn out. I mostly feel gut-wrenching sadness for doing this to the person I love most in the world.

THERAPIST: [Softly] So even though on the outside [*pause*] you seem worn out and you show frustration and anger, to the point of yelling at him and saying that he deserved this pain, [*pause*] deep down you're feeling desperate and so much sadness, [*pause*] so much regret, [*pause*] yes? (Criterion 3)

PARTNER 2: [Very sad] I do.

THERAPIST: [Softly] I wonder if you could share this last point with your husband. How would it be to turn to him now [*pause*] and to open up and show him how beneath your frustration and your anger, [*pause*] beneath the overwhelming sense of hopelessness, [*pause*] there is also so much sadness for hurting the one you love? [*pause*] Tell him about the sadness and the regret you feel. [*pause*] Tell him about this in your own words. (Criterion 4)

EXAMPLE RESPONSES TO ADVANCED-LEVEL DIALOGUE 3

PARTNER 1: [Upset] When my partner blames me, I cannot count on him to be a team with me. I yell insulting things and even go so far as to break and throw things. I feel I am basically all alone in this relationship.
THERAPIST: [Softly] You can't count on him [*pause*] to be your true partner; you feel basically [*pause*] all alone in this relationship. (Criterion 1)
PARTNER 1: [Softly] Right.
THERAPIST: [Softly] What do you feel deep down [*pause*] when you say to yourself [*pause*] "I am basically all alone in this relationship"? (Criterion 2)
PARTNER 1: [Sad] [*pause*] I feel overwhelmed with sadness.
THERAPIST: [Softly] So, your partner hears your insult [*pause*] and sees you throwing things but doesn't know that deep down [*pause*] you are feeling sad. (Criterion 3)
PARTNER 1: [Softly] I guess so.
THERAPIST: [Softly] I'd like to ask you [*pause*] to please turn to your partner [*pause*] and in your own words [*pause*] tell him about your overwhelming sadness. [*pause*] Tell him how this sadness sometimes comes out in the desperate form of insults and throwing things. (Criterion 4)

EXAMPLE RESPONSES TO ADVANCED-LEVEL DIALOGUE 4

PARTNER 2: [Upset] When I remember how my partner throws things and insults me, I just end up feeling so very alone in this relationship. I tend to shut down and feel destroyed on the inside. He never takes responsibility for what he does. I am so frightened he will leave me.

THERAPIST: [Softly] You feel so alone in this relationship. [*pause*] You can't count on him to take responsibility for what he does. [*pause*] He seems so out of control, [*pause*] sometimes you feel you deserve his insults. (Criterion 1)

PARTNER 2: [Sad, nodding] Right.

THERAPIST: [Softly] What do you feel deep down [*pause*] when you say to yourself, "I am alone in this relationship"? (Criterion 2)

PARTNER 2: [Sad] [*pause*] I feel sad and really anxious about him leaving me.

THERAPIST: [Softly] So, your partner sees you shut down, [*pause*] but he doesn't know that deep down [*pause*] you are feeling sad and anxious—worried that he might leave you. (Criterion 3)

PARTNER 2: [Head hung] Umm-hmm. Yeah.

THERAPIST: [Softly] I'd like to ask you [*pause*] to please turn to your partner [*pause*] and in your own words [*pause*] tell him about your sadness. [*pause*] Tell him how you are worried that he will leave you, [*pause*] that maybe you deserve his insults, [*pause*] and this sometimes causes you to shut down. (Criterion 4)

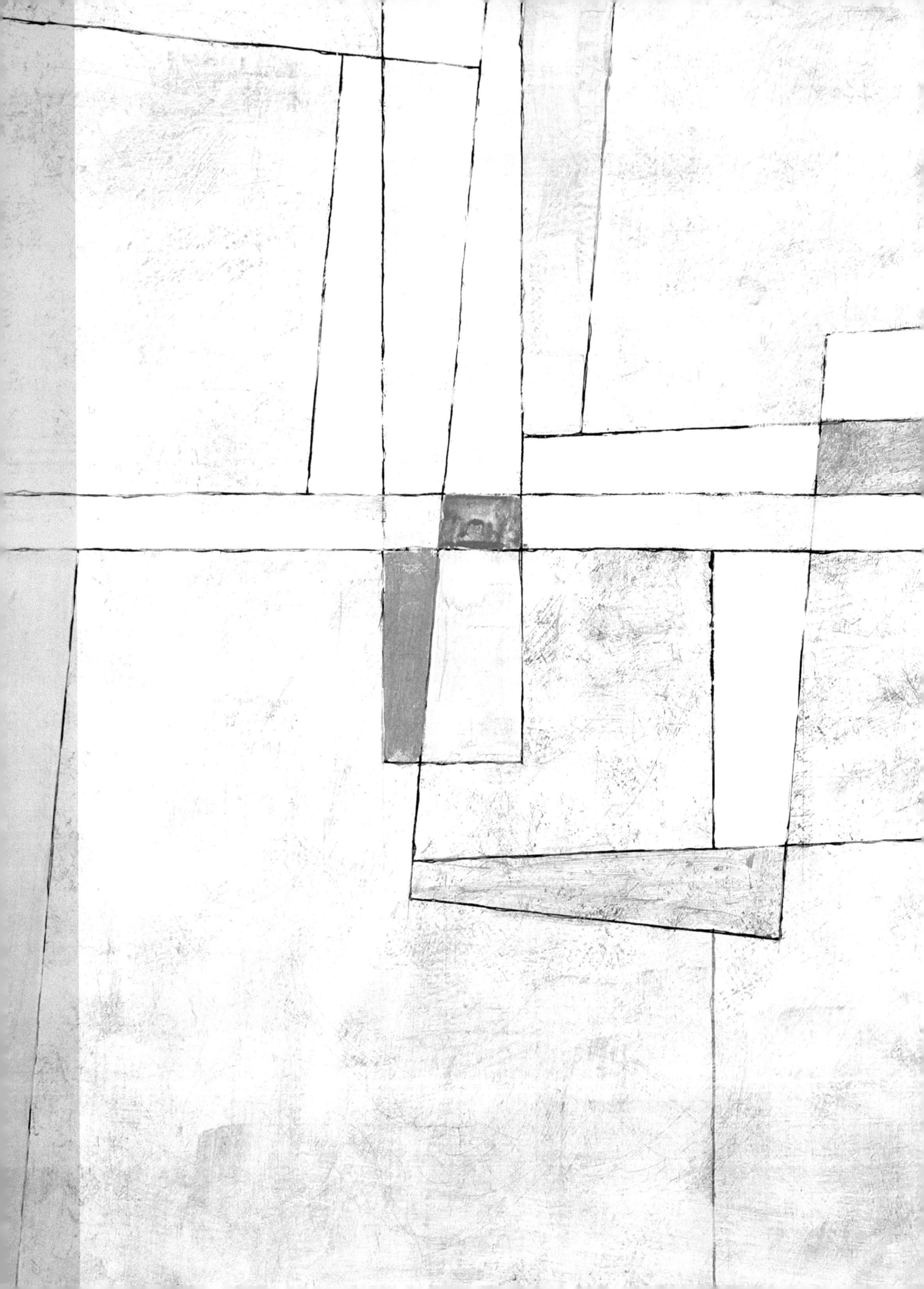

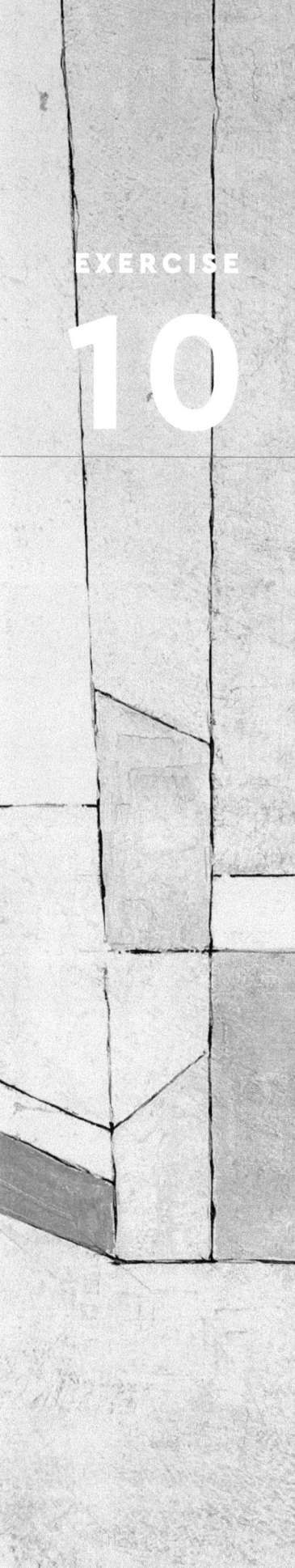

Slicing the Risk Thinner: Helping Partners Express Difficult Emotions

Preparations for Exercise 10

1. Read the instructions in Chapter 2.

2. Download the Deliberate Practice Reaction Form and the Deliberate Practice Diary Form at https://www.apa.org/pubs/books/deliberate-practice-emotionally-focused-couple-therapy (see the "Resources" tab; also available in Appendixes A and B, respectively).

Exercise Format

For this skill, you will need two trainees: one role-playing the therapist and one role-playing both partners in a couple, speaking as only one partner for each dialogue. The context for the skill is a couple therapy session where you will imagine that both partners are present, with only one partner speaking at a time.

Skill Description

Skill Difficulty Level: Advanced

This exercise is the last part of the tripartite procedure that begins with gathering and assembling emotion (Exercise 8) and setting up an enactment (Exercise 9). This exercise starts where Exercise 9 leaves off, following the same couples as the previous two exercises. In Exercise 9, the therapist invites the partners to turn toward each other and talk directly about their own vulnerable fears and longings that are happening beneath the surface—a choreographed enactment. Sometimes in EFCT, a partner refuses to follow the therapist's directive; this is when "slicing the risk thinner" (this exercise) comes into play.

https://doi.org/10.1037/0000436-012

Deliberate Practice in Emotionally Focused Couple Therapy, by H. Levenson, S. Jinich, A. Vaz, and T. Rousmaniere

"Slicing the risk thinner" is used when a client experiences resistance to engaging their partner in a vulnerable manner during a choreographed encounter or enactment. In a typical enactment, the therapist asks one partner to turn to the other and talk about their attachment fears or longings that are vulnerable primary emotions. For example, "Could you please turn to your partner and let them know how lost you would feel without them in your life?" However, sometimes the partner refuses the therapist's invitation. There are many possibilities as to why a member of the couple might feel it is too risky to comply with the therapist's directive. For some, it is dangerous to be seen as fragile; others might feel shame to be "weak" or not worthy of such emotional expression. Others are afraid that what they say will not be understood or responded to empathically. Or perhaps they have no experience being vulnerable in this way, or their culture and/or family has prohibitions about voicing certain emotions.

In such cases, the therapist can "slice the risk thinner" by asking them to express their *fear* of being vulnerable and being rejected if they revealed their vulnerable primary emotions directly. This allows the partner to communicate their emotions indirectly (i.e., by talking about their fears of direct communication) in a slightly safer ("more thinly sliced") way. This approach is designed to create a space not only for the partner to talk about their fears but also for the other member of the couple to hear their partner's underlying attachment fears and longings. For example, the therapist might ask, "Could you turn to your partner and let them know that you fear that if you let them know how you would feel lost without them, they will reject you because you seem too needy?" Using this skill, both people in the couple have taken a step closer, ultimately facilitating deeper emotional connection and growth within the therapeutic process.

As in the previous two exercises, the trainee playing the client will alternate between playing Partner 1 and Partner 2 within a couple. For instance, Partner 1 of a couple speaks in Beginner Dialogue 1, then Partner 2 of the same couple speaks in Beginner Dialogue 2. The therapist should improvise a response to each client statement following these skill criteria:

1. **Ask the client why they are reluctant to share how they feel with their partner, repeating what they have said.** This question will help the therapist understand the partner's reluctance to share from a vulnerable place. That information will be used in a validating way in the next step (Criterion 2).

2. **Validate the client's reason not to share and invite them to explain their reluctance to their partner in their own words.** This invitation is the therapist's use of slicing the risk thinner by asking the client to say something to their partner in a way that seems less vulnerable.

Note: The phrasing of the opening client statements can sound a little "clunky." We are writing them that way on purpose to create the best conditions for you to practice this exercise.

SKILL CRITERIA FOR EXERCISE 10
Note: Do both of these criteria in a soft, slow, and simple manner.
1. Ask the client why they are **reluctant** to share how they feel with their partner, repeating what they have said.
2. **Validate** the client's reason not to share and invite them to **explain** their reluctance to their partner in their own words.

Example of Therapist Slicing the Risk Thinner

Note: Underlined text is to be read aloud by the person playing the client to provide context. Pauses are indicated in brackets, but the therapist should pause in places that seem natural for them.

This is Partner 1 of a couple who is stuck in a pursue–withdraw cycle.

PARTNER 1: [*reluctant*] So you want me to turn to my partner and tell them that when I yell about their messiness, what I'm really feeling is sadness that I don't seem to matter to them. Well, no, I just can't say that to them.

THERAPIST: So, you don't want to tell your partner that the thought of being unimportant to them [*pause*] makes you feel like yelling, but underneath you are really very sad. [*pause*] What makes it so difficult to say that to your partner? (Criterion 1—**Reluctant**)

PARTNER 1: [*ashamed*] It sounds so cheesy and weak and vulnerable.

THERAPIST: I get it; why would you want to do something that would put you in a bad light? (Criterion 2—**Validate**) Can you tell them this important part, [*pause*] that you don't want to open up about how sad you feel at times [*pause*] because you would just sound too weak and vulnerable [*pause*] and who wants a partner like that? Can you tell them that part [*pause*] in your own words? (Criterion 2—**Explain**)

INSTRUCTIONS FOR EXERCISE 10

Step 1: Role-Play and Feedback

- The partner says the first beginner client statement and reads the therapist prompt for Criterion 1. The therapist **improvises** a response based on the skill criterion.
- The trainer (or, if not available, the partner) provides **brief** feedback based on the skill criterion. If the criterion is not met, the partner then repeats the same statement, and the therapist again improvises responses until it is too easy to meet the skill criterion.
- The partner reads the second beginner partner statement in the same dialogue, followed by the therapist prompt for Criterion 2. The therapist improvises a response.
- This continues until the dialogue has been completed.

Step 2: Repeat

- Repeat Step 1 for all the dialogues **in the current difficulty level** (beginner, intermediate, or advanced).

Step 3: Assess and Adjust Difficulty

- The therapist completes the Deliberate Practice Reaction Form (see Appendix A) and decides whether to make the exercise easier or harder or to repeat the same difficulty level.

Step 4: Repeat for Approximately 15 Minutes

- Repeat Steps 1 to 3 for at least 15 minutes.
- The trainees then switch therapist and client roles and start over.

Now it's your turn! Follow Steps 1 and 2 from the exercise instructions.

Remember: The goal of the role-play is for trainees to practice improvising responses to the client statements in a manner that (a) uses the skill criteria and (b) feels authentic for the trainee. **Example therapist responses for each client statement are provided at the end of this exercise. Trainees should attempt to improvise their own responses before reading the examples.**

BEGINNER-LEVEL DIALOGUE 1: COUPLE 1, PARTNER 1 (THIS IS PARTNER 1 OF A COUPLE WHO ARE STUCK IN A PURSUE–WITHDRAW CYCLE.)
PARTNER 1: [Anxious] You want me to turn to my partner and let them know that my yelling is a cover for my sadness, but I don't think I'm ready to do that.
THERAPIST PROMPT (CRITERION 1): Ask Partner 1 why they don't want to share how they feel with Partner 2, repeating what they have said.
PARTNER 1: [Thoughtful] In my family, you could never be sad. I feel strongest when I show my anger. If I let my partner know that I am sad, I won't feel strong, and they won't see me as strong.
THERAPIST PROMPT (CRITERION 2): Validate their reason not to share and invite them to explain their reluctance to Partner 2 in their own words.

BEGINNER-LEVEL DIALOGUE 2: **COUPLE 1, PARTNER 2 (THIS IS PARTNER 2 OF A COUPLE WHO** **ARE STUCK IN A PURSUE–WITHDRAW CYCLE.)**
PARTNER 2: [Hesitant] You really want me to tell my partner that when I withdraw, deep down I am really sad and believe I'm a big disappointment to them? I really can't do that. I just can't imagine saying that to them.
THERAPIST PROMPT (CRITERION 1): Ask Partner 2 why they don't want to share how they feel with Partner 1, repeating what they have said.
PARTNER 2: [Frank] I'll be criticized or judged or disbelieved, and I just don't want to have to put myself out there like that.
THERAPIST PROMPT (CRITERION 2): Validate their reason not to share and invite them to explain their reluctance to Partner 1 in their own words.

BEGINNER-LEVEL DIALOGUE 3:
COUPLE 2, PARTNER 1 (THIS IS A COUPLE WHO HAVE BEEN LIVING TOGETHER FOR 1 YEAR. PARTNER 1 IS EXPLORING THE SADNESS SHE FEELS WHEN HER PARTNER WANTS TO TALK ABOUT THEIR SEXUAL RELATIONSHIP.)

PARTNER 1: [Irritated] So you want me to tell my partner that there is a lot of sadness and loneliness behind my tears. Well, he just heard me talk about it with you. I don't want to have to say it again to him.

THERAPIST PROMPT (CRITERION 1): Ask Partner 1 why she doesn't want to share how she feels with Partner 2, repeating what she has said.

PARTNER 1: [Earnest] We don't talk that way. It just feels strange, and I feel kind of silly.

THERAPIST PROMPT (CRITERION 2): Validate her reason not to share and invite her to explain her reluctance to Partner 2 in her own words.

BEGINNER-LEVEL DIALOGUE 4: COUPLE 2, PARTNER 2 (THIS IS PARTNER 2 OF THE SAME COUPLE.)
PARTNER 2: **[Adamant]** So you want me to turn to my partner and tell her I'd rather disconnect than tell her I feel guilty that my sexual needs upset her? I don't want to say it again. It was bad enough to say it to you.
THERAPIST PROMPT (CRITERION 1): Ask Partner 2 why he doesn't want to share how he feels with Partner 1, repeating what he has said.
PARTNER 2: **[Sad]** I'm afraid that she will get quiet and cry again, and I just can't bear it.
THERAPIST PROMPT (CRITERION 2): Validate his reason not to share and invite him to explain his reluctance to Partner 1 in his own words.

🛑 **Assess and adjust the difficulty before moving to the next difficulty level (see Step 3 in the exercise instructions).**

INTERMEDIATE-LEVEL DIALOGUE 1:
COUPLE 3, PARTNER 1 (THIS IS A COUPLE WHO HAVE BEEN MARRIED FOR
4 YEARS. THEY ARE STUCK IN A PURSUE–WITHDRAW CYCLE.)

PARTNER 1: [Embarrassed] So you want me to turn toward my wife and tell her that although I come across as critical and yell at her, deep down I feel empty and sad? That just feels too hard to say to her. Maybe later I'll feel like I can, but not now.
THERAPIST PROMPT (CRITERION 1): Ask Partner 1 why he doesn't want to share how he feels with Partner 2, repeating what he has said.
PARTNER 1: [Ashamed] I don't know. I guess I feel embarrassed and maybe ashamed that I have treated her so badly. She's a good person.
THERAPIST PROMPT (CRITERION 2): Validate his reason not to share and invite him to explain his reluctance to Partner 2 in his own words.

INTERMEDIATE-LEVEL DIALOGUE 2:
COUPLE 3, PARTNER 2 (WIFE, COUPLE MARRIED 4 YEARS, STUCK IN A PURSUE–WITHDRAW CYCLE.)
PARTNER 2: **[Embarrassed]** So you want me to turn to my husband and tell him how my being afraid he may want to leave our marriage causes me to withdraw to quiet myself down. That's hard for me!
THERAPIST PROMPT (CRITERION 1): Ask Partner 2 why she doesn't want to share how she feels with Partner 1, repeating what she has said.
PARTNER 2: **[Sad]** I don't want to say that to him because it makes me sound so needy.
THERAPIST PROMPT (CRITERION 2): Validate her reason not to share and invite her to explain her reluctance to Partner 1 in her own words.

🛑 **Assess and adjust the difficulty before moving to the next difficulty level (see Step 3 in the exercise instructions).**

ADVANCED-LEVEL DIALOGUE 1: **COUPLE 4, PARTNER 1 (THIS IS A COUPLE WHO HAVE BEEN MARRIED FOR** **4 YEARS. THEY ARE STUCK IN A PURSUE–WITHDRAW CYCLE.)**
PARTNER 1: **[Upset]** You want me to tell my partner that I really need reassurance—that my asking a lot of questions comes from my need to be reassured that she will never cheat again? I don't want to have to say it.
THERAPIST PROMPT (CRITERION 1): Ask Partner 1 why he doesn't want to share how he feels with Partner 2, repeating what he has said.
PARTNER 1: **[Hesitant]** I am a strong person, you know? And what you're asking me to do makes me seem so weak. I don't feel safe being that vulnerable ever again.
THERAPIST PROMPT (CRITERION 2): Validate his reason not to share and invite him to explain his reluctance to Partner 2 in his own words.

ADVANCED-LEVEL DIALOGUE 2: COUPLE 4, PARTNER 2 (WIFE, MARRIED 4 YEARS, STUCK IN A PURSUE–WITHDRAW CYCLE.)
PARTNER 2: **[Hesitant]** So you want me to turn to my partner and tell him that I am deeply sad for hurting him by having this affair and that it is easier for me to get defensive and angry than to say all that. No, I don't think I can say that to him.
THERAPIST PROMPT (CRITERION 1): Ask Partner 2 why she doesn't want to share how she feels with Partner 1, repeating what she has said.
PARTNER 2: **[Plaintive]** It won't make a difference. I've lost all credibility given my past lies.
THERAPIST PROMPT (CRITERION 2): Validate her reason not to share and invite her to explain her reluctance to Partner 1 in her own words.

ADVANCED-LEVEL DIALOGUE 3:
COUPLE 5, PARTNER 1 (PARTNER 1 OF A COUPLE WHO IS DEALING WITH THE AFTERMATH OF A TRAUMATIC INCIDENT.)

PARTNER 1: [Annoyed] You want me to turn to my partner and tell him I am overwhelmingly sad that we are not a team and that what is underneath my insulting and aggressive behavior is this sadness? I'd rather eat glass than say that to him right now.

THERAPIST PROMPT (CRITERION 1): Ask Partner 1 why he doesn't want to share how he feels with Partner 2, repeating what he has said.

PARTNER 1: [Defensive] Well, I think if I say that, I might just get blamed again and then I'll be doubly sad because I don't want to be the bad guy in his eyes.

THERAPIST PROMPT (CRITERION 2): Validate his reason not to share and invite him to explain his reluctance to Partner 2 in his own words.

ADVANCED-LEVEL DIALOGUE 4: COUPLE 5, PARTNER 2 (PARTNER 2 OF A COUPLE WHO IS DEALING WITH THE AFTERMATH OF A TRAUMATIC INCIDENT.)
PARTNER 2: **[Annoyed]** So you want me to tell my partner about how I shut down because I am sad. I really don't want to say that to him.
THERAPIST PROMPT (CRITERION 1): Ask Partner 2 why he doesn't want to share how he feels with Partner 1, repeating what he has said.
PARTNER 2: **[Looking down, long pause]** Sometimes I feel I deserve his insults and the negative things he says about me. It makes me sad and scares me too that he will leave me. And I don't want that!
THERAPIST PROMPT (CRITERION 2): Validate his reason not to share and invite him to explain his reluctance to Partner 1 in his own words.

Assess and adjust the difficulty here (see Step 3 in the exercise instructions). If appropriate, follow the instructions to make the exercise even more challenging (see Appendix A).

Example Therapist Responses: Slicing the Risk Thinner

Remember: Trainees should attempt to improvise their own responses before reading the examples. **Do not read the following responses verbatim unless you are having trouble coming up with your own!**

EXAMPLE RESPONSES TO BEGINNER-LEVEL DIALOGUE 1
PARTNER 1: [Anxious] You want me to turn to my partner and let them know that my yelling is a cover for my sadness, but I don't think I'm ready to do that.
THERAPIST: [Softly] This sounds important to understand [*pause*]. You don't feel ready to talk about your sadness. Can you tell me why you are not ready [*pause*] to say that to them? (Criterion 1)
PARTNER 1: [Matter-of-fact] In my family, you could never be sad. I feel strongest when I show my anger. If I let my partner know that I am sad, I won't feel strong, and they won't see me as strong.
THERAPIST: [Softly] OK. I can better understand why you are reluctant to tell your partner about your sadness. Can you tell your partner this part? [*pause*] "It's hard for me to talk about my sadness because I would feel too weak, and I don't think you'll see me as strong." Please tell them in your own words. (Criterion 2)

EXAMPLE RESPONSES TO BEGINNER-LEVEL DIALOGUE 2

PARTNER 2: [Hesitant] You really want me to tell my partner that when I withdraw, deep down I am really sad and believe I'm a big disappointment to them? I really can't do that. I just can't imagine saying that to them.

THERAPIST: [Softly] I see [*pause*] so this part is challenging. You can't imagine telling them that underneath you feel sad, and like a disappointment to them. Can you tell me more about why this is so hard for you to imagine telling them? (Criterion 1)

PARTNER 2: [Frank] I'll be criticized or judged or disbelieved, and I just don't want to have to put myself out there like that.

THERAPIST: [Softly] So I understand why your fear that you will be judged or criticized keeps you from letting them know about your sadness. Could you please turn to your partner and let them know this part—the fear you have that makes it hard to share? (Criterion 2)

EXAMPLE RESPONSES TO BEGINNER-LEVEL DIALOGUE 3

PARTNER 1: [Irritated] So you want me to tell my partner that there is a lot of sadness and loneliness behind my tears. Well, he just heard me talk about it with you. I don't want to have to say it again to him.

THERAPIST: [Softly] Right, he just heard us discuss it, [*pause*] and yet somehow [*pause*] saying it directly to him is difficult. Can you tell me [*pause*] what is difficult about saying directly to him that behind the tears, [*pause*] there is sadness deep down? (Criterion 1)

PARTNER 1: [Uncomfortable] We don't talk that way. It just feels strange, and I feel kind of silly.

THERAPIST: [Softly] So it's not how you typically talk. It makes sense that to do so would feel strange or silly. I wonder [*pause*] if you could just say that to him? [*pause*] Maybe just say to him how it feels silly or uncomfortable to talk about your feelings of sadness. Can you turn to him and share that much with him? (Criterion 2)

EXAMPLE RESPONSES TO BEGINNER-LEVEL DIALOGUE 4
PARTNER 2: **[Adamant]** So you want me to turn to my partner and tell her I'd rather disconnect than tell her I feel guilty that my sexual needs upset her? I don't want to say it again. It was bad enough to say it to you.
THERAPIST: **[Softly]** Yes, I can see it's not easy. Help me understand [*pause*] what is so difficult about saying this [*pause*] directly to her? (Criterion 1)
PARTNER 2: **[Sad]** I'm afraid that she will get quiet and cry again, and I just can't bear it.
THERAPIST: **[Softly]** Yes, of course, you don't want to see her cry again. I'd like to ask you to take an easier step. [*pause*] Turn to your partner [*pause*] and tell her how hard it is for you [*pause*] to say that deep down, [*pause*] when you pull away and disconnect, [*pause*] you feel guilty, [*pause*] and yet it feels hard to talk about this part [*pause*] because you really don't want to see her cry again. Would you please share this part with her? (Criterion 2)

EXAMPLE RESPONSES TO INTERMEDIATE-LEVEL DIALOGUE 1

PARTNER 1: [Embarrassed] So you want me to turn toward my wife and tell her that although I come across as critical and yell at her, deep down I feel empty and sad? That just feels too hard to say to her. Maybe later I'll feel like I can, but not now.

THERAPIST: [Softly] So you acknowledge that deep down you really feel empty and sad, but that sometimes your sadness gets expressed in a critical way. Can you tell me why you don't want to say that directly to your wife right now? (Criterion 1)

PARTNER 1: [Ashamed] I don't know. I guess I feel embarrassed and maybe ashamed that I have treated her so badly. She's a good person.

THERAPIST: [Softly] I can understand how your embarrassment [*pause*] and shame [*pause*] for saying harsh things to your wife [*pause*] could cause you to refrain from letting her know [*pause*] that what drove your saying those things was [*pause*] your sadness at not having the marriage you wanted with her. Could I have you turn to her now [*pause*] and let her know that your embarrassment keeps you from telling her about your sadness? (Criterion 2)

EXAMPLE RESPONSES TO INTERMEDIATE-LEVEL DIALOGUE 2
PARTNER 2: **[Embarrassed]** So you want me to turn to my husband and tell him how my being afraid he may want to leave our marriage causes me to withdraw to quiet myself down. That's hard for me.
THERAPIST: **[Softly]** So you don't want to let your husband know that your fears he may want to leave you cause you to withdraw [*pause*] to quiet yourself down. Can you tell me why you don't want to say that directly to your husband right now? (Criterion 1)
PARTNER 2: **[Sad]** I don't want to say that to him because it sounds so needy.
THERAPIST: **[Softly]** I am wondering then [*pause*] if you wouldn't mind turning toward your husband [*pause*] and letting him know that you are reluctant [*pause*] to tell him what is going on [*pause*] because he might think you sound too needy and insecure. (Criterion 2)

EXAMPLE RESPONSES TO ADVANCED-LEVEL DIALOGUE 1

PARTNER 1: [Upset] You want me to tell my partner that I really need reassurance—that my asking a lot of questions comes from my need to be reassured that she will never cheat again? I don't want to have to say it.

THERAPIST: [Softly] Please help me understand what makes it difficult for you to share with your wife that your needs for reassurance that you will not be betrayed again leads to asking a lot of questions. (Criterion 1)

PARTNER 1: [Hesitant] I am a strong person, you know? And what you're asking me to do makes me seem so weak. I don't feel safe being that vulnerable ever again.

THERAPIST: [Softly] I get it [*pause*] and that makes so much sense to me. [*pause*] I wonder though [*pause*] if you could help her understand this part of you. [*pause*] Can you tell her? [*pause*] Would you be willing to tell her how hard it is to let yourself be vulnerable again? You never ever want to [*pause*] experience such pain ever again. (Criterion 2)

EXAMPLE RESPONSES TO ADVANCED-LEVEL DIALOGUE 2
PARTNER 2: [Hesitant] So you want me to turn to my partner and tell him that I am deeply sad for hurting him by having this affair and that it is easier for me to get defensive and angry than to say all that. No, I don't think I can say that to him.
THERAPIST: [Softly] I see that you are reluctant to say all this to him, but I'm not sure I fully understand it. Can you tell me what stops you? (Criterion 1)
PARTNER 2: [Plaintive] It won't make a difference. I've lost all credibility given my past lies.
THERAPIST: [Softly] You are doing such an amazing job [pause] of exploring your experience right now. Can you let your husband know [pause] how hard it is to talk about your sadness [pause] and your fears that you will never be believed again? (Criterion 2)

EXAMPLE RESPONSES TO ADVANCED-LEVEL DIALOGUE 3
PARTNER 1: **[Annoyed]** You want me to turn to my partner and tell him I am overwhelmingly sad that we are not a team and that what is underneath my insulting and aggressive behavior is this sadness? I'd rather eat glass than say that to him right now.
THERAPIST: **[Softly]** OK. [*pause*] I understand that you are really sad underneath your aggressive behavior [*pause*] and that you are really against telling your partner that right now. Can you help me understand what makes it uncomfortable [*pause*] for you to share your sadness with him? (Criterion 1)
PARTNER 1: **[Defensive]** Well, I think if I say that, I might just get blamed again and then I'll be doubly sad because I don't want to be the bad guy in his eyes.
THERAPIST: **[Softly]** Perhaps you can tell him this part. [*pause*] "It's hard for me to talk about my sadness [*pause*] because I fear you'll blame me again and that will make me even sadder." Can you tell him that in your own words? (Criterion 2)

EXAMPLE RESPONSES TO ADVANCED-LEVEL DIALOGUE 4
PARTNER 2: **[Annoyed]** So you want me to tell my partner about how I shut down because I am sad. I really don't want to say that to him.
THERAPIST: **[Softly]** I hear you don't want to let your partner know how sad [*pause*] you are [*pause*] when you shut down. Can you tell me why you don't want to turn to your partner and tell him this? (Criterion 1)
PARTNER 2: **[Looking down, long pause]** Sometimes I feel I deserve his insults and the negative things he says about me. It makes me sad and scares me too that he will leave me. And I don't want that!
THERAPIST: **[Softly]** OK. I understand how you could fear telling him that [*pause*] because it might confirm the negative things he sometimes says about you. Then, instead, [*pause*] could I have you turn to your partner [*pause*] and tell him that it is really difficult to say your truth to him [*pause*] because it might precipitate his leaving you, [*pause*] and that would be horrific for you? (Criterion 2)

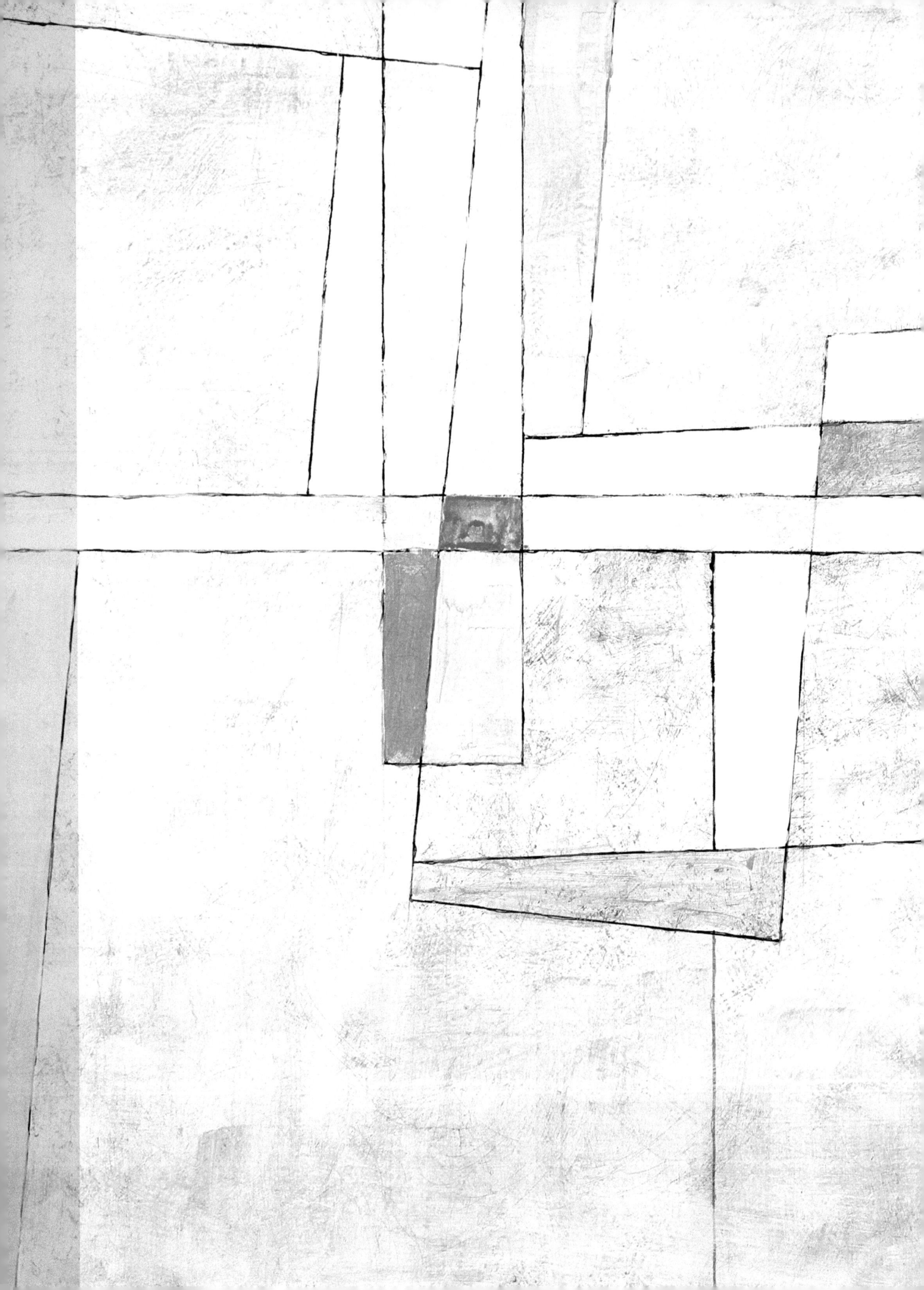

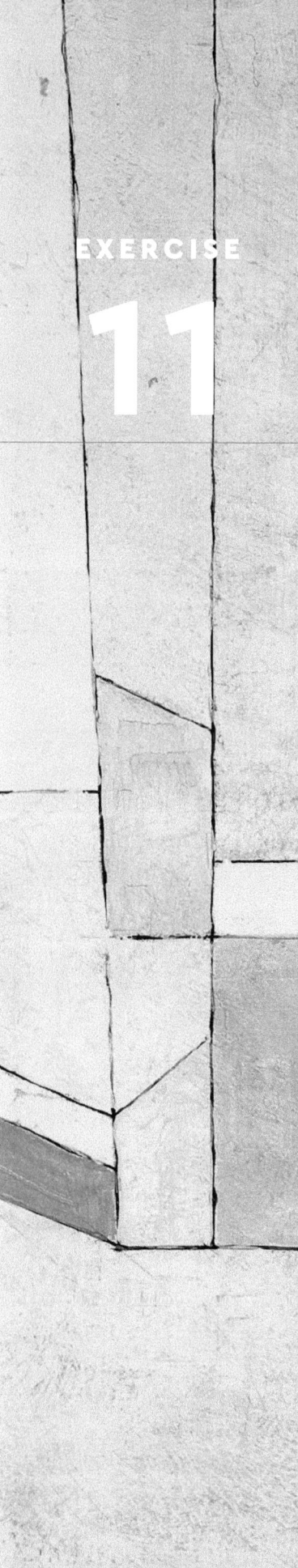

Interrupting Negative Process Early in Therapy: Catching the Bullet I

Preparations for Exercise 11

1. Read the instructions in Chapter 2.

2. Download the Deliberate Practice Reaction Form and the Deliberate Practice Diary Form at https://www.apa.org/pubs/books/deliberate-practice-emotionally-focused-couple-therapy (see the "Resources" tab; also available in Appendixes A and B, respectively).

Exercise Format

For this skill, you will need two trainees: one role-playing the therapist and one role-playing the client, who is one partner of the couple. The context for the skill is a couple therapy session where you can imagine both partners are present, but only one partner is speaking.

Skill Description

Skill Difficulty Level: Advanced

"Catching a bullet" is a metaphor used to describe the therapist's role in intercepting and redirecting ("catching") negative or critical statements ("bullets") between partners during a therapy session. It is an active intervention to prevent harmful communication patterns and create a safe space for more productive emotional exploration. The so-called catching involves softening the emotional blow of a person's aggressive remark on their partner to avoid triggering that partner's reactive, self-protective move of distancing or attacking back, thus fueling another negative interactional cycle.

https://doi.org/10.1037/0000436-013

Deliberate Practice in Emotionally Focused Couple Therapy, by H. Levenson, S. Jinich, A. Vaz, and T. Rousmaniere

There are two ways of handling bullets depending on when they occur in the therapy. In this exercise, we cover how the therapist "catches the bullet" in an early stage of EFCT. In the next exercise (Exercise 12), we present how to deal with bullets that occur in later Stage 2 work. Early in therapy catching bullets focuses on the therapist's getting control of the session by validating the feelings that prompted the bullet, while setting limits on what is acceptable behavior in session. This skill can be used with any couple when one member of the couple says something provocatively negative about their partner (e.g., "She is just like her mother—so wrapped up in herself"). It is particularly useful when high-conflict couples first enter therapy because both partners are used to shooting off rounds of bullets fast and furiously as part of their cycle (where one partner fires the bullet at their partner, who gets triggered and fires back, inciting the original partner to fire again, etc.). If the therapist does not take prompt action, the beginning of therapy can be completely undermined.

Several goals are achieved with successful implementation of this skill: (a) The therapist can prevent (or at least lessen) bullets from setting off a rapidly escalating behavior cycle in-session; (b) it informs the couple of behavior that is not acceptable in therapy; (c) it promotes a positive alliance through validation and empathy; and (d) it builds hope by allowing the therapist to be seen as a take-charge person (e.g., a choreographer), who will not be passive in the face of antitherapeutic behavior.

The therapist should improvise a response to each client statement following these skill criteria:

1. **Interrupt the interaction, matching Partner 1's vocal intensity.** For high-conflict or escalated couples, you may need to do something more dramatic than asking them politely to stop. For example, Sue Johnson often touches one partner on the leg and looks them in the eye. One colleague puts a notebook between the partners, telling them, "You have to stop!" Another calls a partner by name to get their attention. Working online presents its own unique challenges and possibilities; one therapist puts escalated couples on mute and if that doesn't work, puts them into an online "waiting room." Basically, the therapist should do whatever they are comfortable with that gets the couple or partner to stop the undesirable and harmful behavior (within the bounds of reasonableness, of course). Modulate your vocal tone (e.g., loud, forceful, if they are high energy; firm if their tone is more matter-of-fact).

2. **Track what Partner 2 said to cause Partner 1 to become reactive and validate the reasonableness of that reactivity.** Tracking is always a critical part of understanding the couple's cycle. The therapist names what Partner 2 said and links it to Partner 1's reaction. Then the therapist needs to indicate that they can understand the emotion driving Partner 1's reaction. For example, "When your partner said something you felt was untrue, it was hurtful to you." The therapist makes the assumption, based on attachment theory, that the bullet is a way Partner 1 can protest a threat to connection with Partner 2.

3. **Inform Partner 1 of an in-session boundary.** Letting the partners say unkind and aggressive things erodes trust for the therapeutic process in general and in the therapist in particular. Sessions (especially early ones) need to build hope and investment in the therapy. When the therapist does not permit antitherapeutic behavior to go on in session, the couple feels reassured that they are in good hands, even though they might feel annoyed that they are temporarily prevented from venting. Here are some examples of what an emotionally focused couple therapist might say to set appropriate boundaries in session: "I can't work with you if you are verbally jabbing at each other

in here," "Things are happening too quickly and get too escalated for me to be of help," "I can only hear one person at a time," "Criticisms that trigger your partner are not helpful," "I want to understand what is behind that frustration," "Thank you for showing me how things can get so heated, but here we are going to try to do something different."

SKILL CRITERIA FOR EXERCISE 11

1. **Interrupt** the interaction, matching Partner 1's vocal intensity.
2. Track what Partner 2 said to cause Partner 1 to become reactive and **validate** the reasonableness of that reactivity.
3. **Inform** Partner 1 of an in-session boundary.

HELPFUL HINT

If doing all three criteria is too demanding at the beginning, you could try titrating the criteria—only doing Criterion 1 to start (i.e., just practice interrupting), then graduating to doing Criteria 1 *and* 2, and finally all three.

Examples of Therapists Catching the Bullet Early in Therapy

Note: Underlined text is to be read aloud by the person playing the client to provide context.

In all these examples, Partner 1 starts off talking to Partner 2.

Example 1

PARTNER 1: [*fast-paced, energetic*] How dare you go snooping in my phone? It's private. Besides it was no big deal that I texted with my ex. And so what if an old friend and I have a little fun banter back and forth? You are never fun anymore!

THERAPIST: [*fast-paced, energetic*] OK, OK—hang on. Let me stop you here! (Criterion 1— **Interrupt**) [*more measured*] You are upset because your partner looked at your phone and accused you of doing something inappropriate with an ex. I get it. (Criterion 2—**Validate**) But when you attack back and throw out an accusation that your partner is never any fun, it prevents us from doing any meaningful work here. (Criterion 3—**Inform**)

Example 2

PARTNER 1: [*loud*] You're calling me out as dishonest and as not remembering things as they actually happened? Why don't you start being more honest with our therapist and let them know how you think this therapy is a big waste of time and money?

THERAPIST: [*matching volume*] Please . . . let me interrupt you for a second. (Criterion 1— **Interrupt**) [*more measured*] I can imagine that being called out as dishonest feels terrible to you, so of course you are upset, (Criterion 2—**Validate**) but can you see how accusing your partner of the same thing is just going to bog us down in our work? I'd like us to try to avoid that here. (Criterion 3—**Inform**)

Example 3

PARTNER 1: [*harsh, assertive tone*] This has nothing to do with me doing less around the house. I believe this all goes back to your early childhood years when your parents were getting a divorce, and all of the kids were emotionally and physically neglected. [*sarcastic*] It's not my fault that you took on way more than your fair share.

THERAPIST: [*assertive*] Please stop. (Criterion 1—**Interrupt**) Let me be the one to be the therapist here. (Criterion 3—**Inform**) [*more measured*] You're clearly upset about being criticized for not doing enough around the house and I understand your feeling blamed. I really do. (Criterion 2—**Validate**)

INSTRUCTIONS FOR EXERCISE 11

Step 1: Role-Play and Feedback

- The client says the first beginner client statement. The therapist **improvises** a response based on the skill criteria.
- The trainer (or, if not available, the client) provides **brief** feedback based on the skill criteria.
- The client then repeats the same statement, and the therapist again improvises a response. The trainer (or client) again provides brief feedback.

Step 2: Repeat

- Repeat Step 1 for all the statements **in the current difficulty level** (beginner, intermediate, or advanced).

Step 3: Assess and Adjust Difficulty

- The therapist completes the Deliberate Practice Reaction Form (see Appendix A) and decides whether to make the exercise easier or harder or to repeat the same difficulty level.

Step 4: Repeat for Approximately 15 Minutes

- Repeat Steps 1 to 3 for at least 15 minutes.
- The trainees then switch therapist and client roles and start over.

Now it's your turn! Follow Steps 1 and 2 from the exercise instructions.

Remember: The goal of the role-play is for trainees to practice improvising responses to the client statements in a manner that (a) uses the skill criteria and (b) feels authentic for the trainee. **Example therapist responses for each client statement are provided at the end of this exercise. Trainees should attempt to improvise their own responses before reading the examples.**

BEGINNER-LEVEL CLIENT STATEMENTS FOR EXERCISE 11
Beginner Client Statement 1
[Fast-paced, energetic] How dare you go snooping in my phone? It's private. Besides it was no big deal that I texted with my ex. And so what if an old friend and I have a little fun banter back and forth? You're never fun anymore!
Beginner Client Statement 2
[Sharp tone] Ha! Really? Now it's my fault you feel scared when I point out that you did something wrong that upset me? Maybe you are actually failing. Ever consider that?
Beginner Client Statement 3
[Aggressive, interrupting] Well maybe if you didn't ruin our evenings every night by recalling our entire lives over and over again, always blaming me for everything, I too could be the one to approach and try to make the peace between us. I need to sleep. I need to get away from you. Who would want—
Beginner Client Statement 4
[Ironic] Really? You just learned that when I shut down, I'm just trying to calm down, manage my emotions, and not make things worse? Unbelievable. That's what I've been telling you for years. [*rolls eyes*]
Beginner Client Statement 5
[Indignant, loudly] You think that was a joke? You don't even get how insulting and bigoted you are! You are so stupid!

 Assess and adjust the difficulty before moving to the next difficulty level (see Step 3 in the exercise instructions).

INTERMEDIATE-LEVEL CLIENT STATEMENTS FOR EXERCISE 11

Intermediate Client Statement 1

[Angry, suddenly volatile] Fine. Then quit the therapy. As a husband, you've never been committed to our marriage, or to me, or to much of anything in your life. I'm a fool for hoping for something different from you. You are such a coward!

Intermediate Client Statement 2

[Belittling and sarcastic] She wants me to wear a collar so she can put a leash on me! I'm tired of being questioned about my exact whereabouts and my cell phone use.

Intermediate Client Statement 3

[Sarcastic] Oh, so you're finally beginning to see that when you shut me out and refuse to speak to me, it scares me. And you've never thought about it this way. You're unbelievable. Are you serious?

Intermediate Client Statement 4

[Exasperated] I am from a culture where we aren't dramatic with our emotions. When you cry and rant, I think of you as a spoiled kid. You need to grow up!

Intermediate Client Statement 5

[Interrupting, smug] Well, what do you expect? Planning our holiday family dinner is a once-a-year occasion. It's not so simple to plan everything. You never help and just are such a pain in the ass about everything.

Assess and adjust the difficulty before moving to the next difficulty level (see Step 3 in the exercise instructions).

ADVANCED-LEVEL CLIENT STATEMENTS FOR EXERCISE 11
Advanced Client Statement 1
[Detached] I know you are really sad right now about the distance between us, and I know I am supposed to listen and to understand you. So I know I'm being a jerk for saying this, but who would want to be close to you when you are such an aggressive person?
Advanced Client Statement 2
[Shocked] You think things are better between us? Things aren't better. I just stopped pointing out things that upset me! My keeping my mouth shut isn't "intimacy." [*Partner does air quotes with their fingers.*] You don't have a clue! As a partner, you're a joke. Just as I'm giving up on us, you feel like we're better.
Advanced Client Statement 3
[Monotone and defensive] You feel invisible? Really? I think this happens because your brother was always getting in trouble and all the attention in the home went to him and you were always like the invisible little girl. So now, when I'm going through a hard time at work, you think you are invisible, but this has nothing to do with me!
Advanced Client Statement 4
[Angry and loud] I made an innocent comment about thinking our kids could go into town by themselves, and suddenly you think I can't be trusted as a parent. It's not my fault that you are overly strict and have zero flexibility. I think you suck as a parent!
Advanced Client Statement 5
[Angry] I don't want to hear it. Your apologies about calling me fat and ugly over the years come too little too late. I begged you not to be so hurtful to me. It's like you just want me to say "all is forgiven" now? I'm going to be just as cruel to you as you were to me. Just wait and see!

⬯ **Assess and adjust the difficulty here (see Step 3 in the exercise instructions). If appropriate, follow the instructions to make the exercise even more challenging (see Appendix A).**

Example Therapist Responses: Catching the Bullet Early in Therapy

Remember: Trainees should attempt to improvise their own responses before reading the examples. **Do not read the following responses verbatim unless you are having trouble coming up with your own!**

EXAMPLE RESPONSES TO BEGINNER-LEVEL CLIENT STATEMENTS FOR EXERCISE 11
Example Response to Beginner Client Statement 1
[Matching pace/loudness] OK, OK—hang on. Let me stop you here! (Criterion 1) You are upset because your partner looked at your phone and accused you of doing something inappropriate with an ex. I get it. (Criterion 2) But when you attack back and throw out an accusation that your partner is never any fun, it prevents us from doing any meaningful work here. Right? (Criterion 3)
Example Response to Beginner Client Statement 2
[Matching pace/loudness] Let me stop you here! (Criterion 1) I can understand that you feel unjustly accused. (Criterion 2) But when you attack back, it is just going to intensify that dysfunctional cycle we have been talking about. Can you see that? (Criterion 3)
Example Response to Beginner Client Statement 3
[Matching pace/loudness] Alright. Please, pause for a moment. (Criterion 1) You have a lot of feelings around this, and I get how badly it feels to be blamed like that. (Criterion 2) Can you see that when you respond in this way and say how you need to get away, you're just going to trigger your partner to be upset, and that won't help us? (Criterion 3)
Example Response to Beginner Client Statement 4
[Matching pace/loudness] Let me stop you there. (Criterion 1) It's not helpful to use sarcasm in our work in here. (Criterion 3) I can imagine that you are frustrated with how long you have tried to explain things to your partner. (Criterion 2)
Example Response to Beginner Client Statement 5
[Matching pace/loudness] Woah. Stop. (Criterion 1) I understand that you got very hurt. There was nothing you found funny about what your partner said. (Criterion 2) But you cannot say things like that in here because it's just going to trigger you both back into a fight, and it's really important to give the two of you a chance to be with each other without the fighting. Let's all take a moment to catch our breath. (Criterion 3)

EXAMPLE RESPONSES TO INTERMEDIATE-LEVEL CLIENT STATEMENTS FOR EXERCISE 11

Example Response to Intermediate Client Statement 1

[Matching pace/loudness] Please stop. (Criterion 1) I know it's disappointing to hear your husband talk about not being sure he wants to keep coming to therapy, (Criterion 2) but when you say things like calling him cowardly, it's really not helpful, and I need you not to say things like that here, OK? (Criterion 3)

Example Response to Intermediate Client Statement 2

[Matching pace/loudness] Let me interrupt here. (Criterion 1) I understand that it's very difficult to have your whereabouts questioned all the time. You feel like you never catch a break, and that doesn't feel good. (Criterion 2) However, using sarcasm is a way of avoiding and invalidating your partner's fears and it only makes things worse between you. (Criterion 3)

Example Response to Intermediate Client Statement 3

[Matching pace/loudness] Let me stop you for a second. Wow. (Criterion 1) I can understand how you are skeptical about whether your partner is really beginning to understand how scared you get. (Criterion 2) However, speaking to him sarcastically and calling what he says "unbelievable" is not going to help matters. (Criterion 3)

Example Response to Intermediate Client Statement 4

[Matching pace/loudness] Whoa, slow down. I need you to stop. (Criterion 1) I get how off-putting it can be to deal with behaviors that are so alien to you, (Criterion 2) but when you add fuel to the fire by ordering your partner to "grow up," you're going to start another cycle and I want to help the two of you avoid doing that. (Criterion 3)

Example Response to Intermediate Client Statement 5

[Matching pace/loudness] Wait a minute. (Criterion 1) You clearly just got quite triggered. I get how it's not so simple to plan everything without your partner's help. (Criterion 2) However, when you get defensive and you say something in a global condemning way, it's going to trigger your partner and derail our conversation. Does that make sense? (Criterion 3)

EXAMPLE RESPONSES TO ADVANCED-LEVEL CLIENT STATEMENTS FOR EXERCISE 11
Example Response to Advanced Client Statement 1
[Matching pace/loudness] Let me interrupt you. (Criterion 1) I get that it is hard to be close when you feel attacked or spoken to aggressively. (Criterion 2) But can you see that framing your partner's aggressive behavior towards you as a character flaw has an element of name-calling? That will not help our work. (Criterion 3)
Example Response to Advanced Client Statement 2
[Matching pace/loudness] I'm going to interrupt. I'd like to stay here for a second. (Criterion 1) It makes sense to me that you feel upset when your reality doesn't match your partner's. (Criterion 2) It doesn't help to name-call or to use sarcasm. (Criterion 3)
Example Response to Advanced Client Statement 3
[Matching pace/loudness] Hang on! Let me interrupt here. (Criterion 1) Your partner was just beginning to explore how she feels invisible, and you shifted the attention to her family history. While family history is important, shifting the focus away from your partner's feelings isn't going to be helpful. (Criterion 3) I can imagine it must be hard for you to hear her talk about feeling invisible and just listen. (Criterion 2)
Example Response to Advanced Client Statement 4
[Matching pace/loudness] Please stop. That's enough. (Criterion 1) Obviously, it must feel terrible to get the message you cannot be trusted as a parent. I get it. (Criterion 2) But to then retaliate in this damning way will only bring the two of you back into the negative cycle. (Criterion 3)
Example Response to Advanced Client Statement 5
[Matching pace/loudness] Pause, please. I really want to understand what just happened. (Criterion 1) You're doing a good job of expressing that you don't want to hear apologies now when you've been so hurt. Of course, it's not easy to just let go of the hurt now. (Criterion 2) However, if you want to be heard, you need to make it safe for your partner to hang in there—threatening to be cruel in return will have the opposite effect. (Criterion 3)

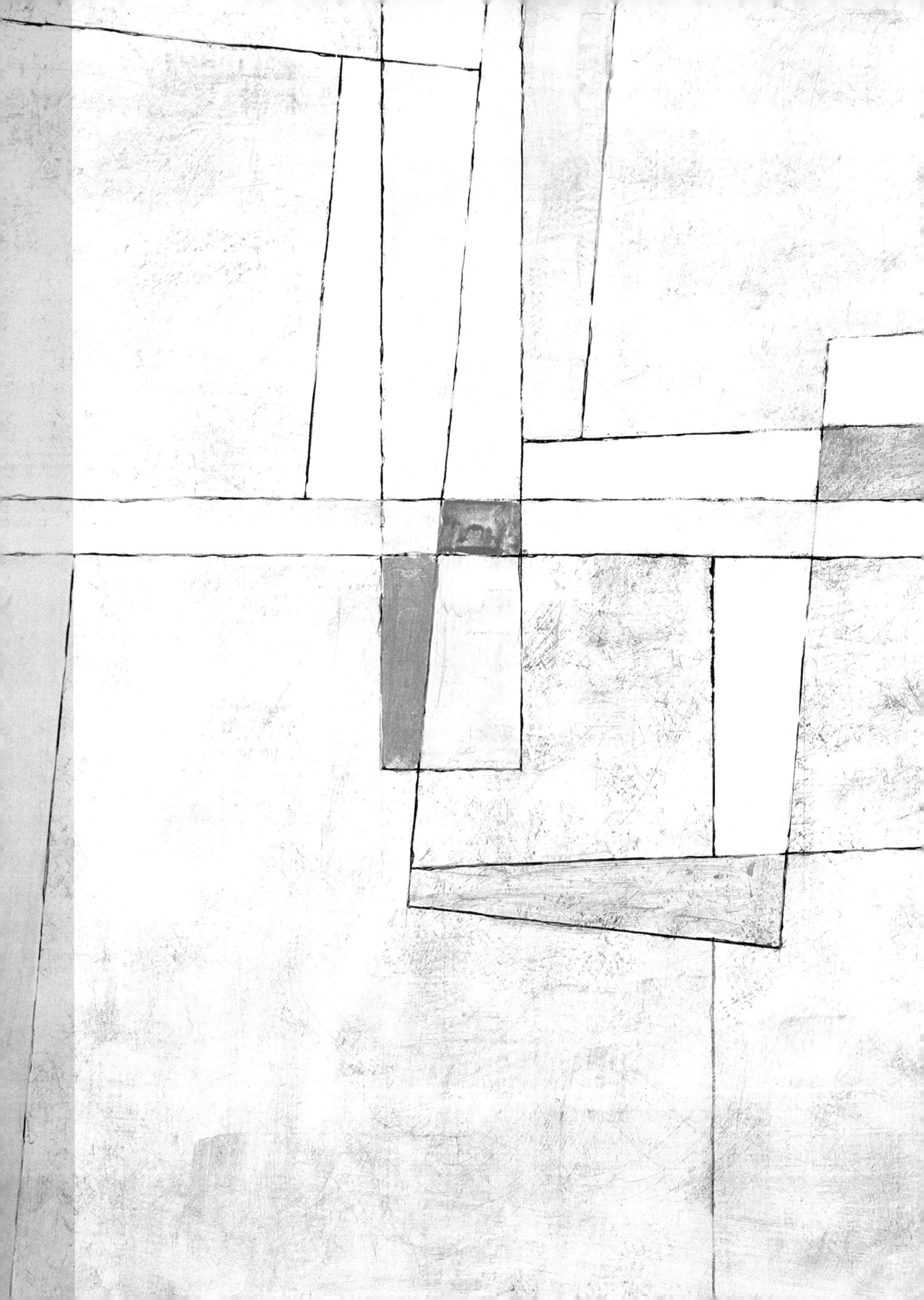

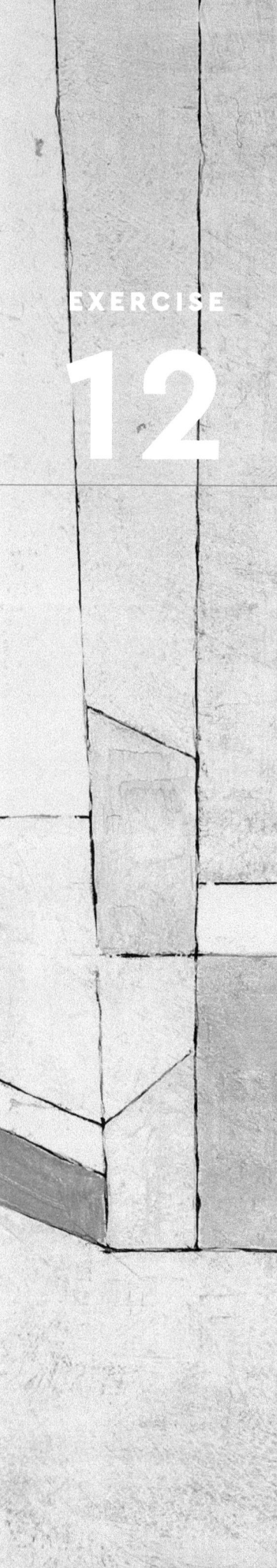

Interrupting Negative Process Later in Therapy: Catching the Bullet II

Preparations for Exercise 12

1. Read the instructions in Chapter 2.

2. Download the Deliberate Practice Reaction Form and the Deliberate Practice Diary Form at https://www.apa.org/pubs/books/deliberate-practice-emotionally-focused-couple-therapy (see the "Resources" tab; also available in Appendixes A and B, respectively).

Exercise Format

For this skill, you will need three trainees: one role-playing the therapist, one role-playing Partner 1 and one role-playing Partner 2. The context is a couple therapy session where both partners are present.

Skill Description

Skill Difficulty Level: Advanced

In Exercise 11, we covered catching bullets in early sessions of therapy, when one member of the couple says something provocatively negative about their partner. The goal of that exercise was to prevent bullets from setting off the dysfunctional dance that typically leads to conflict and disconnection and to set limits in the session while trying to build a positive alliance through validation and empathy.

In this exercise, we are going to focus on another occasion where the therapist needs to catch a particularly painful bullet. This is when one member of the couple says something from a place of vulnerability, and their partner mistrusts or minimizes what was said.

https://doi.org/10.1037/0000436-014

Deliberate Practice in Emotionally Focused Couple Therapy, by H. Levenson, S. Jinich, A. Vaz, and T. Rousmaniere

An example of such minimization at a time of partner vulnerability is "Yeah you say you love me and wonder if you are worthy of me, but that's too little, too late!" These types of bullets most often appear in Stage 2 work, where the couple is no longer escalated and they understand the relevance of their cycle and see it as a common enemy. In Stage 2, the partners are, with the help of their therapist, taking vulnerable risks with each other, exploring unmet attachment longings, reviewing attachment histories, and shifting their internal working models (view of self–other) in order to have an engaged encounter where attachment fears are shared with each other.

In Stage 2, the therapist is working on restructuring the partners' positions. This is commonly known as withdrawer reengagement and/or blamer softening. As part of this process, one partner expresses emotional vulnerability. The bullet occurs when their partner, who has longed to hear such vulnerability and softness for so long, doubts it could really be happening. And if it is happening, they fear it will soon be snapped away. This partner is caught off guard, overwhelmed, or disbelieving, and, in these dysregulated states, fires off a bullet from pent-up unresolved longing. It is a form of attachment protest.

The emotionally focused couple therapist needs to be aware that this protest occurs at a particularly tender time when the vulnerable partner is emotionally exposed. To catch the bullet before it pierces the vulnerable partner, the therapist must interrupt the speaking partner, empathize with the vulnerable partner's experience, comment on the process, and ask the person firing the bullet what was happening for them. Sometimes the therapist can conjecture that the harmful words (the bullet) came from a place of disorientation, disbelief, or overwhelm that their partner could say something so vulnerable. Here the therapist can bring up attachment longings to explain the seemingly paradoxical behavior of saying something so rejecting (the bullet) when responding to something they have actually longed to hear.

In this exercise, Partner 1 will begin by saying something from a place of vulnerability that triggers a negative response (a bullet) from Partner 2 that the therapist must then catch. The therapist should improvise a response to each client statement following these skill criteria:

1. **[Interrupt Partner 2 and speak to Partner 1] Empathize with the conjectured experience of Partner 1 as a result of hearing the bullet.** This first step is critical in stopping Partner 2's negative comments from continuing (bullet) and helping ameliorate Partner 1's negative emotional reaction to hearing those negative comments. The therapist's tone should be soft and compassionate, given Partner 1's vulnerable state.

2. **[Speak to Partner 2] Mention something important has just happened and track Partner 1's vulnerable comment and Partner 2's hurtful response (the bullet).** ("Something important just happened. When your partner said X [something vulnerable], I noticed you responded negatively [bullet].") Tracking is always a critical part of understanding the couple's cycle (see Exercise 3); informing the couple about what leads to what helps the partners understand their own and their partner's roles in maintaining the cycle. The therapist's tone is softer than in Exercise 11. It is expected that the therapist has a good alliance by this point, and the couple is de-escalated and understands their cycle and some of their unmet attachment longings.

3. **Inquire about Partner 2's feelings:**

   • **Option 1:** Ask Partner 2 an open-ended question about what was happening for them at that moment when they responded with a bullet.

- **Option 2:** Conjecture that Partner 2's hurtful response (the bullet) is due to their disorientation, disbelief, or overwhelm upon seeing their partner's vulnerability. For example, "You can't believe their softness right now, after you have wished to hear that softness for such a long time." Conjecture that Partner 2's bullet is actually a protest about having unmet attachment needs.

SKILL CRITERIA FOR EXERCISE 12

1. **[Interrupt Partner 2 and speak to Partner 1] Empathize** with the conjectured experience of Partner 1 as a result of hearing the bullet.
2. **[Speak to Partner 2]** Mention something important has just happened and **track** Partner 1's vulnerable comment and Partner 2's hurtful response (the bullet).
3. Inquire about Partner 2's feelings:
   - **Option 1: Ask** an open-ended question about what was happening for Partner 2 at the moment when they responded with a bullet.
   - **Option 2: Conjecture** that Partner 2's hurtful response (bullet) is due to disorientation, disbelief, or overwhelm upon seeing their partner's vulnerability.

HELPFUL HINTS

1. If you find yourself favoring one option over another, try the other option.
2. As with the previous exercise, if you find doing all three criteria together too difficult, try titrating them. You could start off by practicing Criterion 1 (i.e., interrupting) alone, and adding Criteria 2 and then 3 as the task becomes easier.

Examples of Therapists Catching the Bullet Later in Therapy

Note: The therapist initially interrupts Partner 2 and then quickly turns to Partner 1, eventually returning to Partner 2.

Example 1

PARTNER 1 TO PARTNER 2: [*soft*] I really deeply desire and need your love.

PARTNER 2 TO PARTNER 1: [*snapping back aggressively*] After all these years of ignoring me, *now* you tell me you need my love!

THERAPIST: [To Partner 2] I need to interrupt you here. **[To Partner 1]** Wow! That must be really hard to hear right now, given that you just said how you deeply desire and need your partner's love. (Criterion 1—**Interrupt and Empathize**) **[To Partner 2]** And yet, for you, something important just happened. When your partner said they really do need your love, you responded pretty quickly with some forceful, pushback words. (Criterion 2—**Track**) I'm wondering what happened to you when you heard those words. (Criterion 3, Option 1—**Ask**)

or

I'm wondering if you can hardly let in that your partner really needs your love, when you have wished to hear that for so long. (Criterion 3, Option 2—**Conjecture**)

Example 2

PARTNER 1 TO PARTNER 2: [*sad*] I feel alone in this relationship. Sometimes you don't seem interested in doing things with me. Maybe I disappoint you.

PARTNER 2 TO PARTNER 1: [*disparaging*] Why would I want to do things with you? You don't really care about anyone else but yourself.

THERAPIST: **[To Partner 2]** Let me interrupt you for a moment. **[To Partner 1]** That must be painful to hear just as you expressed feeling lonely in the relationship and wondering if you are a disappointment to your partner. (Criterion 1—**Interrupt and Empathize**) **[To Partner 2]** And yet for you, something important just happened. So when your partner said they feel lonely and are afraid they disappoint you, you responded with some pretty strong criticism. (Criterion 2—**Track**) I'm wondering what was going on for you just before you responded? (Criterion 3, Option 1—**Ask**)

or

I'm wondering if you were a bit disoriented hearing how much your partner misses you. You've wanted to hear that for so long but have rarely heard it. (Criterion 3, Option 2—**Conjecture**)

Example 3

PARTNER 1 TO PARTNER 2: [*ashamed*] I don't feel that I deserve you. I feel completely inadequate in the relationship.

PARTNER 2 TO PARTNER 1: [*accusing*] Are you even trying?

THERAPIST: **[To Partner 2]** Can I interrupt here? **[To Partner 1]** I imagine this accusation is hard for you just now, especially after vulnerably saying that you feel inadequate in the relationship. (Criterion 1—**Interrupt and Empathize**) **[To Partner 2]** I think something important just happened. So when your partner said they feel so undeserving and inadequate, you accused them of not working on the relationship. (Criterion 2—**Track**) What was happening for you right then? (Criterion 3, Option 1—**Ask**)

or

Could it be that you can't believe what they are saying—that they feel inadequate and that they don't deserve you? You've never heard them so open like that before, although you've wanted to hear how they really feel for so long. (Criterion 3, Option 2—**Conjecture**)

INSTRUCTIONS FOR EXERCISE 12

Step 1: Role-Play and Feedback

- Partner 1 reads their lines out loud, then Partner 2 reads their lines. The therapist **improvises** a response based on the skill criteria.
- The trainer (or, if not available, the partners) provides **brief** feedback based on the skill criteria.
- The partners then repeat the same statements, and the therapist again improvises a response. The trainer (or the partners) again provides brief feedback.

Step 2: Repeat

- Repeat Step 1 for all the statements **in the current difficulty level** (beginner, intermediate, or advanced).

Step 3: Assess and Adjust Difficulty

- The therapist completes the Deliberate Practice Reaction Form (see Appendix A) and decides whether to make the exercise easier or harder or to repeat the same difficulty level.

Step 4: Repeat for Approximately 15 Minutes

- Repeat Steps 1 to 3 for at least 15 minutes.
- The trainees then switch therapist and client roles and start over.

> **Now it's your turn! Follow Steps 1 and 2 from the exercise instructions.**

Remember: The goal of the role-play is for trainees to practice improvising responses to the client statements in a manner that (a) uses the skill criteria and (b) feels authentic for the trainee. **Example therapist responses for each client statement are provided at the end of this exercise. Trainees should attempt to improvise their own responses before reading the examples.**

BEGINNER-LEVEL CLIENT STATEMENTS FOR EXERCISE 12
Beginner Client Statement 1
PARTNER 1 TO PARTNER 2: [Ashamed] When you criticize me, I feel ashamed. My withdrawing is just my way to not feel badly about all the ways I've disappointed you.   **PARTNER 2 TO PARTNER 1: [Critical]** Now it's my fault? How am I supposed to react when you don't do the most basic things that I ask for?
Beginner Client Statement 2
PARTNER 1 TO PARTNER 2: [Meek] When you get very upset with me, I feel completely helpless and inadequate—and so scared that you'll want to break up with me that I shut down and just wait for the storm to pass.   **PARTNER 2 TO PARTNER 1: [Critical]** You think I'm the storm? How do you think I feel when you shut me out? You keep all your feelings under tight control or on the surface, and you never talk to me about anything.
Beginner Client Statement 3
PARTNER 1 TO PARTNER 2: [Ashamed] My whole life I've been afraid of being seen as "a weakling," as my grandfather would say, and now, whenever I don't meet your expectations, I feel like a weakling, and all I can do is shut down and withdraw.   **PARTNER 2 TO PARTNER 1: [Pleading]** Look, when you do things right, I tell you so. Don't make me out to be such a hard ass.
Beginner Client Statement 4
PARTNER 1 TO PARTNER 2: [Sad] Even though we rarely get into arguments like we used to, I've been feeling sad that you don't seem as committed to the relationship anymore. I don't feel as important to you as I used to feel, and I get scared and wonder if you still want me.   **PARTNER 2 TO PARTNER 1: [Critical]** Here we go again. Things are better, but somehow you always find a way to focus on the negatives.
Beginner Client Statement 5
PARTNER 1 TO PARTNER 2: [Embarrassed] I feel lonely in the relationship and desperately need you to reassure me that I matter. I've never risked telling you about this in this way because I'm fearful that you'll see me as weak or as too needy and dependent.   **PARTNER 2 TO PARTNER 1:** [*Sighs and shakes head in disbelief*]

 Assess and adjust the difficulty before moving to the next difficulty level (see Step 3 in the exercise instructions).

INTERMEDIATE-LEVEL CLIENT STATEMENTS FOR EXERCISE 12
Intermediate Client Statement 1
PARTNER 1 TO PARTNER 2: [Ashamed] My cardiac condition makes it impossible for me to help you with most things at home, and it's so painful for me to disappoint you in any way, especially since I was always such a disappointment to my father. **PARTNER 2 TO PARTNER 1: [Critical]** The last thing I need is to be told that I'm just like your father.
Intermediate Client Statement 2
PARTNER 1 TO PARTNER 2]: [Anxious] I get scared when you get angry with me and then I seize up and get paralyzed. I'm ashamed of becoming paralyzed. **PARTNER 2 TO PARTNER 1: [Matter-of-fact]** Don't be such a scaredy-cat!
Intermediate Client Statement 3
PARTNER 1 TO THERAPIST: [Worried] My partner's family seems more important to him than I am. I get worried that I'm not that important to him any longer—or maybe I never was. In fact, I'm downright scared. **PARTNER 2 TO PARTNER 1: [Critical]** I think that's absurd.
Intermediate Client Statement 4
PARTNER 1 TO PARTNER 2: [Sad] Since the baby was born, I feel so lonely. If I disappeared, I don't think you would miss me or maybe even notice. **PARTNER 2 TO PARTNER 1: [Critical]** You don't get to be the center of attention now. What did you think would happen after the baby was born?
Intermediate Client Statement 5
PARTNER 1 TO PARTNER 2: [Ashamed] I always feel so needy compared to you. You seem so self-sufficient and sturdy, and I don't feel that way a lot of the time—especially compared to you. I'm afraid you'll tire of me and see me as too dependent on you. **PARTNER 2 TO PARTNER 1: [Matter-of-fact]** What did you say?

🛑 **Assess and adjust the difficulty before moving to the next difficulty level (see Step 3 in the exercise instructions).**

ADVANCED-LEVEL CLIENT STATEMENTS FOR EXERCISE 12

Advanced Client Statement 1

PARTNER 1 TO PARTNER 2: [Soft] When you're disappointed or dissatisfied with me, [*pause*] I need you to tell me in a soft, kind manner. I need to know that in your eyes, I am still special and valued and that even if I make mistakes, I can still be seen this way. Honestly, if you could do this, I think I would feel more loved and cared for, and I'd be much more engaged.

PARTNER 2 TO PARTNER 1: [Irritated] You're always wanting more.

Advanced Client Statement 2

PARTNER 1 TO PARTNER 2: [Hesitant] This is hard for me to admit, you know? Even if I have not always lived up to your expectations, I hoped you'd still want me as I want you.

PARTNER 2 TO PARTNER 1: [Ambivalent] All I can promise is that I'll try. Will you really listen to what I need?

Advanced Client Statement 3

PARTNER 1 TO PARTNER 2: [Pleading] I have a terror of finding out that I will never matter to you, and that I will always be kept on the outside. Please don't keep me at such a distance.

PARTNER 2 TO PARTNER 1: [Harsh] You keep me at such a distance! You put it on me, but it's always been you.

Advanced Client Statement 4

PARTNER 1 TO PARTNER 2: [Assertive] What I need the most from you is to be told that "I am wanted, needed, that I am enough and that I belong to you."

PARTNER 2 TO PARTNER 1: [Complaining] And what about what I have asked for from you? For years I have practically begged you for the least bit of affection and touch.

Advanced Client Statement 5

PARTNER 1 TO PARTNER 2: [Nervous] So this is hard for me, OK? When I get scared that I'll end up all alone, I need you to tell me that you love me. I need to know that I'm not alone.

PARTNER 2 TO PARTNER 1: [Argumentative] I already do that.

Assess and adjust the difficulty here (see Step 3 in the exercise instructions). If appropriate, follow the instructions to make the exercise even more challenging (see Appendix A).

Example Therapist Responses: Catching the Bullet Later in Therapy

Remember: Trainees should attempt to improvise their own responses before reading the examples. **Do not read the following responses verbatim unless you are having trouble coming up with your own!**

EXAMPLE RESPONSES TO BEGINNER-LEVEL CLIENT STATEMENTS FOR EXERCISE 12
Example Response to Beginner Client Statement 1
[To Partner 2] Let me step in for a moment. **[To Partner 1]** I imagine that this is hard to hear again, especially when you just said that criticism leads you to feel shame and then need to withdraw. (Criterion 1) **[To Partner 2]** Something important happened for you just now. As your partner was just beginning to explore feeling ashamed and disappointing, you reacted pretty quickly there and pushed back. (Criterion 2) I'm wondering what happens on the inside when your partner starts focusing on feeling ashamed? (Criterion 3, Option 1) or I wonder if it's somehow hard to believe that your partner feels ashamed since you rarely hear about that? (Criterion 3, Option 2)
Example Response to Beginner Client Statement 2
[To Partner 2] Can I interrupt you? **[To Partner 1]** I imagine you might be feeling helpless and inadequate even now and that must be hard, especially after just sharing this. (Criterion 1) **[To Partner 2]** It seems like something important just happened, and I don't want us to move past it too quickly. Your partner was just beginning to open up about fears of losing you and of feelings of inadequacy, and yet you just criticized them for not sharing feelings. (Criterion 2) What happened there? (Criterion 3, Option 1) or I imagine that one never knows when one will finally receive the very things we have been asking for, and it can be rather disorienting. Did that happen to you? (Criterion 3, Option 2)
Example Response to Beginner Client Statement 3
[To Partner 2] Let's me interrupt here. **[To Partner 1]** You just took a vulnerable risk and I imagine you feel a bit taken aback and unheard, (Criterion 1) **[To Partner 2]** so let's slow things down a bit here since this is new territory and it seems like something really meaningful just happened for you. You just chastised your partner right after they talked about feeling like a weakling. (Criterion 2) Can you tell me what just happened inside of you? (Criterion 3, Option 1) or It must be rather confusing for you when your partner finally opens up about feeling like a weakling when they don't meet your expectations. What they are saying is so different from what you usually hear. (Criterion 3, Option 2)

**EXAMPLE RESPONSES TO BEGINNER-LEVEL
CLIENT STATEMENTS FOR EXERCISE 12**

Example Response to Beginner Client Statement 4

[To Partner 2] Let me interrupt you please. **[To Partner 1]** This must be hard for you to hear at this moment, especially because you were focusing on your sadness and your fears of not seeming as important to your partner anymore. (Criterion 1) **[To Partner 2]** And for you something important just happened here. Your partner was just saying that they wonder if you still want them, and then you criticized them. Even though you feel better about the relationship, you reacted in a way that seems judgmental and blocks any further exploration of feelings between you. (Criterion 2) Can you tell me what just happened inside of you? (Criterion 3, Option 1)

or

It must be confusing to feel like things are finally better and to hear your partner talking about their lingering sadness and fears you don't want them. (Criterion 3, Option 2)

Example Response to Beginner Client Statement 5

[To Partner 2] OK, I think I need to jump in here to try to understand what just happened. **[To Partner 1]** You just took a very vulnerable step and I imagine seeing your partner's reaction must feel quite bad. (Criterion 1) **[To Partner 2]** This is important. Tell me what just happened for you? (Criterion 3, Option 1) When, as your partner began to speak about feeling lonely and in need of some reassurance, you sighed and shook your head. (Criterion 2)

or

Maybe it's hard to believe that your partner is fearful that you'll see them as too needy. It just doesn't compute given what they've said in the past? (Criterion 3, Option 2)

EXAMPLE RESPONSES TO INTERMEDIATE-LEVEL CLIENT STATEMENTS FOR EXERCISE 12

Example Response to Intermediate Client Statement 1

[To Partner 2] Let me interrupt for a second. **[To Partner 1]** This is hard, yes? I imagine it feels hurtful not to have your vulnerability understood by your partner just now. (Criteria 1) **[To Partner 2]** And yet it is clear to me that something important got stirred up in you, and I'd like to explore it. Your partner was speaking about how it is painful for them to disappoint you when they can't help out at home, especially since they were always disappointing their father. And then you retorted that they shouldn't compare you to their father. (Criterion 2) Can you tell me what just happened for you? (Criterion 3, Option 1)

or

I wonder if perhaps it's difficult to hear how incapacitated your partner is due to their cardiac condition. Perhaps you feel badly that on top of doing so much more around the house, you also have to take care of their fears of disappointing you? (Criterion 3, Option 2)

Example Response to Intermediate Client Statement 2

[To Partner 2] Let me step in and slow us down. **[To Partner 1]** I wonder if you are feeling hurt by being called a scaredy-cat when you just revealed that your partner's anger *is* scary to you (Criterion 1) **[To Partner 2]** and yet something important just happened for you. Your partner was talking about feeling ashamed of becoming paralyzed when they get scared, and then you admonished them for being a "scaredy-cat." (Criterion 2) What were you thinking or feeling just now as you heard them speak about feeling ashamed? (Criterion 3, Option 1)

or

I wonder if you were confused in some way, when you heard your partner was ashamed of becoming paralyzed. You always thought they were closing themselves off from you. (Criterion 3, Option 2)

Example Response to Intermediate Client Statement 3

[To Partner 2] Let me step in and let's take this slower. **[To Partner 1]** I wonder if you are feeling a bit invalidated just now. (Criterion 1) **[To Partner 2]** And yet, I think something important just happened for you. Your partner is opening up about feeling afraid that they don't rank as high with you as your family does and is worried they are not important to you any longer. And after they said this, you dismissed what you heard as absurd. (Criterion 2) Can you tell me what was happening for you as you heard their feelings of fear? (Criterion 3, Option 1)

or

I wonder if it feels overwhelming to hear your partner talk about feeling worried and scared that they are no longer important to you. You wanted to let them know that these fears are not warranted. Yes? (Criterion 3, Option 2)

Example Response to Intermediate Client Statement 4

[To Partner 2] Let me interrupt you please. **[To Partner 1]** Wow, it must feel hurtful to open up vulnerably about feeling less relevant or important to your partner to be told that you don't get to feel this way. (Criterion 1) **[To Partner 2]** And yet, I think what happened is quite important. Your partner was opening up about feeling sad and lonely for your attention, and you responded in a dismissive manner. (Criterion 2) Can you tell me what got triggered in you just now? (Criterion 3, Option 1)

or

I wonder when you respond in this dismissive way if you feel helpless to resolve your partner's lonely feelings. (Criterion 3, Option 2)

**EXAMPLE RESPONSES TO INTERMEDIATE-LEVEL
CLIENT STATEMENTS FOR EXERCISE 12**

Example Response to Intermediate Client Statement 5

[To Partner 2] OK, so let's slow things down a bit. **[To Partner 1]** It must be hurtful to open up with such vulnerability and speak about your fear of being too much, and then feel unheard. (Criterion 1) **[To Partner 2]** This is new territory, and it's important to understand what is going on with you. You apparently just couldn't let in what your partner said about feeling needy compared to seeing you as self-sufficient. (Criterion 2) Can you tell me what just happened inside of you? (Criterion 3, Option 1)

or

In moments like these when your partner is opening up to you in such a vulnerable way, I wonder if it feels uncomfortable for you or if it's hard to focus on what is being said? You seemed a bit disoriented. (Criterion 3, Option 2)

EXAMPLE RESPONSES TO ADVANCED-LEVEL CLIENT STATEMENTS FOR EXERCISE 12

Example Response to Advanced Client Statement 1

[To Partner 2] Woah, let me step in here for a moment as this is important. **[To Partner 1]** You just did such an amazing job of vulnerably asking for what you need that it must be so hurtful to be seen as dissatisfied with what you do have. (Criterion 1) **[To Partner 2]** And yet something important just came up for you too just now. Your partner took a big risk to ask you what they need the most from you, deep down, is to feel loved and valued, and your response was rather blaming. (Criterion 2) We were exploring things on a pretty deep level up until now, and things were going pretty well, so what happened inside of you just then? (Criterion 3, Option 1)

or

I wonder if this particular request was hard for you to let in or even believe, given how long you have wanted your partner to anticipate and respond to your needs and understand your disappointment. (Criterion 3, Option 2)

Example Response to Advanced Client Statement 2

[To Partner 2] OK, let me slow this down. **[To Partner 1]** I can imagine that your partner's response just now is hard to hear. (Criterion 1) **[To Partner 2]** Something important seems to have just happened. As your partner was beginning to express their hopes that you would still choose them as they choose you, you said you'd try, but only if they give you what you need. (Criterion 2) What was going on inside of you just then? (Criterion 3, Option 1)

or

I wonder if you just can't trust that your partner really wants you after all of the things they have said over the years? (Criterion 3, Option 2)

Example Response to Advanced Client Statement 3

[To Partner 2] Let me interrupt you, please. **[To Partner 1]** I imagine it's painful to be accused of the very thing that you are trying to say has been hurtful to you. (Criterion 1) **[To Partner 2]** And yet for you something pretty big just happened. Your partner was just talking about wanting to be closer to you, when you pushed back defensively accusing them of creating distance. (Criterion 2) What just happened there? (Criterion 3, Option 1)

or

I wonder if it's confusing to hear your partner pleading to be close when you have felt held at arm's length? (Criterion 3, Option 2)

Example Response to Advanced Client Statement 4

[To Partner 2] OK, hang on, [*pause*] let's stop for a minute. **[To Partner 1]** You have just taken a big risk in asking for what you need and so it must be painful to not be heard and responded to. (Criterion 1) **[To Partner 2]** Something big just got triggered here. Your partner was beginning to take a big leap and was asking to feel more wanted and needed and to feel like you really belong to each other, and then suddenly you started arguing with them. (Criterion 2) Can you tell me what was going on with you, on the inside? (Criterion 3, Option 1)

or

You have been wanting to feel closer and to hear this for so long, and it finally comes. I wonder if it all feels a bit overwhelming and you needed to slow it down somehow— to catch your breath or something. (Criterion 3, Option 2)

EXAMPLE RESPONSES TO ADVANCED-LEVEL
CLIENT STATEMENTS FOR EXERCISE 12

Example Response to Advanced Client Statement 5

[**To Partner 2**] Hang on, let's pause for a second to explore what just happened. [**To Partner 1**] It must not feel so good to open up vulnerably and to say what you need, only to hear back that they already give you what you need. (Criterion 1) [**To Partner 2**] It seems like something important happened for you. Your partner was taking a big risk confessing that they deeply need your reassurance and commitment when they get scared and feel all alone. Then you replied by denying the validity of their request. (Criterion 2) What was going on with you that led you to respond in such a way? (Criterion 3, Option 1)

or

I wonder if you got overwhelmed when you were asked for reassurance and so responded in an argumentative manner. Is that what happened here? (Criterion 3, Option 2)

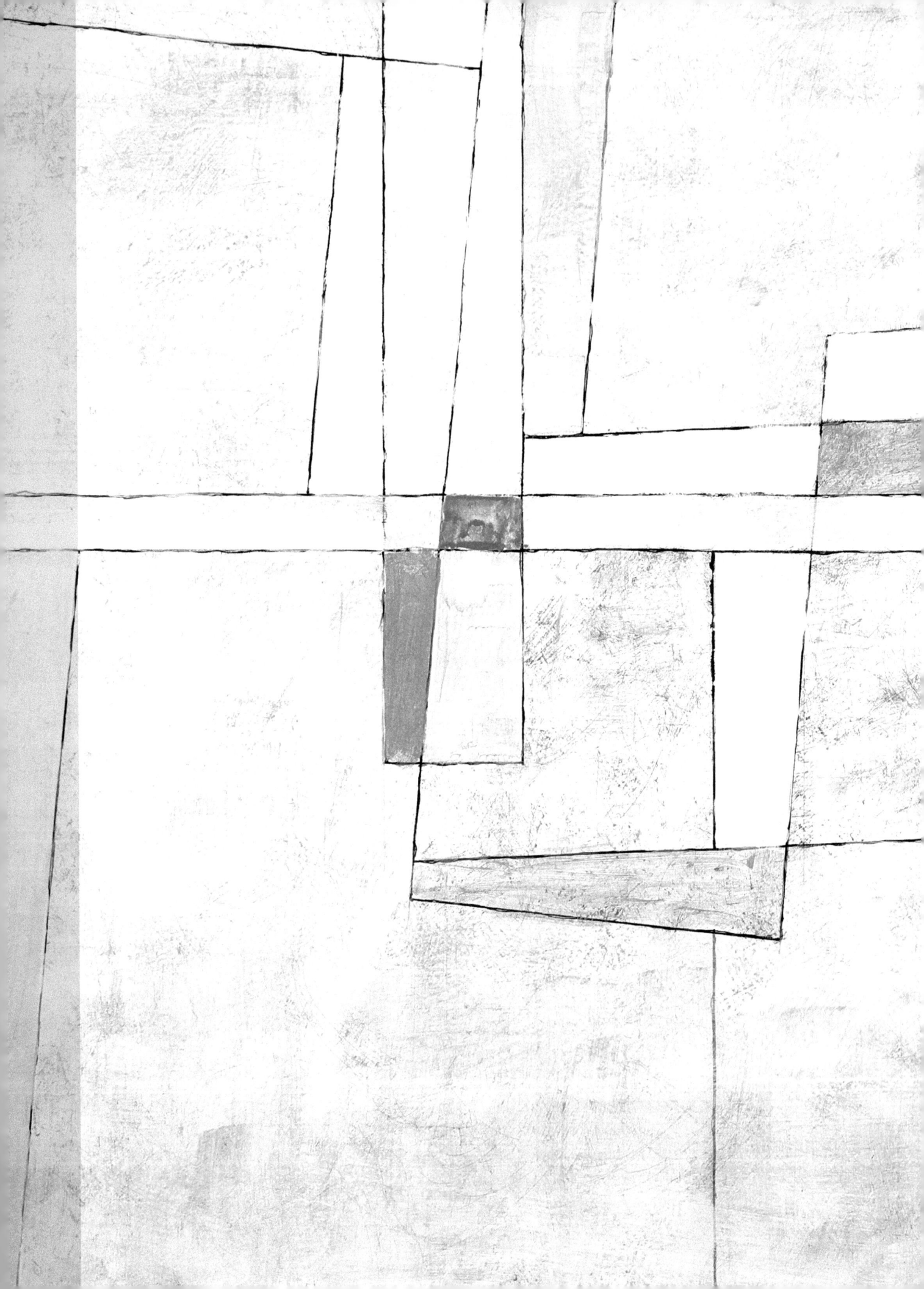

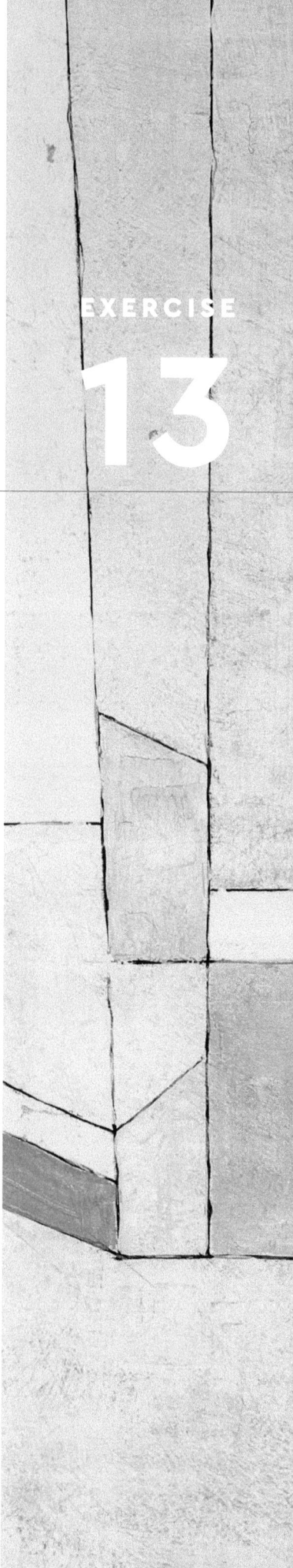

Annotated Emotionally Focused Couple Therapy Practice Session Transcript

It is now time to put all the skills you have learned together! This transcript is a hypothetical example of what a typical emotionally focused couple therapy (EFCT) session might look like, using the skills discussed across this book. Each therapist statement is annotated to indicate which EFCT skill from Exercises 1 through 12 is used. This transcript provides an example of how therapists can interweave many different EFCT skills in response to clients.

Instructions

In doing this exercise, one trainee can play the therapist while the other plays the client, displaying a tone and affect congruent with the material. Both participants can read line-by-line from the transcript. As with all deliberate practice exercises, try it again! The purpose of this transcript is to provide you with an opportunity to experience how it feels to offer all the EFCT skills we have discussed in the context of a session that mimics live therapy.

Note to Therapists

Remember to be aware of your vocal quality. Much of how EFCT works has to do with the way interventions are said, not simply the words used. Match your tone to the client's presentation. Thus, if the clients present in a soft, vulnerable manner, soften your tone to be soothing and calm. If, on the other hand, clients are aggressive and angry, match your tone to be firm and solid. Attunement to the client is paramount.

Annotated Emotionally Focused Couple Therapy Transcript

Note: Francisco and Monique came to therapy initially because they are planning on getting married and felt there were "a few places in our interactions that don't go well." The therapist has been seeing them for 2 months. They are in Stage 1 of EFCT.

https://doi.org/10.1037/0000436-015

Deliberate Practice in Emotionally Focused Couple Therapy, by H. Levenson, S. Jinich, A. Vaz, and T. Rousmaniere

The therapist is in Step 3 of the model where the focus is on using the EFT tango to access underlying vulnerable emotions and to choreograph an engaged encounter. Throughout, the therapist is using RISSSSC (R standing for repeat, I for images, S for simple, S for slow, S for soft, S for specific, and C for client's words), attuning the prosody of the partners' voices to deepen their affect. This case has been significantly altered to protect the confidentiality of the clients.

MONIQUE 1: Last night we had a conversation related to our wedding, and it was really hard. I didn't sleep all night.

THERAPIST 1: The wedding is coming up in [*pause*]?

MONIQUE 2: Six weeks. [*pause*] I don't know if you're interested in hearing about that?

THERAPIST 2: It makes sense to me especially if you had a hard time last night. Yeah, absolutely. (Skill 3: Validating Partners' Experiences and Tracking Dysfunctional Patterns)

MONIQUE 3: And it's directly related to what we have been talking about with you. Right before we went to bed, I told Francisco that even though you've been saying that it's really normal for us to be having a lot of fears coming up and that it might become more challenging around this time, that I have been feeling really super delighted and excited about our wedding. And I just wanted him to know that, so I said that to Francisco, and he said something like, "Oh" or "Yeah."

FRANCISCO 1: I think I said, "Thank you, babe."

MONIQUE 4: Oh, yeah, he said, "Thank you." And then, I didn't realize how vulnerable I would feel after that and I was like, I wish I hadn't said that because he didn't say, "Me too." And so I said, "Are you excited?" And he said, "Yeah. I'm excited." Everything about his tone and body language was like, "No, I'm not excited."

THERAPIST 3: So that is the message that you got—that Francisco was not excited? (Skill 8: Gathering and Assembling Elements of Emotion)

MONIQUE 5: Not at first, but then I was able to get out of him that he really hasn't been that excited about it.

THERAPIST 4: That's what you heard? (Skill 8: Gathering and Assembling Elements of Emotion)

MONIQUE 6: Yeah. And then he said, "I'm feeling really stressed and I feel like we're not spending a lot of time together, and it's been too stressful," and blah, blah, blah.

THERAPIST 5: OK. Let's start with that. Let's slow down a little bit. Maybe you can help me understand how that landed for you? When you first felt that sense of vulnerability of like, "Wow, I just showed him what I was feeling and then I didn't get back what I was hoping to hear." (Skill 1: Evocative Inquiry; Skill 8: Gathering and Assembling Elements of Emotion)

MONIQUE 7: It felt horrible.

THERAPIST 6: Tell me about that horrible feeling. (Skill 8: Gathering and Assembling Elements of Emotion)

MONIQUE 8: It just felt like, I don't know, it felt like the worst possible thing, in terms of what it leads me to think, which is that he's not going to be happy on the day of our wedding. And that feels really lonely and sad and scary.

THERAPIST 7: So, in that moment when you don't get the mirroring back of your own excitement, that moment, the way that you said it, what comes up for you is some loneliness and some fear and some sadness. (Skill 8: Gathering and Assembling Elements of Emotion) Maybe we can just explore those a little bit. Tell me about that sense of loneliness that you feel. (Skill 2: Evocative Reflection)

MONIQUE 9: It just feels like essentially—and I know there's part of this that Francisco's excited about. I mean I know it's not like he's dreading marrying me, but I know it's layered. It feels like I'll be standing up there alone—essentially, I'll know I am standing next to someone who doesn't want to be there.

THERAPIST 8: So the feeling of loneliness comes when you imagine that in the moment of being at the altar, at the wedding itself, that you'll be alone? (Skill 1: Evocative Inquiry; Skill 8: Gathering and Assembling Elements of Emotion)

MONIQUE 10: Yeah. And I've been feeling more and more excited as it leads up to it, and so I think it feels lonely now too.

THERAPIST 9: It feels lonely just as the wedding is approaching and just as you were really feeling more excited about it. Is that right? I can understand your lonely feeling. (Skill 3: Validating Partners' Experiences and Tracking Dysfunctional Patterns)

MONIQUE 11: Yeah.

THERAPIST 10: Since Francisco is so important to you, you would like him to share in that excitement with you. (Skill 2: Evocative Reflection; Skill 4: Attachment-Reframed Validation)

MONIQUE 12: Yeah.

THERAPIST 11: So when you get the sense that he's not as excited or isn't expressing his joy about it, then that's when you start to feel really lonely? (Skill 8: Gathering and Assembling Elements of Emotion) Help me understand what that's like inside, that feeling, what's that feeling? [*pause*] (Skill 1: Evocative Inquiry; Skill 5: Deepening Emotions With RISSSSC)

MONIQUE 13: I just right now feel heavy and tense in my heart and dark. [*places hand on chest*]

THERAPIST 12: Dark. It's dark and it's heavy, there's some tension in your chest? [*places hand on own chest*] (Skill 8: Gathering and Assembling Elements of Emotion; Skill 5: Deepening Emotions With RISSSSC)

MONIQUE 14: Yeah. I just felt anxious all night.

THERAPIST 13: Tell me about the feeling in your chest and that sense of anxiety (Skill 8: Gathering and Assembling Elements of Emotion) [*pause*] Is it like a fear? (Skill 1: Evocative Inquiry)

MONIQUE 15: I am anxious and scared. The pressure in my chest feels heavy and like [*pause*] what am I doing?

THERAPIST 14: Let's slow this down a bit. [*pause*] Francisco let you know that a part of him isn't excited, and then you started feeling pressure in your chest, yes? And an anxious feeling. [*pause*] What did you say to yourself in that moment? When you heard him express a lack of joy or excitement like you have been feeling, [*pause*] what's the meaning that it has for you? What are you saying on the inside? (Skill 8: Gathering and Assembling Elements of Emotion)

MONIQUE 16: That once again I'm the one driving everything in our relationship and that I am really alone and it's scary to be alone. I have felt alone a lot in my life, and it's so scary to think that here we are, weeks away from taking this huge step and it's supposed to be happy and exciting and the beginning of something beautiful, and I know we have had a lot of fights and all but we have worked so, so hard to get to this point. [*pause*] Can't we just finally both be on the same page for once?

THERAPIST 15: It makes so much sense to me that you felt afraid. It is scary to think that you're alone in this, given how important he is to you [*pause*] and that he is "agreeing to" take this step instead of thrilled and excited about taking this step with you, [*pause*] yes? (Skill 4: Attachment-Reframed Validation) Am I getting it, Monique? Last night you were feeling afraid and alone, [*pause*] alone in the excitement? (Skill 1: Evocative Inquiry) Like he won't share the experience with you. [*pause*] Like he won't be there, and he won't feel anything like what you are feeling, [*pause*] alone in your experience. [*pause*] Am I getting it? (Skill 2: Evocative Reflection; Skill 5: Deepening Emotions With RISSSSC)

MONIQUE 17: Right. And that's what we were talking about yesterday, that I don't feel like I'm necessarily going to be physically alone, but I will be emotionally, I guess.

THERAPIST 16: Emotionally alone. (Skill 5: Deepening Emotions With RISSSSC) And tell me, when you say to yourself that you'll end up emotionally alone and you feel this heavy pressure in your chest, and you say to yourself, "Once again I'm alone in driving things between us," [*pause*] what happens? What do you say or do in that moment? (Skill 8: Gathering and Assembling Elements of Emotion)

MONIQUE 18: I have a really hard time with it. I get stuck in the thought pattern, and that's what was going on last night. It just feels miserable. I felt angry and I just went to our bedroom and, well, I just have a hard time. [*pause*]

THERAPIST 17: A hard time?

MONIQUE 19: Thinking about something else or seeing an alternative or reassuring myself.

THERAPIST 18: Because in that moment all that is really present, really up and running for you, is just how scary that would be and how alone it would feel? (Skill 2: Evocative Reflection)

MONIQUE 20: Yeah.

THERAPIST 19: That makes a lot of sense to me, especially given how challenging it has been to finally arrive at this special moment in your life and how much you want to be with Francisco. It is especially hard to imagine feeling emotionally alone on that day from the person you love the most. (Skill 4: Attachment-Reframed Validation) Do you, in those moments, especially in such difficult moments, do you ever turn to him and let him in a little bit about how scary it feels when you imagine being alone in that situation, [*pause*] how alone it feels, even just coming up to the day of the wedding [*pause*] all the while as you experience your own excitement, not feeling him with you, how scary and lonely that feels for you? Do you turn to him and tell him that? (Skill 9: Enactments)

MONIQUE 21: No, I didn't. I mean, we're going to sleep. It's like I'm already feeling in pain and vulnerable and that feels like more [*pause*] making myself more vulnerable.

THERAPIST 20: More vulnerable. Right. I get it. (Skill 3: Validating Partners' Experiences and Tracking Dysfunctional Patterns) You know, I see Francisco looking at you very intently right now, and I'm wondering whether you could look in his eyes for a moment and maybe tell him about that fear of ending up alone. (Skill 9: Enactments) I know you fear you will make yourself *more* vulnerable, but could you try to tell him about how lonely it feels for you? (Skill 3: Validating Partners' Experiences and Tracking Dysfunctional Patterns)

MONIQUE 22: [*turning toward Francisco*] It feels really scary to think about us doing this together and you being there physically but not being there emotionally and not feeling excited and happy, and that to me feels just as lonely as being physically alone.

THERAPIST 21: What's it like right now for you Monique to say that to him, that you feel scared to be taking such an important step together and yet feeling emotionally alone, as if you were physically alone? How is it to share this with him in this way? (Skill 1: Evocative Inquiry)

MONIQUE 23: It's OK. It feels true.

THERAPIST 22: It feels OK to say? It's what you truly feel?

MONIQUE 24: Yeah.

THERAPIST 23: And how about for you, Francisco? What's it like right now to hear her just really open her heart like that and share that with you? (Skill 5: Deepening Emotions With RISSSSC)

FRANCISCO 2: It's the biggest part of my experience right now too—this fear that we're each going to be emotionally alone. It's a very familiar feeling.

THERAPIST 24: It's familiar for you too?

FRANCISCO 3: Yes.

THERAPIST 25: So you can hear this from her, this fear and this loneliness, and it also taps into some of your own experience? In a moment we can explore how that is for you as well, but just now, [*pause*] how is it inside of you, for her to open up to you in this way? (Skill 1: Evocative Inquiry)

FRANCISCO 4: [*reaching over and holding his partner's hand*] Yeah. I feel badly about it. I don't want her to feel that. It's something we both share.

THERAPIST 26: So when you hear her tell you this, you can let that in?

FRANCISCO 5: Yeah. I can let it in. It doesn't change the fear that I see. I absolutely see her fear.

THERAPIST 27: I'm just very impressed already with your ability to turn to each other and share something so deep and so vulnerable, really. It's very courageous, especially when you said, Monique, it's hard to be more vulnerable when you already feel so vulnerable and so nervous about exposing the vulnerability. But you just did that, it shows a lot of strength and courage on your part, and for you, Francisco, I saw as you reached over and held her hand as she was sharing this. (Skill 3: Validating Partners' Experiences and Tracking Dysfunctional Patterns)

FRANCISCO 6: Well, we love each other a lot.

THERAPIST 28: Yeah. And I can see that. I can see how in those moments of vulnerability when you share your vulnerability, you actually get closer. (Skill 3: Validating Partners' Experiences and Tracking Dysfunctional Patterns)

MONIQUE 25: It's hard translating that to home, because we think we're doing it, but it doesn't go in the same direction.

THERAPIST 29: Is that right?

MONIQUE 26: Or I think I'm doing it. I think Francisco thinks he is, sometimes.

THERAPIST 30: So that's maybe when it's hard to do because maybe you get caught up in your negative cycle and then in those moments when you're going into a—I don't know [*pause*] like a tailspin, it's hard to grab onto something to steady yourself so that you can turn to each other and share the vulnerability. Especially when you're so scared. This is really scary and of course it makes so much sense to me that it would be hard to want to talk about it. (Skill 2: Evocative Reflection; Skill 4: Attachment-Reframed Validation)

MONIQUE 27: Yeah. I think part of me doesn't want to know more. I'm scared of hearing more about how [*pause*]

THERAPIST 31: Right. Especially if you're already not sensing, he's not reflecting back what you're feeling and so you're like, "I should take care of myself. I should protect myself. [*therapist softens voice and slows down*] It's too scary. [*pause*] I'll hear something I don't want to hear [*pause*] and it'll only hurt me further." (Skill 5: Deepening Emotions With RISSSSC). Can you tell me about that? [*Monique is nodding*] What's the scary thing you fear you might hear? What's scary? (Skill 1: Evocative Inquiry)

MONIQUE 28: [*voice quivering*] Just more about him telling me how unhappy he is, as if this whole thing has been my sole production. [*pause*] Like I forced this on him. [*pause*] Maybe he regrets that we're getting married and all the time my wishing it was different.

THERAPIST 32: So you take it to a place where you feel like, more than the timing of it, that maybe it's more about how he feels toward you? Does it go to a place like that? (Skill 1: Evocative Inquiry)

MONIQUE 29: Probably. So when we first got engaged, he wanted to wait to get married much farther out obviously than I did, and my immediate feeling was like, he must not actually want to marry me. He's not sure he wants to be with me.

THERAPIST 33: [*slowly, softly*] What was [*pause*] the feeling associated with that? (Skill 1: Evocative Inquiry; Skill 5: Deepening Emotions With RISSSSC; Skill 8: Gathering and Assembling Elements of Emotion)

MONIQUE 30: A dread sort of a feeling.

THERAPIST 34: [*slowly, simply*] Dread. [*pause*] Yeah. Absolutely. [*pause*] (Skill 3: Validating Partners' Experiences and Tracking Dysfunctional Patterns) The dread is, "He doesn't love me? [*pause*] He doesn't want to be with me? [*pause*] He probably doesn't want to marry me," right? (Skill 2: Evocative Reflection; Skill 5: Deepening Emotions With RISSSSC)

MONIQUE 31: [*tearful*] Right. It's not safe to feel joyful about being engaged.

THERAPIST 35: I see tears welling up. (Skill 2: Evocative Reflection)

MONIQUE 32: Yeah.

THERAPIST 36: Yeah. [*pause*] Tell me about this. Tell me about these tears, this dread. (Skill 1: Evocative Inquiry)

MONIQUE 33: I think my whole life there's been a need for me not to relax or not let myself feel comfortable or happy. I have always needed to be on the lookout for something bad happening. I think of myself as jumpy, you know, [*pause*] like hypervigilant. Growing up everything was always ruined in some way. My mother's alcoholism, and my father's disappearing when I was a baby. It was impossible to be happy as a kid. I felt like I was too much for my father, so he left. And I spent most of my time watching out for my mother, so she didn't die choking on her own vomit. It was always that way. I never felt that I was entitled to want something, you know? I could never count on things just being nice because nothing ever lasted. Something good would inevitably get ruined. I could never count on anything good just staying that way. I always have had to justify or fight for everything that I want, and it always feels like I want everything just a little more than others, especially because to me, good things don't last, it's hard to hold on to it [*pause, and more tears*] and so that makes me the needy one or the difficult one.

THERAPIST 37: So you're on edge, on the lookout for a sign that someone will withdraw their love, [*pause*] that good things won't last [*pause*]—that Francisco will pull away, back away, and withdraw his love [*pause*] because you fear you are too needy. (Skill 2: Evocative Reflection; Skill 5: Deepening Emotions With RISSSSC) Sounds like this was something you dealt with a lot in childhood. (Skill 1: Evocative Inquiry)

MONIQUE 34: Yeah.

THERAPIST 38: So you got really good at looking out for the signs of people pulling back, I bet. That must have been so painful. [*pause*] I can see you are emotionally moved, Monique. [*pause*] You so need to be enough just as you are [*pause*] and to have your needs be OK, especially by those who you love and who love you. Am I getting it? (Skill 4: Attachment-Reframed Validation; Skill 5: Deepening Emotions With RISSSSC)

MONIQUE 35: It is painful. [*Monique pauses and begins to sob. The therapist pauses 20 seconds, leans forward, and hands her a tissue. The therapist was aware at this moment of feeling so much sadness for this person, who has longed for love throughout her life.*] (Skill 6: Tracking the Therapist's Inner Experience)

THERAPIST 39: [*very softly and soothingly*] How was it then, [*pause*] when that love would disappear? What happened for you [*pause*] when all of a sudden [*pause*] you would feel like someone was either unkind [*pause*] or unavailable, [*pause*] like they were withdrawing their love from you? [*pause*] Or that what you wanted [*pause*] was too much [*pause*] just because you wanted it. (Skill 5: Deepening Emotions With RISSSSC) What would that be like then? (Skill 1: Evocative Inquiry)

MONIQUE 36: It feels cruel. What I feel is like the ground is opening up, and not only is the ground opening up, but Francisco or whoever, my mom for example, is well aware that the ground is opening up underneath me, and then Francisco just turns around and walks away, like not helping. Like I don't matter. I have told him how scary this is for me. [*continues to cry*]

THERAPIST 40: Oh, Monique [*pause*] what a painful image you are sharing with me. [*pause*] Stepping away from you [*pause*] when you most need him to step forward, [*pause*] he steps back. [*pause*] The ground is opening up, and you can fall into it. You need him to reach for you so you won't fall, and he walks [*pause*] away. (Skill 2: Evocative Reflection; Skill 4: Attachment-Reframed Validation; Skill 5: Deepening Emotions With RISSSSC)

MONIQUE 37: It's really horribly scary.

THERAPIST 41: [*softly*] That seems terrifying to me, in a moment of such fear and such loneliness to look to him, and turn to him and to not see him there for you. (Skill 4: Attachment-Reframed Validation) And something else that you just said, which strikes me as really important, you said, "And he knows [*pause*], he knows that the ground opens up under my feet [*pause*]. I've told him. [*pause*] It's even more important for me [*pause*] if he really knows that it's happening to me, [*pause*] that he not step away," right? (Skill 5: Deepening Emotions With RISSSSC)

MONIQUE 38: Yeah. The feeling that I've had my whole life is like this deep anger, it's like a trap, like the strongest anger at the person that I desperately need to be close. I'm like, I hate you and I love you at the same time. You're making my life miserable, but I need you.

THERAPIST 42: That makes so much sense to me, because what I'm hearing from you, it's like you're saying, "Where are you? Where are you? Where are you? You're the person who I love the most. You're the person who's supposed to love me the most. Why won't you come to me and be there for me, catch me before I fall in. You're supposed to do that," and he doesn't. Francisco doesn't turn to you when you most need him; [*pause*] you experience him move away. He doesn't respond in that moment, so of course you get angry. It's that double feeling of hating and loving, like you talked about. Right? (Skill 4: Attachment-Reframed Validation; Skill 8: Gathering and Assembling Elements of Emotion)

MONIQUE 39: Mmm-hmm. [*nods, looks down at her feet*]

THERAPIST 43: Like so angry, because you feel he should be so aware of what is happening to you in the moment and he's not reaching for you [*pause*] as if you don't matter. [*pause*] I think I am really understanding the feeling of fear, loneliness, and anger that you were telling me about earlier. What's that like when you hear me say that? (Skill 2: Evocative Reflection; Skill 1: Evocative Inquiry)

MONIQUE 40: That resonates. It sounds [*pause*]

THERAPIST 44: It sounds right?

MONIQUE 41: Yeah. I'm nervous that Francisco is going to think that all my anger is toward him.

THERAPIST 45: You're worried right now . . . [*pause*]

MONIQUE 42: Yeah.

THERAPIST 46: [*pause*] . . . about how he's hearing this? (Skill 8: Gathering and Assembling Elements of Emotion)

MONIQUE 43: Yeah.

THERAPIST 47: And that he will hear this how? (Skill 8: Gathering and Assembling Elements of Emotion)

MONIQUE 44: That I really, truly think he's causing all of my hurt and that he's doing a bad job by not helping.

THERAPIST 48: I see.

MONIQUE 45: I don't want him to think that. I don't want to hurt him.

THERAPIST 49: You don't want him to think that or to feel hurt by you saying this. (Skill 2: Evocative Reflection)

MONIQUE 46: Right.

THERAPIST 50: So, it seems to me like now you have another fear, right? This is what happens to all of us, OK? We have so many layers to our emotions, so many, and it's complicated. And you're doing an amazing job of exploring all the different layers inside of you. (Skill 2: Evocative Reflection) At the same time, you want to open up and you want to explore your heart and your hurt, and at the same time you care about how he hears this and you don't want him to hear that it's all because of him. Because you have a history of needing a father and a mother, and having to deal with not getting their attention and love. These are experiences that you grew up with, right? (Skill 2: Evocative Reflection; Skill 3: Validating Partners' Experiences and Tracking Dysfunctional Patterns)

MONIQUE 47: [*gently nodding head*] Yeah.

THERAPIST 51: Yeah. So tell me about that fear that you're going to hurt Francisco. Tell me about that fear that he's going to get hurt. He's going to hear it like you are blaming him and it's all his fault. (Skill 1: Evocative Inquiry)

MONIQUE 48: Well, I think that's part of what keeps me from talking to him about stuff. [*tears well up again*]

THERAPIST 52: I see. Tell me about these tears that I'm seeing right now.

MONIQUE 49: I don't know.

THERAPIST 53: What happens inside when you think he's going to get hurt by what you say? Take your time. (Skill 8: Gathering and Assembling Elements of Emotion)

MONIQUE 50: I just think . . . I don't know. It feels sad.

THERAPIST 54: You feel sad? It is sad. (Skill 3: Validating Partners' Experiences and Tracking Dysfunctional Patterns)

MONIQUE 51: It's like we're in this weird bind.

THERAPIST 55: Tell me what you mean by that?

MONIQUE 52: Well, I want to be able to express my fears and stuff.

THERAPIST 56: So that he can be there for you. (Skill 4: Attachment-Reframed Validation)

MONIQUE 53: Yeah.

THERAPIST 57: And what's the dilemma here? The other side of it is that if you do, what could happen? (Skill 8: Gathering and Assembling Elements of Emotion)

MONIQUE 54: I think it's really hard for Francisco and for me when either one of us does that. We feel like we're being blamed, or like we're failing and in my case, like I am ruining things by voicing my needs or my excitement, or my need for his excitement.

THERAPIST 58: So there's two parts here. There's a part of you that really wants him to see that "the ground is opening up [*pause*] underneath my feet, [*pause*] stay with me, [*pause*] be with me," right? And there's another part of you that says, [*pause*] "I can't tell him, [*pause*] because if I tell him, [*pause*] he'll feel bad. He'll feel blamed or hurt. He'll move away from me [*pause*] I will be left and I will fall" And then? (Skill 5: Deepening Emotions With RISSSSC, Skill 3: Validating Partners' Experiences and Tracking Dysfunctional Patterns)

MONIQUE 55: And I'll feel worse.

THERAPIST 59: "I'll feel worse and then maybe he'll even move further away." (Skill 2: Evocative Reflection) Is that what happens?

MONIQUE 56: Yeah.

THERAPIST 60: So then you get your confirmation, right, that he'll be upset, "I'll feel worse. If I share with him my sadness or my fears or my anger [*pause*] and he goes away, [*pause*] now I really don't have him. I shouldn't have said anything. I should have kept it to myself." [*pause*] What do you say to yourself in those moments? (Skill 8: Gathering and Assembling Elements of Emotion)

MONIQUE 57: What do I say to myself?

THERAPIST 61: Yeah. What do you do with that?

MONIQUE 58: Oh, I say to myself, "Why do you always mess it up? Why do you want too much?" I tell myself, "Never say this again."

THERAPIST 62: "I should just keep it to myself." You know, that makes a lot of sense to me, Monique—especially because he's your person, right? He's who is supposed to catch you especially when you're hurting, and you risk letting him in and letting him know what you are really feeling deep down [*pause*] when you are scared or lonely. It's Francisco that you most want to turn to and it's him you most need in those moments, [*pause*] so it's especially risky to trust, and then [*pause*] you're reminded [*pause*] he won't be there. He'll move away [*pause*] "I'm messing it up again." And you know what I'm hearing then is "I should just accept my fate of being alone. I should just get better at just accepting that, because if I say something, it's worse. So I should just keep it to myself. Keep it on the inside. And if the ground opens and I fall into this scary lonely place, well, so be it." [*pause*] Am I getting you? (Skill 4: Attachment-Reframed Validation; Skill 8: Gathering and Assembling Elements of Emotion)

MONIQUE 59: [*crying*] Yes [*pause*] that's it.

THERAPIST 63: Yeah. I hear you. And you're in a dilemma. "I want to be able to reach out to him. [*pause*] He is whom I need right now [*pause*] but if I were to really tell him how I feel, he won't like it, he won't like it." Yes? He won't want to hear this, is that right? (Skill 2: Evocative Reflection)

MONIQUE 60: It'll just scare him and piss him off. Yeah. I think he won't want to hear it.

THERAPIST 64: Do you ever tell him about this fear? This fear that "If I tell you when I need you, and if I tell you what I fear, if I tell you how scary it is for me when I imagine the ground opening up, and if I really take that risk and show you my biggest vulnerabilities, my deepest vulnerability, you won't like it and you'll step away from me and leave me there [*pause*] and I'll end up feeling even more alone." Do you ever say that? (Skill 9: Enactments)

MONIQUE 61: Not that way.

THERAPIST 65: That would be hard to do?

MONIQUE 62: He won't like it. He'll just think of me as too needy and weak.

THERAPIST 66: So you don't risk it. It would be too hard, [*pause*] too painful and risky to show him this part? I see him looking at you intently [*pause*]; he seems to be really present right now. [*turning to Francisco*] Francisco, are you here? Would you be able to hear her talk to you about this fear of turning to you when she feels scared or lonely and how afraid she gets when she imagines that you won't care? That you'll just walk away? (Skill 9: Enactments)

FRANCISCO 7: I want to hear it. I really want to hear *all* of it. [*turning to Monique*] It's OK to tell me. Really.

THERAPIST 67: Monique, here's an opportunity because he's right here with you. He's paying a lot of attention, and I'm wondering whether you could look at him, look at his eyes, and share a little bit of that fear with him? Tell him how scary it feels at times to open up to him [*pause*] to really let him in [*pause*], scared that he will freeze up or step away [*pause*], not catch you. [*pause*] Tell him. (Skill 9: Enactments)

MONIQUE 63: I don't think I want to risk doing this right now. It seems too hard to open up like that. And besides he heard it. Why do I need to say it again?

THERAPIST 68: I know it's hard and that Francisco has been listening intently to our conversation. In the kind of therapy that we are doing, it makes a big difference to say something directly to one's partner. It somehow goes in, in a deeper kind of way because when you say it, it is a vulnerable communication that has a greater chance to speak to Francisco's heart. (Skill 7: Providing a Rationale for EFCT) [*pause*] So can you tell me [*pause*]—help me understand the hard part about telling him how scary it feels to open up to him and the fear that he won't be there? (Skill 10: Slicing the Risk Thinner)

MONIQUE 64: I'm feeling it now. [*pause*] I don't think he'll know what to say or what I need. I don't like this needy part about myself, and I know he doesn't like this about me either.

THERAPIST 69: It's scary to take this risk right now? I understand; he is so important to you. (Skill 4: Attachment-Reframed Validation)

MONIQUE 65: [*nods and looks down at her feet*]

THERAPIST 70: I'd like to ask you to just say that part. Just tell him about how scary it is to talk about this because you don't like this part of you, and you don't think he'll like hearing this part either. Can you tell him just the part about this, that is so scary to talk about? (Skill 10: Slicing the Risk Thinner; Skill 9: Enactments)

MONIQUE 66: Well, [*pauses, takes a deep breath; pauses again, then turns to Francisco*] it's really scary to talk to you about this—I feel scared talking about what I'm afraid of because it feels like . . . [*turning to therapist*] I [*pauses*] don't know if this is what you want me to get at. [*therapist nods, and Monique turns back to Francisco*] I'm afraid you'll feel pressured or blamed and that you'll get cloudy and won't know how to help me. I'm scared just talking to you about this. I fear it is going to push you away and make us further apart, and so it just feels like a scary trap and where I'll end up feeling even more alone.

FRANCISCO 8: I think we've gotten closer when we're talking about that stuff, usually.

THERAPIST 71: [*to Francisco*] Hang on for a little longer Francisco [*pause*] I promise I will turn to you in a moment. [*pauses, turns to Monique*] So right now Monique, as you say that to him, as you tell him, "I fear if I really tell you how I am feeling, it is going to push you away and make us further apart, and so it just feels like a scary trap," [*pause*] what was it like to look at him and to share that fear? (Skill 1: Evocative Inquiry)

MONIQUE 67: Before he talked, it was good.

FRANCISCO 9: [*throws his hands in the air, exasperated*] What did I say that was bad? You always do this Monique! [*pause*] You're impossible.

THERAPIST 72: [*to Francisco*] Woah! [*pause*] Let's slow down here! [*pause*] Something just happened. Francisco, you're upset because Monique said all was well until you spoke up. [*pause*] Is that it? (Skill 11: Catching a Bullet Early in Therapy)

FRANCISCO 10: All I said was something positive. But it's never good enough for her.

THERAPIST 73: I get that. It makes sense to me that that would upset you. (Skill 3: Validating Partners' Experiences and Tracking Dysfunctional Patterns) It was something positive, [*pauses; softens voice and slows down, then pauses again*] but when you say things like "you're impossible," it sounds like it could easily provoke Monique into a strong reaction, or even confirm her fears that if she opens up, you'll get upset, and then the two of you are back in your negative cycle and that prevents us from doing any meaningful work in here, right? (Skill 11: Catching a Bullet Early in Therapy)

MONIQUE 68: [*to Francisco*] It's OK, don't worry about it. I was feeling sensitive, [*pause*] and you're right, you didn't do anything wrong. I'm sorry I said what I said.

FRANCISCO 11: [*to Monique*] I'm sorry too. [*pause*] Please I really want to hear what you have to say, Monique. Please go on.

THERAPIST 74: [*to Monique*] Can we go back to where we were? You were taking a big risk there and sharing something really important, and although it was scary to say your fears, you did it. Did that feel OK in that moment? (Skill 1: Evocative Inquiry)

MONIQUE 69: That felt OK. And actually, [*pause*] his eyes and face looked very warm and sweet and caring. [*to Francisco*] I'm sorry I triggered you, babe. [*pause*]

THERAPIST 75: Yeah. I saw that too, [*pause*] like he was letting it in. (Skill 3: Validating Partners' Experiences and Tracking Dysfunctional Patterns) And you so very much need for him to let it in, right? I get that. (Skill 4: Attachment-Reframed Validation)

MONIQUE 70: Yeah. I don't know why when he spoke, it pulled me out of what I was feeling, scared to hear it, maybe I was anticipating him pulling away or something but . . . [*to Francisco*] really, babe, it felt good to be able to say it and to have you hang in there with me.

THERAPIST 76: Over time we will explore your past experiences with this, OK? You did a lovely job of opening up to him in a very vulnerable way, [*pause*] and I am wondering, Francisco, with just the words that she shared and the way that she looked to you and shared her vulnerability, how she opened it up for you to look inside, what was that like for you in that moment? (Exercise 1: Evocative Inquiry)

FRANCISCO 12: My experience is that when we really can have those heartfelt discussions of what goes on for her inside, it isn't traumatic, or scary, or painful, or something I don't want to hear.

THERAPIST 77: That, in fact, it feels OK?

FRANCISCO 13: Uh huh. Yes.

THERAPIST 78: It feels better?

FRANCISCO 14: Yeah. Sometimes a little bit hard, but that's . . .

THERAPIST 79: Of course it is hard. She is so important to you. (Skill 4: Attachment-Reframed Validation)

FRANCISCO 15: The reason we're together is because when we get down underneath it, the soul connection is really good.

THERAPIST 80: Did you just say the soil or the soul?

FRANCISCO 16: I could have said soil. I meant soul, though.

THERAPIST 81: You said soul, and I heard soil. Like fertile soil. That's good. Maybe it means the same thing. (Skill 2: Evocative Reflection)

FRANCISCO 17: Yeah.

THERAPIST 82: Yeah. There's a lot of growth that can come out of that. (Skill 2: Evocative Reflection)

FRANCISCO 18: A lot of growth, and we share a lot of very similar pain. And when she shares her pain, I don't feel cloudy or helpless. That's when I feel like I know what to do because that's what I am here for. When she shares like this, it all feels much easier.

THERAPIST 83: That's amazing. [*pause*] So when she can open up to you in a vulnerable way like this, it doesn't make you feel like pulling away? You want to step toward her? (Skill 1: Evocative Inquiry; Skill 8: Gathering and Assembling Elements of Emotion)

FRANCISCO 19: That's when I feel like I have tools I know how to use. When she's angry and hostile or confusing, then everything gets cloudy for me. It's so ironic because we have very similar pains.

THERAPIST 84: Is that right?

FRANCISCO 20: Yeah.

THERAPIST 85: We'll make sure to explore that next time, [*pause*] but before we end, I just want to tell you that it impresses me, Monique, how you can really connect to that deeper part of you and share that with Francisco. (Skill 6: Tracking the Therapist's Inner Experience) It takes courage. It takes really having a real sense of yourself, and I'm just very impressed by it. And I can really understand what you said, Francisco, which is that when Monique comes toward you in that vulnerable way, you actually find that it is easier to step forward, to move toward her instead of away and it helps to make a deeper connection with her. The soul connection is good, right? It's fertile and produces more growth. (Skill 4: Attachment-Reframed Validation; Skill 2: Evocative Reflection)

FRANCISCO 21: Yeah.

THERAPIST 86: Right. I totally get that from your eyes and the gentle steadiness of your voice. (Skill 3: Validating Partners' Experiences and Tracking Dysfunctional Patterns)

FRANCISCO 22: Yeah. Thank you.

THERAPIST 87: You both did lovely, courageous work today. I look forward to our next session.

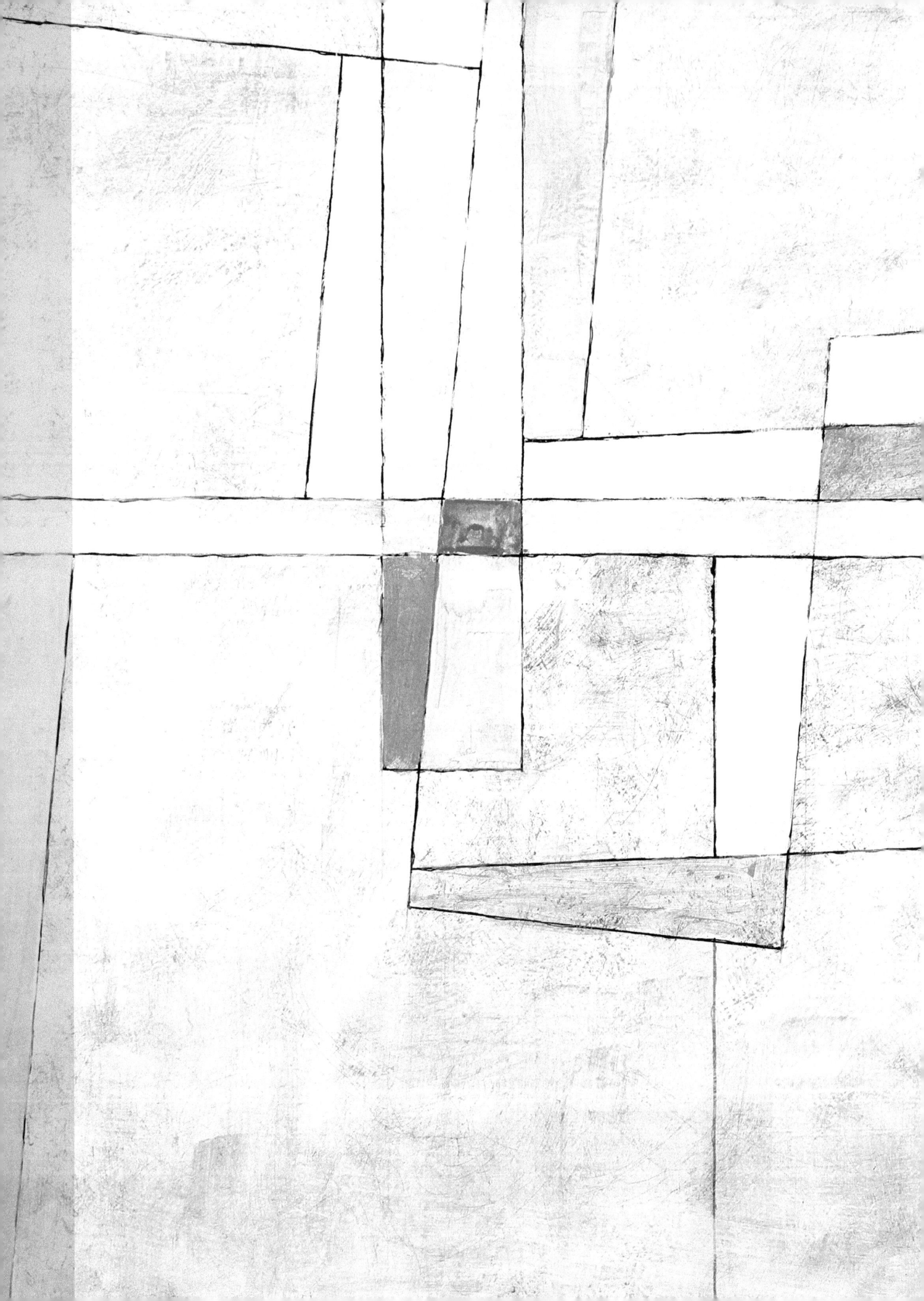

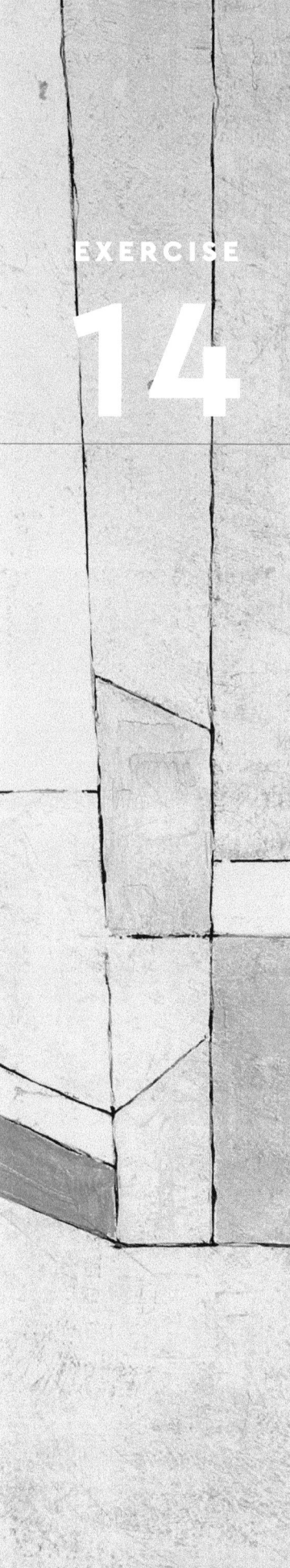

Mock Emotionally Focused Couple Therapy Sessions

In contrast to highly structured and repetitive deliberate practice exercises, a mock emotionally focused couple therapy (EFCT) session is an unstructured and improvised role-play therapy session. Like a jazz rehearsal, mock sessions let you practice the art and science of *appropriate responsiveness* (Hatcher, 2015; Stiles & Horvath, 2017), putting your psychotherapy skills together in a way that is helpful to your mock clients. This exercise outlines the procedure for conducting a mock EFCT session. It offers different couple profiles that you may choose to adopt when role-playing clients.

Mock sessions are an opportunity for trainees to practice the following:

- using psychotherapy skills responsively
- navigating challenging choice-points in therapy
- choosing which interventions to use
- tracking the arc of a therapy session and the overall big-picture therapy treatment
- guiding treatment in the context of the partners' preferences
- determining realistic goals for therapy in the context of the partners' capacities
- knowing how to proceed when the therapist is unsure, lost, or confused
- recognizing and recovering from therapeutic errors
- discovering your personal therapeutic style
- building endurance for working with real clients in couple therapy

Mock EFCT Session Overview

For the mock session, **you will perform a role-play of an initial therapy session**. The role-play involves four people: One trainee role-plays the therapist, two other trainees role-play the partners in the couple, and a trainer (a professor or a supervisor) observes and provides feedback. This is an open-ended role-play, as is commonly done in training. However, this differs in two important ways from the role-plays used in more traditional

https://doi.org/10.1037/0000436-016

Deliberate Practice in Emotionally Focused Couple Therapy, by H. Levenson, S. Jinich, A. Vaz, and T. Rousmaniere

training. First, the therapist will use their hand to indicate how difficult the role-play feels. Second, based on this feedback, the partners will attempt to make the role-play easier or harder to ensure the therapist is practicing at the right difficulty level.

Preparation

1. Download the Deliberate Practice Reaction Form and the Deliberate Practice Diary Form from the "Resources" tab at https://www.apa.org/pubs/books/deliberate-practice-emotionally-focused-couple-therapy (also available in Appendixes A and B, respectively). Every student will need their own copy of the Deliberate Practice Reaction Form on a separate piece of paper so they can access it quickly.

2. Designate one student to role-play the therapist and two students to role-play the partners. The trainer will observe and provide corrective feedback.

Mock EFCT Session Procedure

1. The trainees will role-play an initial (first) therapy session. The trainees role-playing the clients select a profile from the end of this exercise.

2. Before beginning the role-play, the therapist raises their hand to their side, at the level of their chair seat (see Figure E14.1). They will use this hand throughout the whole role-play to indicate how challenging it feels to them to help the client. Their starting hand level (chair seat) indicates that the role-play feels easy. By raising their hand, the

FIGURE E14.1. Ongoing Difficulty Assessment Through Hand Level

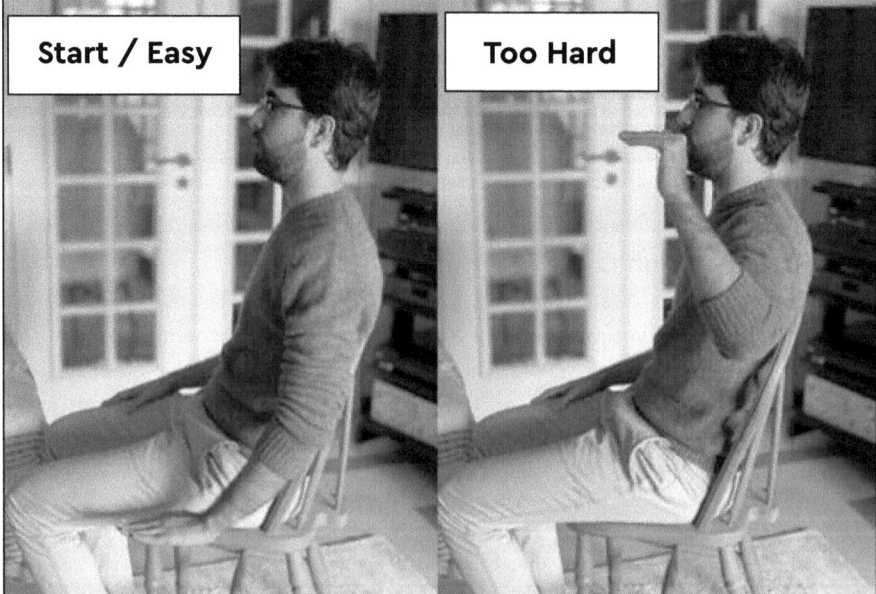

Note. Left: Start of role-play. Right: Role-play is too difficult. From *Deliberate Practice in Emotion-Focused Therapy* (p. 156), by R. N. Goldman, A. Vaz, and T. Rousmaniere, 2021, American Psychological Association (https://doi.org/10.1037/0000227-000). Copyright 2021 by the American Psychological Association.

therapist indicates that the difficulty is rising. If their hand rises above their neck level, it indicates that the role-play is too difficult.

3. The therapist begins the role-play. The therapist and couple should engage in the role-play in an improvised manner, as they would engage in a real therapy session. The therapist keeps their hand out at their side throughout this process. (This may feel strange at first!)

4. Whenever the therapist feels that the difficulty of the role-play has changed significantly, they should move their hand up if it feels more difficult, down if it feels easier. If the therapist's hand drops below the seat of their chair, the clients should make the role-play more challenging; if the therapist's hand rises above their neck level, the clients should make the role-play easier. Instructions for adjusting the difficulty of the role-play are described in the Varying the Level of Challenge section.

Note to Therapists

Remember to be aware of your vocal quality. Match your tone to the clients' presentation. Thus, if the clients present vulnerable, soft emotions behind their words, soften your tone to be soothing and calm. If clients, on the other hand, are aggressive and angry, match your tone to be firm and solid (but never angry). If you choose interventions that are prompting of client exploration, such as evocative reflections, remember to adopt a more querying, exploratory tone of voice.

5. The role-play continues for at least 15 minutes. The trainer may provide corrective feedback during this process if the therapist gets significantly off track. However, trainers should exercise restraint and keep feedback as short and tight as possible, so as not to reduce the therapist's opportunity for experiential training.

6. After the role-play is finished, the therapist and one of the clients can switch roles and begin a new mock session.

7. After the three trainees have completed the mock session as a therapist, the trainees and the trainer discuss the experience.

Varying the Level of Challenge

If the therapist indicates that the mock session is too easy, the trainees enacting the roles of the partners can use the following modifications to make it more challenging (see also Appendix A):

- The clients can improvise with topics that are more evocative or make the therapist uncomfortable, such as expressing currently held strong feelings (see Figure A.2).
- The clients can use a distressed voice (e.g., angry, sad, sarcastic) or unpleasant facial expression. This increases the emotional tone.
- The clients can blend complex mixtures of opposing feelings (e.g., love and rage).
- The clients can become confrontational, questioning the purpose of therapy or the therapist's fitness for the role.

If the therapist indicates that the mock session is too hard:

- The clients can be guided by Figure A.2 to
  - present topics that are less evocative,
  - present material on any topic but without expressing feelings, or
  - present material concerning the future or the past or events outside therapy.

- The clients can ask the questions in a soft voice or with a smile. This softens the emotional stimulus.

- The therapist can take short breaks during the role-play.

- The trainer can expand the "feedback phase" by discussing EFCT or psychotherapy theory.

Mock Session Couple Profiles

Following are six couple profiles for trainees to use during mock sessions, presented in order of difficulty. The choice of couple profile may be determined by the trainees playing the therapist or couple or assigned by the trainer.

The most important aspect of role-plays is for trainees to convey the emotional tone indicated by the couple's profile (e.g., "angry" or "sad"). The demographics of the clients (e.g., age, gender) and specific content of the couple profiles are not important. Thus, trainees should adjust the couple profile to be most comfortable and easy for the trainee to role-play. For example, a trainee may change a client from female to male, from 45 to 22 years old, and so on.

Beginner Profile: Transition to Parenthood

Lara, a 28-year-old, college-educated Jamaican woman who immigrated to the United States at age 12, and her partner Jorge, a 32 year-old physician born in the United States and raised by undocumented, Mexican farmworkers, are seeking EFCT. They have one child, an 8-month-old daughter, Terri. The couple reports that as soon as Terri was born, the couple began to quarrel "like never before." Before her birth, they described their relationship as "best friends" and had a very active sex life. In the past several months, Lara has been feeling increasingly lonely and angry at Jorge for being distant with her. She wishes he would show more interest in how she is doing and be more involved with their child. In the evenings Jorge goes to his study to catch up on paperwork or falls asleep on the couch, leaving her feeling frustrated and hopeless. When she tries to talk about it, he becomes defensive and shuts down.

- **Symptoms:** This couple is experiencing maladaptive adjustment after birth of child. Lara is increasingly feeling depressed and lonely since Terri's birth. Jorge feels frustrated and unappreciated. The more Lara tries to get Jorge's attention or complains about his distancing, the more Jorge becomes defensive and withdraws. The more he feels criticized and withdraws, the lonelier she feels.

- **Clients' goals for therapy:** Both partners report wanting to stop arguing. Lara wants Jorge to be more a part of the family. Jorge would like Lara to give him space when he needs it.

- **Attitude toward therapy:** Lara went to therapy several years ago to deal with issues around her mother's death; she felt it was a positive experience. She is hopeful that this therapy will be helpful. Jorge sees therapy as "too touchy-feely" but recognizes that they need help. He agreed to come to couple therapy but is skeptical it can be helpful. He does not like talking about his feelings.

- **Strengths:** Both are kind and respectful and want to do everything they can to save the relationship. They love Terri and want the best for her. Jorge admits that his defensiveness is a problem in the relationship. Lara can see that her criticizing Jorge only makes him withdraw more.

Beginner Profile: Conflicts Over Household Chores

Keisha and Damian, a Black couple in their 30s, have been together for 4 years. They met during the COVID pandemic and dated for 2 or 3 months before they decided to live together. Damian's primary complaint is that he feels used and disrespected by Keisha when it comes to domestic chores. He states that he contributes more than his fair share of cleaning and shopping. He feels Keisha pays little attention to the housework, leaving him to do the "real cleaning." He already feels burdened by doing all the shopping and repair work in their home. Keisha complains that she does do her share of the household chores but that Damian criticizes her for how she does it and that in his eyes, she "can never do anything good enough. After I've cleaned the kitchen, he'll find the tiniest crumb on the counter and make a big deal about it." Typical fights involve Damian's criticizing Keisha's irresponsible attitude and minimal cleaning efforts, and Keisha's slamming the door and leaving for an hour or so. When she returns, they both avoid talking about what has happened until the next time.

- **Symptoms:** This couple is experiencing conflict, pursue–withdraw patterns. The more Damian complains and criticizes Keisha for not cleaning the home adequately or doing her fair share of the chores, the more Keisha withdraws and at times angrily leaves their home.

- **Clients' goals for therapy:** Damian wants Keisha to do her share of the housework more thoroughly. Keisha wants Damian to stop trying to change her and treat her as an adult.

- **Attitude toward therapy:** This is Keisha and Damian's first time in any kind of therapy, but they are feeling eager for help and have a good alliance with the therapist, although they each pull for the therapist's validation that they are right.

- **Strengths:** Other aspects of their relationship are going well. They have similar interests, a compatible sex life, good support systems, and rewarding work.

Intermediate Profile: Jealousy in a Blended Family

Veronica is a 23-year-old, Latina woman of Chilean background. Patrick is a 32-year-old White man of Irish-Italian background. Patrick divorced his wife, Vera, 3 years ago. He has a 4-year-old daughter from that marriage. Veronica and Patrick have been together for a year. They are very affectionate with each other and enjoy most of their time together. She usually stays at his place 3 days a week and most weekends, including when he has his daughter with him. Veronica feels uncomfortable about photographs and things belonging to Vera that are still in his house. Patrick states that he wants these photos and objects in their home to comfort his daughter who often misses her mother when staying with Patrick. Veronica initially tried, gently and respectfully, to point out to Patrick that he needs to move on and get rid of these objects; recently her complaints have become more forceful. Patrick's response is either silence or comments that he doesn't like to be pressured. Then he shuts down and refuses to talk about it. Veronica's response is to get angry and insult him. On two occasions, she accused him of still loving Vera. Their arguments escalate until he threatens to end the relationship, which causes her to cry and go back to her house. Then they don't talk for days. Patrick eventually reaches out to her to apologize, and the couple has several good days before the cycle starts up again. They both suffer immensely as they see their relationship deteriorating. Veronica threatened to end the relationship if they didn't go to couple therapy to try to "fix his problem."

- **Symptoms:** Veronica is increasingly anxious. Patrick has suffered from depression on and off since adolescence and is currently taking antidepressant medication. The more Veronica complains about not feeling prioritized or understood by Patrick, the more Patrick gets agitated and defensive and eventually shuts down. His depressive symptoms are getting worse.

- **Clients' goals for therapy:** Patrick wants Veronica to understand how dismayed he gets when his daughter misses her mother. Veronica wants to feel like she is Patrick's priority and to feel comfortable in his home.

- **Attitude toward therapy:** Both have had previous therapy and have a positive view of it.

- **Strengths:** The partners each say they love each other very much. They have similar values, good friends who like them as a couple, a healthy sex life, and many shared interests. There seems to be genuine affection between Veronica and Patrick's child. The couple misses each other when apart and want to do whatever they can to be in this relationship.

Intermediate Profile: Discovery of an Emotional Affair

Steve is 45 years old; Yolanda is 46 years old. They have two children (13 and 10 years old). As their interests and friends changed over time, their intimacy declined. A year ago, Steve began a friendship with a female colleague at work. The colleague never knew that Steve was romantically attracted to her and that secretly he had strong feelings of love and erotic desire for her. Six months later, the coworker left the company, and Steve has not seen her since. Instead of talking about it with his wife or a therapist, he wrote about his feelings in a journal. The week before coming to therapy, Yolanda found Steve's hidden diary behind some books. She is terribly hurt and confused. Steve feels lonely and guilty. In the first session, Yolanda tells the therapist that she has never heard her husband of 16 years talk about her with such desire like he wrote about having for this woman.

- **Symptoms:** Both come to therapy feeling sad, confused, and hopeless about the future of their marriage. The more Yolanda wants to talk about what she read and about her fears of not being as important or desirable as she used to feel, the more questions she asks him about his feelings, and the more reactive Steve becomes by trying to stop her or change the subject. On a few occasions Steve has raised his voice and accused her of not understanding that "nothing happened" between him and his former colleague.

- **Clients' goals for therapy:** Steve wants Yolanda to understand what he has been going through. Yolanda wants to know if he will ever feel for her how he felt for the colleague.

- **Attitude toward therapy:** They are committed to the therapy and have a good alliance with the therapist.

- **Strengths:** Steve loves Yolanda and doesn't want to lose her. Yolanda is resilient and willing to put effort toward making a good decision about their relationship. Both are devoted parents who love their children and agree on childrearing practices.

Advanced Profile: Alcohol Abuse and Pornography-Related Sexual Difficulties

Peter and Martin have been together for almost 10 years. They are a gay couple, both in their late 40s. Peter is the son of highly religious parents. He is a self-described work-aholic and tends to stay at work late. Martin contacted the therapist and requested help. The presenting problem is twofold. Peter has told Martin that he no longer has sexual feelings for him, and Martin is drinking more than usual. Their fights are typically around Martin's drinking or about Peter's not initiating sex or, when having sex, losing his erection. Although Martin has no moral issue with pornography, he worries Peter's use of pornography is causing his erectile dysfunction and loss of libido.

- **Symptoms:** Both partners are feeling anxious. Martin states that he is depressed and lonely. The more Martin wants to talk about their sex life, the more Peter tears up and avoids the subject. The more he tries to avoid the subject, the angrier Martin becomes until they have a fight that typically ends with Peter threatening to leave Martin.

- **Clients' goals for therapy:** Peter would like to out if he has fallen out of love with Martin. Martin would like to find a way for them to continue to be together in a more loving way.

- **Attitude toward therapy:** Peter is very ambivalent about therapy, especially after the alliance with the therapist was negatively affected when the therapist mistakenly only texted Martin instead of both of them to let them know that the therapist needed to change the appointment time. Martin has had many years of individual therapy in the past and has a positive alliance with the couple therapist. He is starting to go to AA to address his drinking.

- **Strengths:** Both are highly educated, psychologically sophisticated, and able to explore and verbalize their emotions easily.

Advanced Profile: Increased Verbal Abuse

Susan and Fred have been married for 15 years. They have three children, all in elementary school. Fred always had a tendency to be irritable and short with his wife and kids. Susan accepted his moods as part of his personality; for the most part, the family relationships were satisfactory and secure. For the past 3 years, however, Fred has been devoted to bodybuilding, working out every day and twice a week with a trainer. While he has gotten in better shape, his mood has shifted, and he is not only quick to anger but also has started verbally abusing Susan and being angry with the kids in ways that scare them. Although there is no physical violence, Susan finds herself tiptoeing around him. If she does ask him to "settle down," he becomes more enraged. Susan fears she is falling out of love with her husband. She feels she can't talk to him and is desperate; she is also worried about the effect of all the tension in the house on their children. Susan would like to ask Fred to move into one of his company's apartments but is afraid to do so. Fred feels Susan is micromanaging him and is jealous of how he has gotten himself into shape. He would like her to start going to the gym and losing some weight.

- **Symptoms:** Susan feels trapped and is getting more and more anxious, helpless, and concerned for her children. Fred is highly volatile and reactive. They can barely talk to each another.

- **Clients' goals for therapy:** Susan wants the therapist to figure out what is going on with her husband and get him "back to normal." Fred wants his wife to admire his new body and take better care of the kids so they are not so aggravating when he gets home. He wants help getting his wife to stop lecturing him.

- **Attitude toward therapy:** Susan is feeling desperate and needs things to change in her marriage. She sees this therapy as her only hope. Fred would rather not have to talk to a therapist, but he can't stand the way his wife is treating him. Although he is quite skeptical about therapy, he feels he has no choice but to go.

- **Strengths:** Until recently the couple enjoyed each other's company and were raising three well-adjusted children. Although Fred's irritability always bothered Susan, she was never scared of her husband or felt like she couldn't talk freely. And although Fred's work was difficult, he always felt he had a refuge at home. Despite the severe strain on their marriage, they both seem to care about each another.

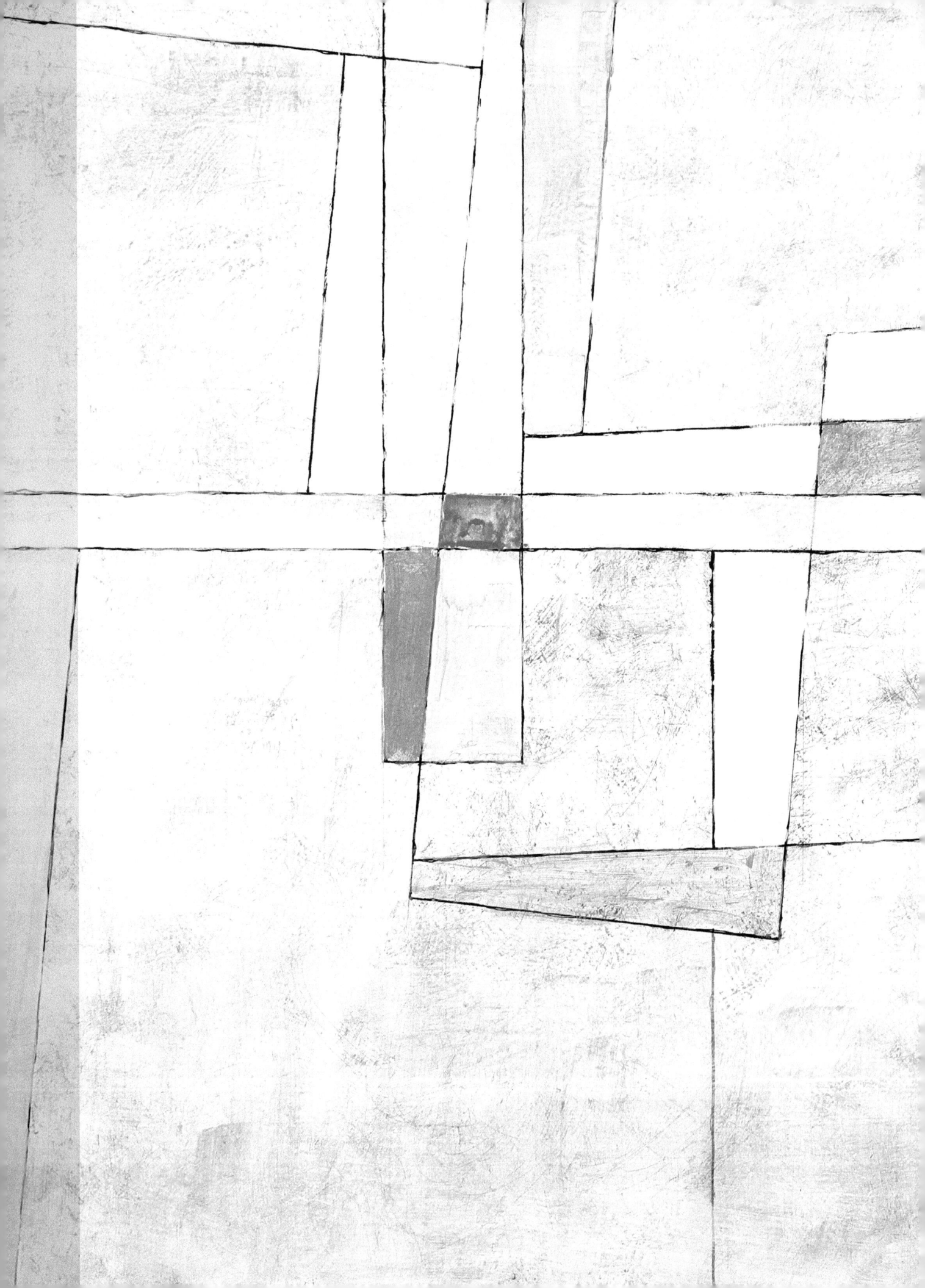

Strategies for Enhancing the Deliberate Practice Exercises

Part III consists of one chapter, Chapter 3, that provides additional advice and instructions for trainers and trainees so that they can reap more benefits from the deliberate practice exercises in Part II. Chapter 3 offers six key points for getting the most out of deliberate practice, guidelines for practicing appropriately responsive treatment, evaluation strategies, methods for ensuring trainee well-being and respecting their privacy, and advice for monitoring the trainer–trainee relationship.

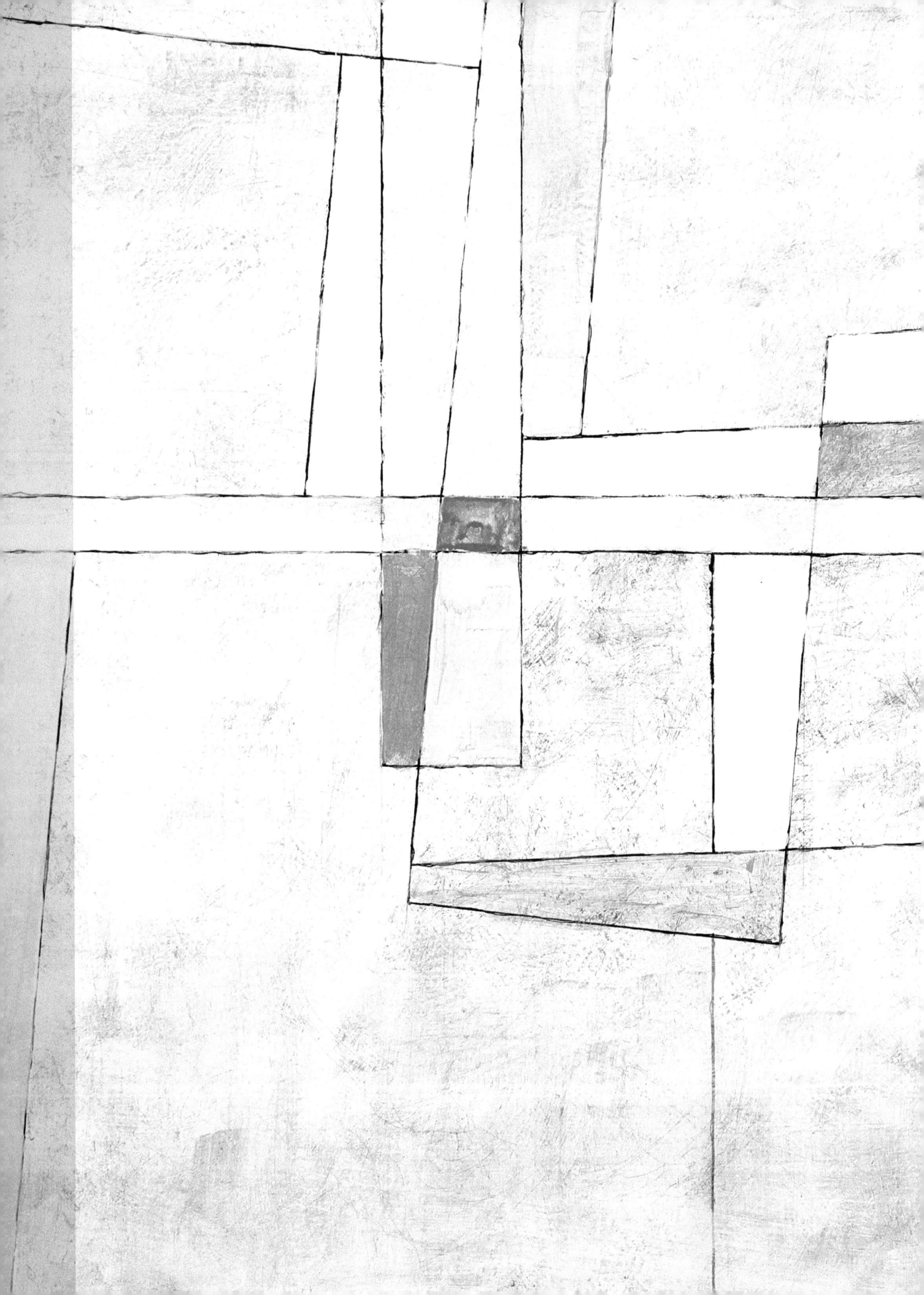

How to Get the Most Out of Deliberate Practice: Additional Guidance for Trainers and Trainees

In Chapter 2 and in the exercises themselves, we have provided instructions for completing these deliberate practice exercises. This chapter provides guidance on big-picture topics that trainers will need to successfully integrate deliberate practice into their training program. This guidance is based on relevant research and the experiences and feedback from trainers at more than a dozen psychotherapy training programs who volunteered to test the deliberate practice exercises in this book. We cover topics including evaluation, getting the most from deliberate practice, trainee well-being, respecting trainee privacy, trainer self-evaluation, responsive treatment, and the trainee–trainer alliance.

Six Key Points for Getting the Most From Deliberate Practice

Following are six key points of advice for trainers and trainees to get the most benefit from the emotionally focused couple therapy (EFCT) deliberate practice exercises. The following advice is gleaned from experiences vetting and practicing the exercises, sometimes in different languages, with many trainees, across many countries.

Key Point 1: Create Realistic Emotional Stimuli

A key component of deliberate practice is using stimuli that provoke similar reactions to challenging real-life work settings. For example, pilots train with flight simulators that present mechanical failures and dangerous weather conditions; surgeons practice with surgical simulators that present medical complications with only seconds to respond. Training with challenging stimuli will increase trainees' capacity to perform therapy effectively under stress, for example with clients they find challenging. The stimuli used for EFCT deliberate practice exercises are role-plays of challenging client statements in therapy. **It is important that the trainee who is role-playing the client perform the script with appropriate emotional expression and maintain eye contact with the therapist.**

https://doi.org/10.1037/0000436-017
Deliberate Practice in Emotionally Focused Couple Therapy, by H. Levenson, S. Jinich, A. Vaz, and T. Rousmaniere

For example, if the client statement calls for sad emotion, the trainee should try to express sadness eye-to-eye with the therapist. We offer the suggestions regarding emotional expressiveness:

1. The emotional tone of the role-play matters more than the exact words of each script. Trainees role-playing the client should feel free to improvise and change the words if it will help them be more emotionally expressive. Trainees do not need to stick 100% exactly to the script. In fact, to read off the script during the exercise can sound flat and prohibit eye contact. Rather, trainees in the client role should first read the client statement silently to themselves, then, when ready, say it in an emotional manner while looking directly at the trainee playing the therapist. This will help the experience feel more real and engaging for the therapist.

2. While adhering to the previous suggestion, we also wish to reiterate (see Chapter 1) that when trainees role-play clients who hold an identity they do not share (e.g., a male reading a female client's statement, a straight person reading a gay client's statement), they should not try to imagine how that person might act or sound. Instead, they need to just follow the descriptors (provided in brackets for every client statement) that suggest what emotional tone the statement is designed to convey (e.g., sad, mad, glad). And when trainees are in the role of the therapist working with clients who hold identities different from their own, they should try to do so in a culturally sensitive and informed manner without making stereotyped or limiting assumptions.

3. Trainees whose first language isn't English may particularly benefit from reviewing and changing the words in the client statement script before each role-play so that they can find words that feel congruent and facilitate emotional expression.

4. Trainees role-playing the client should try to use tonal and nonverbal expressions of feelings. For example, if a script calls for anger, the trainee can speak with an angry voice and make fists with their hands; if a script calls for shame or guilt, the trainee could hunch over and wince; if a script calls for sadness, the trainee could speak in a soft or deflated voice.

5. If trainees are having persistent difficulties acting believably when following a particular script in the role of client, it may help to first do a "demo round" by reading directly from the paper, and then, immediately after, dropping the paper to make eye contact and repeating the same client statement from memory. Some trainees reported this helped them "become available as real clients" and made the role-play feel less artificial. Some trainees did three or four demo rounds to get fully into their role as a client.

Key Point 2: Customize the Exercises to Fit Your Unique Training Circumstances

Deliberate practice is less about adhering to specific rules than it is about using training principles. Every trainer has their own individual teaching style and every trainee their own learning process. Thus, the exercises in this book are designed to be flexibly customized by trainers across different training contexts within different cultures. Trainees and trainers are encouraged to adjust exercises continually to optimize their practice. The most effective training will occur when deliberate practice exercises are customized to fit the learning needs of each trainee and culture of each training site. In our experience with numerous trainers and trainees across many countries, we found that everyone spontaneously customized the exercises for their unique training circumstances. No two trainers followed the exact same procedure. For example:

- One supervisor used the exercises with a trainee who found all the client statements to be too hard, including the "beginner" stimuli. This trainee had multiple reactions in the "too hard" category, including nausea, severe shame, and self-doubt. The trainee disclosed to the supervisor that she had experienced extremely harsh learning environments earlier in her life and found the role-plays to be highly evocative. To help, the supervisor followed the suggestions offered in Appendix A to make the stimuli progressively easier until the trainee reported feeling "good challenge" on the Deliberate Practice Reaction Form. Over many weeks of practice, the trainee developed a sense of safety and was able to practice with more difficult client statements. (Note that if the supervisor had proceeded at the too hard difficulty level, the trainee might have complied while hiding her negative reactions, become emotionally flooded and overwhelmed, leading to withdrawal and thus prohibiting her skill development and risking dropout from training.)

- Supervisors of trainees for whom English was not their first language adjusted the client statements to their own primary language.

- One supervisor used the exercises with a trainee who found all the stimuli to be too easy, including the advanced client statements. This supervisor quickly moved to improvising more challenging client statements from scratch by following the instructions in Appendix A on how to make client statements more challenging.

Key Point 3: Discover Your Own Unique Personal Therapeutic Style

Deliberate practice in psychotherapy can be likened to the process of learning to play jazz music. Every jazz musician prides themselves in their skillful improvisations, and the process of "finding your own voice" is a prerequisite for expertise in jazz musicianship. Yet improvisations are not a collection of random notes but the culmination of extensive deliberate practice over time. Indeed, the ability to improvise is built on many hours of dedicated practice of scales, melodies, harmonies, and so on. Much in the same way, psychotherapy trainees are encouraged to experience the scripted interventions in this book not as ends in themselves but as a means to promote skill in a systematic fashion. Over time, effective therapeutic creativity can be aided, instead of constrained, by dedicated practice in these therapeutic "melodies."

Key Point 4: Engage in a Sufficient Amount of Rehearsal

Deliberate practice uses rehearsal to move skills into procedural memory, which helps trainees maintain access to skills even when working with challenging clients. This only works if trainees engage in many repetitions of the exercises. Think of a challenging sport or musical instrument you learned: How many rehearsals would a professional need to feel confident performing a new skill? Psychotherapy is no easier than those other fields!

Key Point 5: Continually Adjust Difficulty

A crucial element of deliberate practice is training at an optimal difficulty level: neither too easy nor too hard. To achieve this, do difficulty assessments and adjustments with the Deliberate Practice Reaction Form in Appendix A. **Do not skip this step!** If trainees don't feel any of the "good challenge" reactions at the bottom of the Deliberate Practice Reaction Form, then the exercise is probably too easy; if they feel any of the "too hard" reactions then the exercise could be too difficult for the trainee to benefit.

Advanced trainees and therapists may find all the client statements too easy. If so, they should follow the instructions in Appendix A on making client statements harder to make the role-plays sufficiently challenging.

Key Point 6: Putting It All Together With the Practice Transcript and Mock Therapy Sessions

Some trainees may seek greater contextualization of the individual therapy responses associated with each skill, feeling the need to integrate the disparate pieces of their training in a more coherent manner with a simulation that mimics a real therapy session. The annotated transcript in Exercise 13 and the mock therapy sessions in Exercise 14 give trainees this opportunity, allowing them to practice delivering different responses sequentially in a more realistic therapeutic encounter.

Responsive Treatment

The exercises in this book are designed not only to help trainees acquire specific skills of EFCT but also to use them in ways that are responsive to each individual client. Across the psychotherapy literature, this stance has been referred to as *appropriate responsiveness*, wherein the therapists exercise flexible judgment, based in their perception of the client's emotional state, needs, and goals, and integrates techniques and other interpersonal skills in pursuit of optimal client outcomes (Hatcher, 2015; Stiles et al., 1998). The effective therapist is responsive to the emerging context. As Stiles and Horvath (2017) argued, therapists are effective because they are appropriately responsive. Doing the "right thing" may be different each time and means providing each client with an individually tailored response.

Appropriate responsiveness counters a misconception that deliberate practice rehearsal is designed to promote robotic repetition of therapy techniques. Psychotherapy researchers have shown that over-adherence to a particular model while neglecting client preferences reduces therapy effectiveness (e.g., Castonguay et al., 1996; Henry et al., 1993; Owen & Hilsenroth, 2014). Therapist flexibility, on the other hand, has been shown to improve outcomes (e.g., Bugatti & Boswell, 2016; Kendall & Beidas, 2007; Kendall & Frank, 2018). It is important, therefore, that trainees practice their newly learned skills in a manner that is flexible and responsive to the unique needs of a diverse range of clients (Hatcher, 2015; Hill & Knox, 2013). It is thus of paramount importance for trainees to develop the necessary perceptual skills to be able to attune to what the client is experiencing in the moment and form their response based on the client moment-by-moment context (Greenberg & Goldman, 1988).

Supervisors must help the supervisee to attune themselves specifically to the unique and specific needs of the clients during sessions. Process supervision (Greenberg & Tomescu, 2017; Levenson, 1995, 2017)—the practice of supervisor and supervisee listening to tapes, stopping at particular poignant moments and considering client's feelings and meanings—lends itself to teaching appropriate responsiveness. The supervisor can stop the recording, ask the supervisee to reflect on the client's current feelings and meanings, and help the supervisee consider which response would be best in that moment. By enacting responsiveness with the supervisee, the supervisor can demonstrate its value and make it more explicit. In these ways, attention can be given to the larger picture of appropriate responsiveness. Here the trainee and supervisor can work together to help the trainee master not just the techniques but also how the therapist can use their judgment to put the techniques together to foster positive change. Helping trainees keep this overarching goal in mind while reviewing therapy process is a valuable feature of supervision that is difficult to obtain otherwise (Hatcher, 2015).

It is also important that deliberate practice occurs within a context of wider EFCT learning. As noted in Chapter 1, training should be combined with supervision of actual therapy recordings, theoretical learning, observation of competent EFCT psychotherapists, and personal therapeutic work. When the trainer or trainee determines that the trainee is having difficulty acquiring EFCT skills, it is important to assess carefully what is missing or needed. Assessment should then lead to the appropriate remedy, as the trainer and trainee collaboratively determine what is required.

Being Mindful of Trainee Well-Being

Although negative effects that some clients experience in psychotherapy have been well documented (Barlow, 2010), negative effects of training and supervision on trainees have received less attention (Ellis et al., 2014). EFCT has a strong tradition of creating and sustaining safety in training and supervision (Furrow et al., 2022). In keeping with the humanistic tradition, the supervisory and training relationship is built on warmth, empathy, and a validating bond. The trainer must be present (Johnson, 2019) with the trainee and attentive to feelings and needs. Collaboration of goals and tasks of training and supervision is founded on such core relational conditions.

To support strong self-efficacy, trainers must ensure that trainees are practicing at a correct difficulty level. The exercises in this book feature guidance for frequently assessing and adjusting the difficulty level so that trainees can rehearse at a level that precisely targets their personal skill threshold. Trainers and supervisors must be mindful to provide an appropriate challenge. One risk to trainees that is particularly pertinent to this book occurs when using role-plays that are too difficult. The Deliberate Practice Reaction Form in Appendix A is provided to help trainers ensure that role-plays are done at an appropriate challenge level. Trainers or trainees may be tempted to skip the difficulty assessments and adjustments out of their motivation to focus on rehearsal to make fast progress and quickly acquire skills. But across all our test sites, we found that skipping the difficulty assessments and adjustments caused more problems and hindered skill acquisition more than any other error. Thus, trainers are advised to remember that **one of their most important responsibilities is to remind trainees to do the difficulty assessments and adjustments.**

Additionally, the Deliberate Practice Reaction Form serves a dual purpose of helping trainees develop the important skills of self-monitoring and self-awareness (Bennett-Levy, 2019). This will help trainees adopt a positive and empowered stance regarding their own self-care and should facilitate career-long professional development.

Respecting Trainee Privacy

The deliberate practice exercises in this book may stir up complex or uncomfortable personal reactions within trainees, including for example memories of past traumas. Exploring psychological and emotional reactions may make some trainees feel vulnerable. Therapists of every career stage, from trainees to seasoned therapists with decades of experience, commonly experience shame, embarrassment, and self-doubt in this process. Although these experiences can be valuable for building trainees' self-awareness, it is important that training remains focused on professional skill development and not blur into personal therapy (e.g., Ellis et al., 2014). Therefore, one trainer role is to remind trainees to maintain appropriate boundaries.

Trainees must have the final say about what to disclose or not disclose to their trainer. Trainees should keep in mind that the goal is for the trainee to expand their own self-awareness and psychological capacity to stay active and helpful while experiencing uncomfortable reactions. The trainer does not need to know the specific details about the trainee's inner world for this to happen.

Trainees should be instructed to share only personal information that they feel comfortable sharing. The Deliberate Practice Reaction Form and difficulty assessment process is designed to help trainees build their self-awareness while retaining control over their privacy. Trainees can be reminded that the goal is for them to learn about their own inner world. They do not necessarily have to share that information with trainers or peers (Bennett-Levy & Finlay-Jones, 2018). Likewise, trainees should be instructed to respect the confidentiality of their peers.

Trainer Self-Evaluation

The exercises in this book were tested at a wide range of training sites around the world, including graduate courses, practicum sites, and private practice offices. Although trainers reported that the exercises were highly effective for training, some also said that they felt disoriented by how different deliberate practice feels compared with their traditional methods of clinical education. Many felt comfortable evaluating their trainees' performance but were less sure about their own performance as trainers.

The most common concern we heard from trainers was, "My trainees are doing great, but I'm not sure if I am doing this correctly!" To address this concern, we recommend trainers perform periodic self-evaluations along the following five criteria:

1. Observe trainees' work performance.
2. Provide continual corrective feedback.
3. Ensure rehearsal of specific skills is just beyond the trainees' current ability.
4. Ensure that the trainee is practicing at the right difficulty level (neither too easy nor too challenging).
5. Continuously assess trainee performance with real clients in couple therapy.

Criterion 1: Observe Trainees' Work Performance

Determining how well we are doing as trainers means first having valid information about how well trainees are responding to training. This requires that we directly observe trainees practicing skills to provide corrective feedback and evaluation. One risk of deliberate practice is that trainees gain competence in performing therapy skills in role-plays, but those skills do not transfer to trainees' work with real clients. Thus, trainers will ideally also have the opportunity to observe samples of trainees' work with real clients, either live or via recorded video. Supervisors and consultants rely heavily—and, too often, exclusively—on supervisees' and consultees' narrative accounts of their work with clients (Goodyear & Nelson, 1997). EFCT, however, has a long history of not only showing EFCT expert therapists doing couple therapy live or via video recordings but also of observing the role-plays and actual therapeutic work with real clients of therapists or trainees learning EFCT. In fact, to become a certified EFCT therapist (via the International Centre for Excellence in Emotionally Focused Therapy), applicants are required to show their own work through presentation of video-recorded therapy sessions and are judged on how well they perform EFCT skills. Haggerty and Hilsenroth (2011) described this challenge:

> Suppose a loved one has to undergo surgery and you need to choose between two surgeons, one of whom has never been directly observed by an experienced surgeon while performing any surgery. He or she would perform the surgery and return to his or her attending physician and try to recall, sometimes incompletely or inaccurately, the intricate steps of the surgery they just performed. It is hard to imagine that anyone, given a choice, would prefer this over a professional who has been routinely observed in the practice of their craft. (p. 193)

Criterion 2: Provide Continual Corrective Feedback

Trainees need corrective feedback to learn what they are doing well and doing poorly and how to improve their skills. Feedback should be as specific and incremental as possible. The following are examples of specific feedback: "Your voice sounds rushed. Try slowing down by pausing for a few seconds between your statements to the client" and "That's excellent how you are making eye contact with the client." Examples of vague and nonspecific feedback are "Try to build better rapport with the client" and "Try to be more open to the client's feelings."

Criterion 3: Specific Skill Rehearsal Just Beyond the Trainees' Current Ability (Zone of Proximal Development)

Deliberate practice emphasizes skill acquisition via behavioral rehearsal. Trainers should endeavor not to get caught up in client conceptualization at the expense of focusing on skills. For many trainers, this requires significant discipline and self-restraint. It is simply more enjoyable to talk about psychotherapy theory (e.g., case conceptualization, treatment planning, nuances of psychotherapy models, similar cases the supervisor has had) than watch trainees rehearse skills. Trainees have many questions, and supervisors have an abundance of experience; the allotted supervision time can easily be filled sharing knowledge. The supervisor gets to sound smart, while the trainee doesn't have to struggle with acquiring skills at their learning edge. Although answering questions is important, trainees' intellectual knowledge about psychotherapy can quickly surpass their procedural ability to perform psychotherapy, particularly with clients they find challenging. Here's a simple rule of thumb: The trainer provides the knowledge, but the behavioral rehearsal provides the skill (Rousmaniere, 2019).

Criterion 4: Practice at the Right Difficulty Level (Neither Too Easy nor Too Challenging)

Deliberate practice involves *optimal strain*: practicing skills just beyond the trainee's current skill threshold so that they can learn incrementally without becoming overwhelmed (Ericsson, 2006).

Trainers should use difficulty assessments and adjustments throughout deliberate practice to ensure that trainees are practicing at the right difficulty level. Note that some trainees are surprised by their unpleasant reactions to exercises (e.g., dissociation, nausea, blanking out), and may be tempted to "push through" exercises that are too hard. This can happen out of fear of failing a course, fear of being judged as incompetent, or negative self-impressions by the trainee (e.g., "This shouldn't be so hard"). Trainers should normalize the fact that there will be wide variation in perceived difficulty of the exercises and encourage trainees to respect their own personal training process.

Criterion 5: Continuously Assess Trainee Performance With Real Clients

The goal of deliberately practicing psychotherapy skills is to improve trainees' effectiveness at helping real clients. One of the risks in deliberate practice training is that the benefits will not generalize: Trainees' acquired competence in specific skills may not translate into work with real clients. Thus, it is important that trainers assess the impact of deliberate practice on trainees' work with real clients. Ideally, this is done through triangulation of multiple data points:

- Client data (verbal self-report and routine outcome monitoring data)
- Supervisor's report
- Trainee's self-report

If the trainee's effectiveness with real clients is not improving after deliberate practice, the trainer should do a careful assessment of the difficulty. If the supervisor or trainer feels it is a skill acquisition issues, they may want to consider adjusting the deliberate practice routine to better suit the trainee's learning needs or style.

Therapists have traditionally been evaluated from a lens of *process accountability* (Markman & Tetlock, 2000; see also Goodyear, 2015), which focuses on demonstrating specific behaviors (e.g., fidelity to a treatment model) without regard to the impact on clients. We propose that clinical effectiveness is better assessed through a lens tightly focused on client outcomes and that learning objectives shift from performing behaviors that experts have decided are effective (i.e., the competence model) to highly individualized behavioral goals tailored to each trainee's zone of proximal development and performance feedback. This model of assessment has been termed *outcome accountability* (Goodyear, 2015), which focuses on client changes, rather than therapist competence, independent of how the therapist might be performing expected tasks.

Guidance for Trainees

The central theme of this book has been that skill rehearsal is not automatically helpful. Deliberate practice must be done well for trainees to benefit (Ericsson & Pool, 2016). In this chapter and in the exercises, we offer guidance for effective deliberate practice. We would also like to provide additional advice specifically for trainees. That advice is drawn from what we have learned at our volunteer deliberate practice test sites around the world. We cover how to discover your own training process, active effort, playfulness and taking breaks during deliberate practice, your right to control your self-disclosure to trainers, monitoring training results, monitoring complex reactions towards the trainer, and your own personal therapy.

Individualized EFCT Training: Finding Your Zone of Proximal Development

Deliberate practice works best when training targets each trainee's personal skill thresholds. Also termed the *zone of proximal development*, a term first coined by Vygotsky in reference to developmental learning theory (Zaretskii, 2009), this is the area just beyond the trainee's current ability but that is possible to reach with the assistance of a teacher or coach (Wass & Golding, 2014). **If a deliberate practice exercise is either too easy or too hard, the trainee will not benefit.** To maximize training productivity, elite performers follow a "challenging but not overwhelming" principle: Tasks that are too far beyond their capacity will prove ineffective and even harmful, and it is equally true that mindlessly repeating what they already can do confidently will prove fruitless. Because of this, deliberate practice requires ongoing assessment of the trainee's current skill and concurrent difficulty adjustment to target a "good enough" challenge consistently. Thus, if you are practicing Exercise 4, Attachment-Reframed Validation, and it just feels too difficult, consider moving back to a more comfortable skill such as Exercise 3, Validation and Tracking, or Exercise 2, Evocative Reflection, that you may feel you have already mastered.

Active Effort

It is important for trainees to maintain an active and sustained effort while doing the deliberate practice exercises in this book. Deliberate practice really helps when trainees push themselves up to and past their current ability. This is best achieved when trainees take ownership of their own practice by guiding their training partners to adjust roleplays to be as high on the difficulty scale as possible without hurting themselves. This will look different for every trainee. Although it can feel uncomfortable or even frightening, this is the zone of proximal development where the most gains can be made. Simply reading and repeating the written scripts will provide little or no benefit. Trainees are advised to remember that their effort from training should lead to more confidence and comfort in session with real clients.

Stay the Course: Effort Versus Flow

Deliberate practice only works if trainees push themselves hard enough to break out of their old patterns of performance, which then permits growth of new skills (Ericsson & Pool, 2016). Because deliberate practice constantly focuses on the current edge of one's performance capacity, it is inevitably a straining endeavor. Indeed, professionals are unlikely to make lasting performance improvements unless there is sufficient engagement in tasks that are just at the edge of one's current capacity (Ericsson, 2003, 2006). From athletics or fitness training, many of us are familiar with this process of being pushed out of our comfort zones followed by adaptation. The same process applies to our mental and emotional abilities.

Many trainees might be surprised to discover that deliberate practice for EFCT feels harder than psychotherapy with a real client. This may be because when working with a real client a therapist can get into a state of *flow* (Csikszentmihalyi, 1997), where work feels effortless. For example, a trainee at one of our test sites did just fine with most of the beginner exercises, but when it came to using the prosody of her voice (Exercise 5: Deepening Emotions With RISSSSC), something she did not feel proficient at, she felt exhausted doing it. In such cases, it may be wise for trainees to move to offering response formats with which they are more familiar and feel more proficient and try those for a short time, in part to increase a sense of confidence and mastery.

Discover Your Own Training Process

The effectiveness of deliberate practice is directly related to the effort and ownership trainees exert while doing the exercises. Trainers can provide guidance, but it is important for trainees to learn about their own idiosyncratic training processes over time. This will let them become masters of their own training and prepare for a career-long process of professional development. The following are a few examples of personal training processes trainees discovered while engaging in deliberate practice:

- One trainee noticed that she was good at persisting while an exercise is challenging, but also that she required more rehearsal than other trainees to feel comfortable with a new skill. This trainee focused on developing patience with her own pace of progress.

- One trainee noticed that he could acquire new skills rather quickly, with only a few repetitions. However, he also noticed that his reactions to evocative client statements could jump quickly and unpredictably from the "good challenge" to "too hard" categories, so he needed to attend carefully to the reactions listed in the Deliberate Practice Reaction Form.

- One trainee described herself as "perfectionistic" and felt a strong urge to "push through" an exercise even when she had anxiety reactions in the "too hard" category, such as nausea and dissociation. This caused the trainee not to benefit from the exercises and risk getting demoralized. This trainee focused on going slower, developing self-compassion regarding her anxiety reactions, and asking her training partners to make role-plays less challenging.

Trainees are encouraged to reflect deeply on their own experiences using the exercises to learn the most about themselves and their personal learning processes.

Playfulness and Taking Breaks

Psychotherapy is serious work that often involves painful feelings. However, practicing psychotherapy can be playful and fun (Scott Miller, personal communication, 2017). Trainees should remember that one of the main goals of deliberate practice is to experiment with different approaches and styles of therapy. If deliberate practice ever feels rote, boring, or routine, it probably isn't going to help advance trainees' skill. In this case, trainees should try to liven it up. A good way to do this is to introduce an atmosphere of playfulness. For example, trainees can try the following:

- Use different vocal tones, speech pacing, body gestures, or other languages. This can expand trainees' communication range.

- Practice while simulating being blind (with a blindfold). This can increase sensitivity in the other senses.

- Practice while standing up or walking around outside. This can help trainees get new perspectives on the process of therapy.

The supervisor can also ask trainees if they would like to take a 5- to 10-minute break between questions, particularly if the trainees are dealing with difficult emotions and are feeling stressed out.

Additional Deliberate Practice Opportunities

This book focuses on deliberate practice methods that involve active, live engagement between trainees and a supervisor. However, deliberate practice can extend beyond these focused training sessions. This book can be used for individual study and homework. For example, a trainee might read the client stimuli quietly or aloud and practice their responses independently between sessions. In such cases, it is important for the trainee to say their therapist responses aloud, rather than rehearse silently in one's head.

Alternatively, two trainees can practice as a pair, without the supervisor. Although the absence of a supervisor limits one source of feedback, the peer trainee who is playing the client can serve this role. Also, we have had trainees who have used videos of their couple sessions as stimuli, stopping the video at a place of clinical challenge and practicing responses said aloud to the clients on the screen. Doing this for a skill deficit that had been previously identified by a supervisor is particularly beneficial. Using video, in this highly relevant way, is an excellent means to further refine skill performance.

To optimize the quality of the deliberate practice when conducted independently or without a supervisor, we have developed a Deliberate Practice Diary Form that can be found in Appendix B or downloaded from https://www.apa.org/pubs/books/deliberate-practice-emotionally-focused-couple-therapy (see the "Resources" tab). This form provides a template for the trainee to record their experience of the deliberate practice activity, and, ideally, it will aid in the consolidation of learning. This form can be used as part of the evaluation process with the supervisor but is not necessarily intended for that purpose, and trainees are certainly welcome to bring their experience with the independent practice into the next meeting with the supervisor.

Monitoring Training Results

While trainers will evaluate trainees using a competency-focused model, trainees are also encouraged to take ownership of their own training process and look for results of deliberate practice themselves. Trainees should experience the results of deliberate practice within a few training sessions. A lack of results can be demoralizing for trainees and can result in trainees applying less effort and focus in deliberate practice. Trainees who are not seeing results should openly discuss this problem with their trainer and experiment with adjusting their deliberate practice process. Results can include client outcomes and improving the trainee's own work as a therapist, their personal development, and their overall training.

Client Outcomes

The most important result of deliberate practice is an improvement in trainees' client outcomes. This can be assessed via routine outcome measurement (Lambert, 2010; Prescott et al., 2017), qualitative data (McLeod, 2017), and informal discussions with clients. However, trainees should note that an improvement in client outcome due to deliberate practice can sometimes be challenging to achieve quickly, given that the largest amount of variance in client outcome is due to client variables (Bohart & Wade, 2013). For example, a client with severe chronic symptoms may not respond quickly to any treatment, regardless of how effectively a trainee practices. For some clients, an increase in patience and self-compassion regarding their symptoms may be a sign of progress, rather than an immediate decrease in symptoms. Thus, trainees are advised to keep their expectations for client change realistic in the context of their client's symptoms, history, and presentation. It is important that trainees do not try to force their clients to improve in therapy so that the trainee feels like they are making progress in their training (Rousmaniere, 2016).

Trainee's Work as a Therapist

One important result of deliberate practice is change within the trainee regarding their work with clients. For example, trainees at test sites reported feeling more comfortable sitting with evocative clients, more confident addressing uncomfortable topics in therapy, and more responsive to a broader range of clients.

Trainee's Personal Development

Another important result of deliberate practice is personal growth of the trainee. For example, trainees at test sites reported becoming more in touch with their own feelings and having increased self-compassion and enhanced motivation to work with a broader range of clients.

Trainee's Training Process

Another valuable result of deliberate practice is improvement in the training process. For example, trainees at test sites reported becoming more aware of their personal training style, preferences, strengths, and challenges. Over time, trainees should grow to feel more ownership of their training process. Also, training to be a psychotherapist is a complex process that occurs over many years. Experienced, expert therapists still report continuing to grow well beyond their graduate school years (Orlinsky et al., 2005). I (HL) have been doing therapy for almost 50 years, yet it is a rare week when I don't learn something new or am confronted with a situation in which I come up against my own ignorance or skill deficit. Remember, be easy on yourself!

The Trainee–Trainer Alliance: Monitoring Complex Reactions Toward the Trainer

Trainees who engage in difficult deliberate practice often report experiencing complex feelings toward their trainer. For example, one trainee said, "I know this is helping, but I also don't look forward to it!" Another trainee reported feeling both appreciation and frustration toward her trainer simultaneously. Trainees are advised to remember intensive training they have done in other fields, such as athletics or music. When a coach pushes a trainee to the edge of their ability, it is common for trainees to have complex reactions toward them.

This does not necessarily mean that the trainer is doing anything wrong. In fact, intensive training inevitably stirs up reactions toward the trainer, such as frustration, annoyance, disappointment, or anger that coexist with the appreciations they feel. In fact, if trainees do not experience complex reactions, it is worth considering whether the deliberate practice is sufficiently challenging. But what we asserted earlier about rights to privacy apply here as well. Because professional mental health training is hierarchical and evaluative, trainers should not require or even expect trainees to share complex reactions they may be experiencing toward them. Trainers should stay open to their sharing, but the choice always remains with the trainee.

Trainee's Own Therapy

When engaging in deliberate practice, many trainees discover aspects of their inner world that may benefit from attending their own psychotherapy. For example, one trainee discovered that some of the couple situations in the exercises reminded her of her own parents' difficult marriage, which made her recall the blame she placed on herself as a young child for not making them happy. Another trainee found practicing with angry clients stirred up her own painful memories of abuse. Another trainee found himself dissociating while practicing empathy skills, and another trainee started feeling overwhelming shame and self-judgment when she couldn't master skills after just a few repetitions.

Although these discoveries were unnerving at first, they ultimately were very beneficial because they motivated the trainees to seek out their own therapy. Many therapists attend their own therapy. In fact, Norcross and Guy (2005) found in their review of 17 studies that about 75% of the more than 8,000 therapist participants had attended their own therapy. Orlinsky et al. (2005) found that more than 90% of therapists who attended their own therapy reported it to be helpful.

QUESTIONS FOR TRAINEES

1. Are you balancing the effort to improve your skills with patience and self-compassion for your learning process?
2. Are you attending to any shame or self-judgment arising from training?
3. Are you being mindful of your personal boundaries and also respecting any complex feelings you may have toward your trainers?

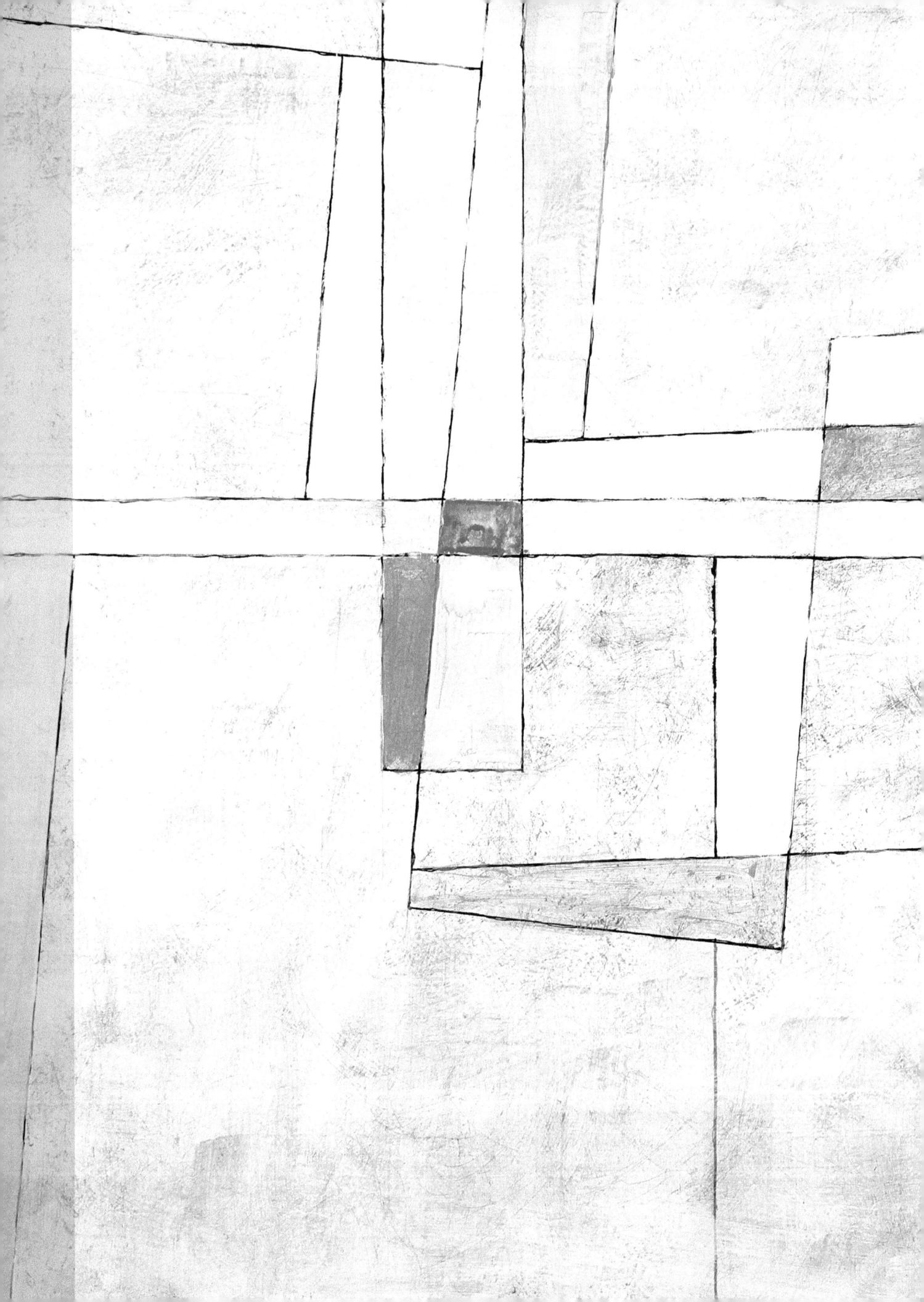

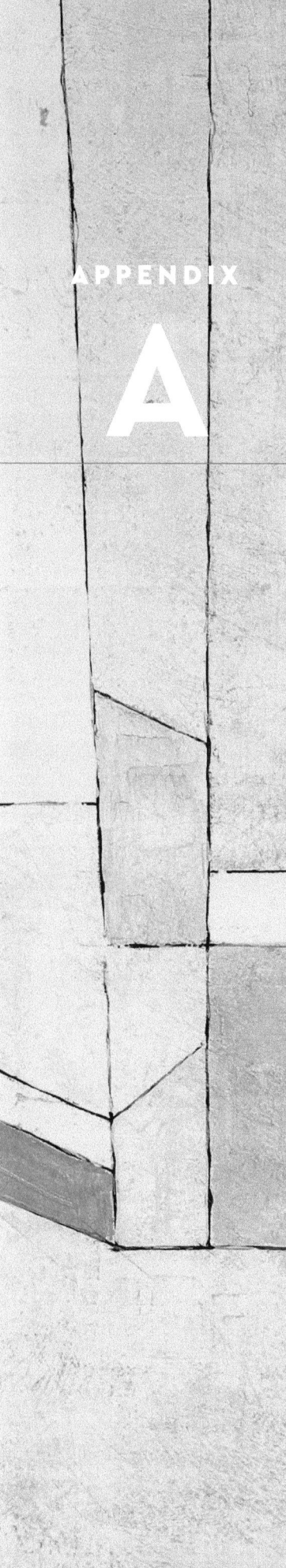

Difficulty Assessments and Adjustments

Deliberate practice works best if the exercises are performed at a good challenge that is neither too hard nor too easy. To ensure that they are practicing at the correct difficulty, trainees should do a difficulty assessment and adjustment after each level of client statement is completed (beginner, intermediate, and advanced). To do this, use the following instructions and the Deliberate Practice Reaction Form (Figure A.1), which is also available in the "Resources" tab online (https://www.apa.org/pubs/books/deliberate-practice-emotionally-focused-couple-therapy). **Do not skip this process!**

How to Assess Difficulty

The therapist completes the reaction form (Figure A.1). If they

- rate the difficulty of the exercise above an 8 or had any of the reactions in the "Too Hard" column, follow the instructions to make the exercise easier;

- rate the difficulty of the exercise below a 4 or didn't have any of the reactions in the "Good Challenge" column, proceed to the next level of harder client statements or follow the instructions to make exercise harder; or

- rate the difficulty of the exercise between 4 and 8 and have at least one reaction in the "Good Challenge" column, do not proceed to the harder client statements but rather repeat the same level.

Making Client Statements Easier

If the therapist ever rates the difficulty of the exercise above an 8 or has any of the reactions in the "Too Hard" column, use the next level easier client statements (e.g., if you were using advanced client statements, switch to intermediate). But if you already were using beginner client statements, use the following methods to make the client statements even easier:

- The person playing the client can use the same beginner client statements but this time in a softer, calmer voice and with a smile. This softens the emotional tone.

261

FIGURE A.1. Deliberate Practice Reaction Form

Question 1: How challenging was it to fulfill the skill criteria for this exercise?

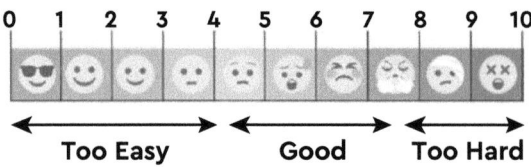

Too Easy　　**Good**　　**Too Hard**

Question 2: Did you have any reactions in "good challenge" or "too hard" categories? (yes/no)					
Good Challenge			**Too Hard**		
Emotions and Thoughts	Body Reactions	Urges	Emotions and Thoughts	Body Reactions	Urges
Manageable shame, self-judgment, irritation, anger, sadness, etc.	Body tension, sighs, shallow breathing, increased heart rate, warmth, dry mouth	Looking away, withdrawing, changing focus	Severe or overwhelming shame, self-judgment, rage, grief, guilt, etc.	Migraines, dizziness, foggy thinking, diarrhea, disassociation, numbness, blanking out, nausea, etc.	Shutting down, giving up

Too Easy	Good Challenge	Too Hard
⬇	⬇	⬇
Proceed to next difficulty level	Repeat the same difficulty level	Go back to previous difficulty level

Note. From *Deliberate Practice in Emotion-Focused Therapy* (p. 180), by R. N. Goldman, A. Vaz, and T. Rousmaniere, 2021, American Psychological Association (https://doi.org/10.1037/0000227-000). Copyright 2021 by the American Psychological Association.

- The client can improvise with topics that are less evocative or make the therapist more comfortable, such as talking about topics without expressing feelings, the future or past (avoiding the here and now), or any topic outside therapy (see Figure A.2).

- The therapist can take a short break (5–10 minutes) between questions.

- The trainer can expand the "feedback phase" by discussing emotionally focused couple therapy or psychotherapy theory and research. This should shift the trainees' focus toward more detached or intellectual topics and reduce the emotional intensity.

Making Client Statements Harder

If the therapist rates the difficulty of the exercise below a 4 or didn't have any of the reactions in the "Good Challenge" column, proceed to next-level harder client statements. If you were already using the advanced client statements, the person playing the client should make the exercise even harder, using the following guidelines:

- The client can use the advanced client statements again with a more distressed voice (e.g., very angry, sad, sarcastic) or unpleasant facial expression. This should increase the emotional tone.

FIGURE A.2. How to Make Client Statements Easier or Harder in Role-Plays

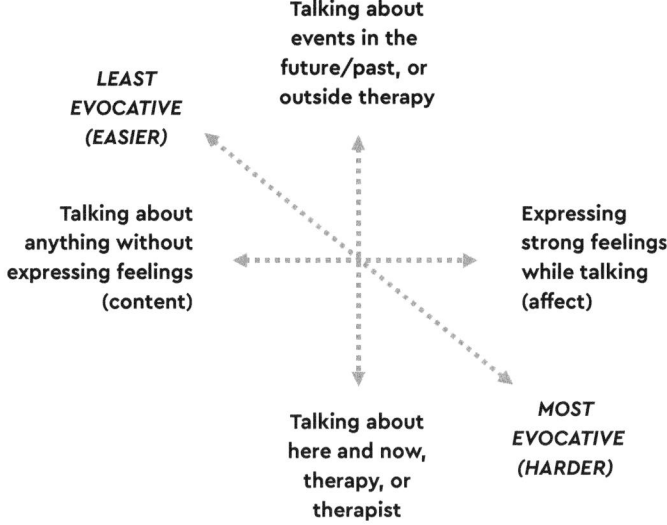

Note. Figure created by Jason Whipple, PhD.

- The client can improvise new client statements with topics that are more evocative or make the therapist uncomfortable, such as expressing strong feelings or talking about the here and now, therapy, or the therapist (see Figure A.2).

Note. The purpose of a deliberate practice session is not to get through all the client statements and therapist responses but rather to spend as much time as possible practicing at the correct difficulty level. This may mean that trainees repeat the same statements and responses many times, which is OK as long as the difficulty remains at the "Good Challenge" level.

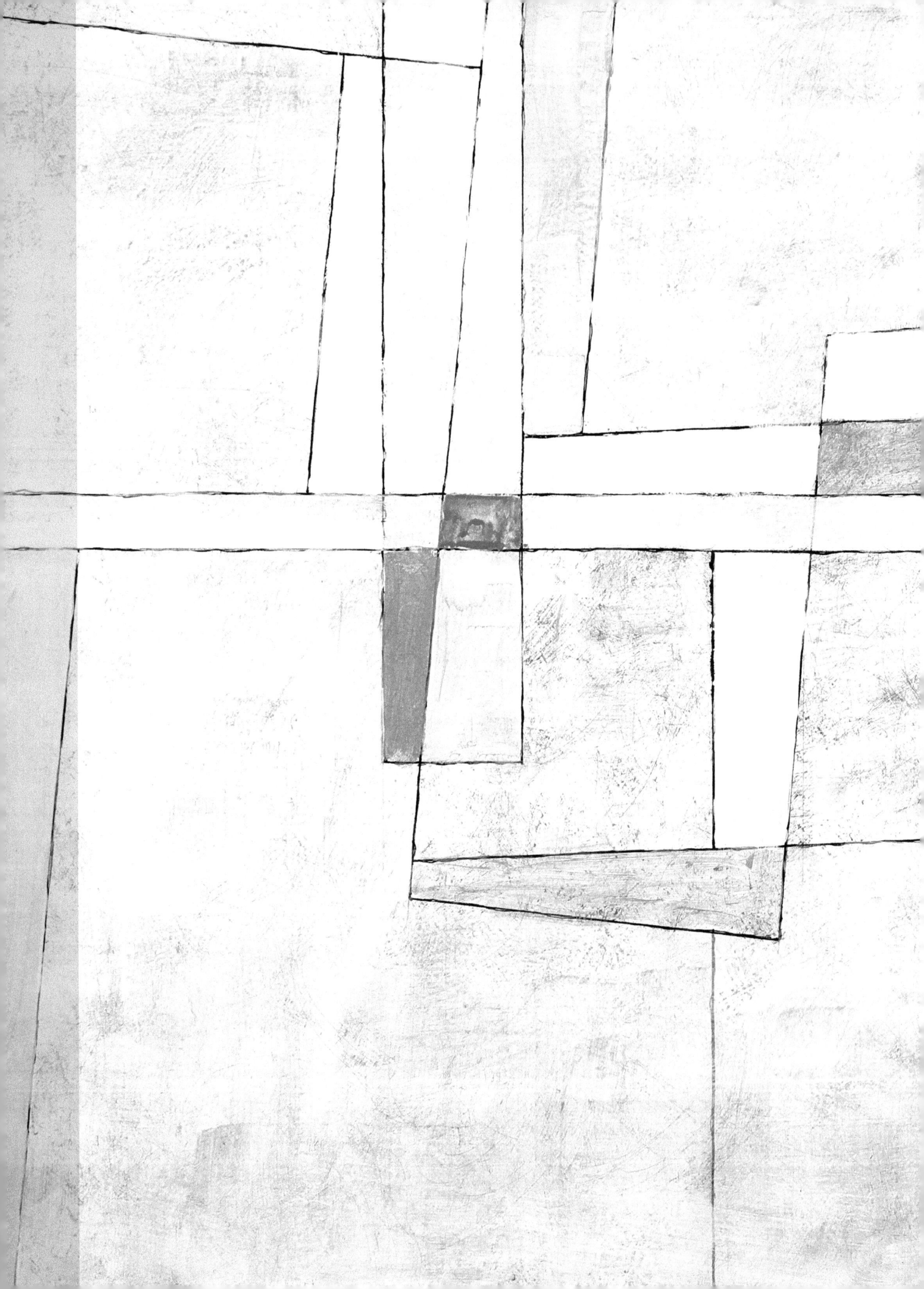

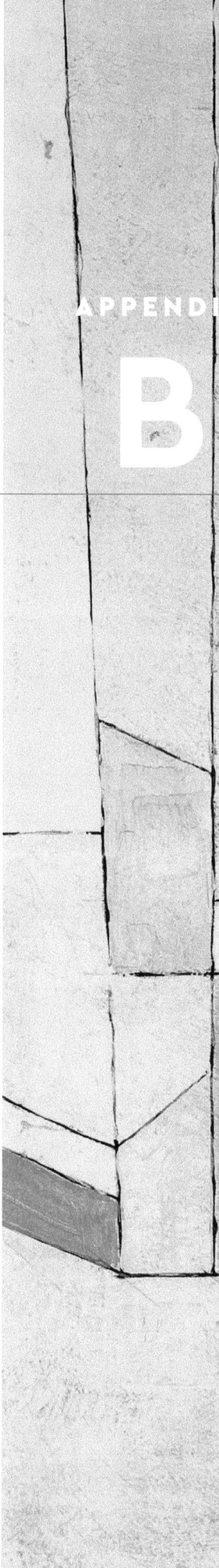

Deliberate Practice Diary Form

This book focuses on deliberate practice methods that involve active, live engagement between trainees and a supervisor. Importantly, deliberate practice can extend beyond these focused training sessions. For example, a trainee might read the client stimuli quietly or aloud and practice their responses independently between sessions with a supervisor. In such cases, it is important for the trainee to speak aloud rather than rehearse silently in one's head. Alternatively, two trainees can practice without the supervisor. Although the absence of a supervisor limits one source of feedback, the peer trainee who is playing the client can serve this role, as they can when a supervisor is present. Importantly, these additional deliberate practice opportunities are intended to take place between focused training sessions with a supervisor. To optimize the quality of the deliberate practice when conducted independently or without a supervisor, we have developed a Deliberate Practice Diary Form that can also be downloaded from the "Resources" tab online (https:// www.apa.org/pubs/books/deliberate-practice-emotionally-focused-couple-therapy). This form provides a template for the trainee to record their experience of the deliberate practice activity and, ideally, will aid in the consolidation of learning. This form can also be used as part of the evaluation process with the supervisor but is not necessarily intended for that purpose, and trainees are certainly welcome to bring their experience with the independent practice into the next meeting with the supervisor.

Deliberate Practice Diary Form

Use this form to consolidate learnings from the deliberate practice exercises. Please protect your personal boundaries by only sharing information that you are comfortable disclosing.

Name: _____ Date: _____

Exercise: _____

Question 1. What was helpful or worked well this deliberate practice session? In what way?

Question 2. What was unhelpful or didn't go well this deliberate practice session? In what way?

Question 3. What did you learn about yourself, your current skills, and skills you'd like to keep improving? Feel free to share any details, but only those you are comfortable disclosing.

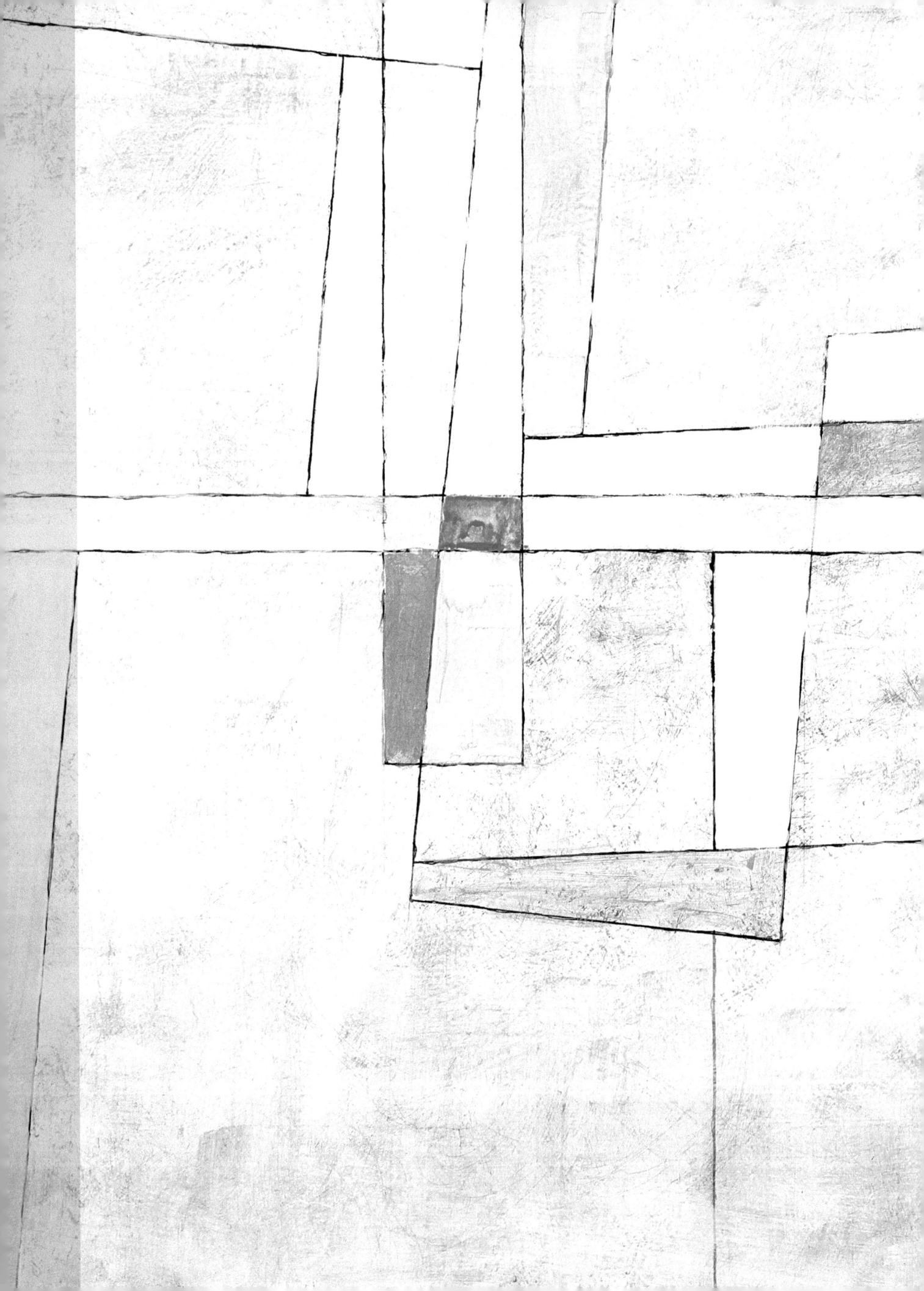

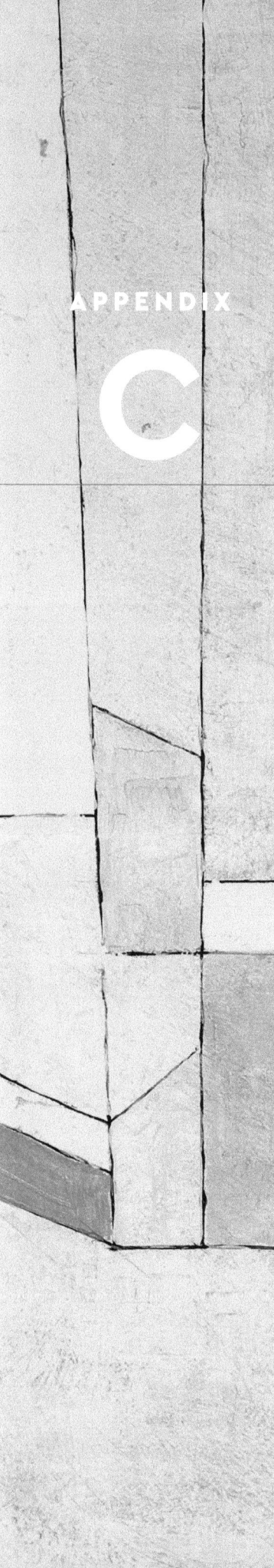

Sample Emotionally Focused Couple Therapy Syllabus With Embedded Deliberate Practice Exercises

This appendix provides a sample one-semester, three-unit course dedicated to teaching emotionally focused couple therapy (EFCT). This course is appropriate for graduate students at all levels of training, including first-year students who have not yet worked with clients. We present it as a model that can be adapted to a specific program's contexts and needs. For example, instructors may borrow portions of it to use in other courses, practica, didactic training events at externships and internships, workshops, and continuing education for postgraduate therapists.

Course Title: Emotionally Focused Couple Therapy: Didactics and Deliberate Practice

Course Description

This graduate-level course provides students with an in-depth understanding of the theory, history, and techniques in EFCT. Through a combination of didactic lectures, independent study and reading, in-class discussions, recorded demonstrations and transcripts of EFCT sessions, mock cases, and experiential learning using deliberate practice exercises, students will begin to develop the necessary skills and knowledge to apply EFCT principles and strategies effectively in couple therapy.

The course will begin with didactic lectures that delve into the theoretical foundations of EFCT. Students will explore the attachment theory underpinnings of EFCT, gaining insight into how attachment patterns influence couples' interactions and emotional experiences. They will also examine the three stages and nine steps of the EFCT process as well as the more process-oriented tango, learning how to identify and work with core emotions and underlying attachment needs within and between the partners, becoming familiar with key psychotherapy change processes.

To deepen their understanding of EFCT, students will engage in independent study and reading. Assigned readings from seminal texts, research articles, and case studies specific to EFCT will provide students with a comprehensive understanding of the model. They will explore topics such as the role of emotion in couple therapy, working with trauma, diversity issues, and the integration of EFCT with other therapeutic approaches.

In-class discussions will provide students with the opportunity to engage actively with the EFCT material, share their insights, and explore real-world case scenarios. Through these discussions, students will develop their critical thinking skills, analyze complex cases, and discuss the nuances of applying EFCT techniques in different therapeutic contexts.

To enhance their learning experience further, students will have the opportunity to observe recorded, expert demonstrations of EFCT sessions. These recordings will showcase experienced EFCT therapists implementing the model's techniques and interventions with real couples. By observing these sessions, students will gain valuable insights into the practical application of EFCT principles, including how to create a safe therapeutic environment, facilitate emotional engagement, and foster secure attachment bonds. The therapist's use of the voice and nonverbal behaviors to deepen emotion and promote new interactions will come alive through the video material.

Experiential exercises using deliberate practice will be a central component of this course, enabling students to experience the power of the model and begin to acquire 12 key EFCT skills. Through these exercises, students will have the opportunity to rehearse EFCT techniques in simulated therapeutic scenarios. They will engage in role-plays as both therapists and clients, practicing interventions such as assembling emotions, enactments, shaping new interactions, and choreographing corrective emotional experiences. Specific, corrective feedback from peers and the instructor will help students refine their therapeutic skills and deepen their understanding of how to use EFCT interventions.

By the end of this course, students will have acquired a comprehensive understanding of beginning, intermediate, and advanced techniques in EFCT. They will have the opportunity to try out the skills necessary to assess and intervene with distressed couples to facilitate emotional engagement and promote secure attachment bonds. Through this didactic and experiential course, students will be able to try out EFCT interventions in their future clinical work with couples.

Course Objectives

Students who complete this course will be able to

1. develop a comprehensive understanding of the theoretical foundations of EFCT, including attachment theory and its application in couple therapy.

2. acquire knowledge of EFCT's three stages, nine steps, and the tango and how they relate to appropriate interventions.

3. identify and work with primary and secondary emotions.

4. gain proficiency in using 12 specific key EFCT skills and begin to see how to combine them appropriately.

5. analyze and critically evaluate complex cases in couple therapy.

6. develop effective communication and collaboration skills through in-class discussions, allowing for the exploration of real-world case scenarios and the integration of EFCT techniques with other therapeutic approaches.

7. demonstrate key EFCT skills and an understanding of how they relate to the EFCT tango.

8. identify key variables when working with diverse clients and begin to develop self-knowledge, comfort, and humility in working with differences.

9. understand how to assess high-risk couples.

10. appreciate applying the principles of deliberate practice for career-long clinical skill development.

Date	Lecture and Discussion	Skills Lab	Assignments to Do Before Class
Week 1	Course overview Historical aspects in couples therapy Theoretical influences in emotionally focused couple therapy (EFCT) Stance of the EFCT therapist Introduction of deliberate practice skills	Exercise 1: Evocative Inquiry Deliberate Practice Diary Form	Johnson (2020, Chapter 1) Furrow et al. (2022, Chapter 2) Explore Sentio site (https://sentio.org/)
Week 2	Basic EFCT microskills The role of emotion Stage 1: de-escalation and stabilization	Exercise 2: Evocative Reflection Deliberate Practice Diary Form	Johnson (2020, Chapters 2 & 3)
Week 3	Basic EFCT microskills Therapeutic alliance Reframing the problem EFCT map	Exercise 3: Validating Partners' Experiences and Tracking Dysfunctional Patterns Deliberate Practice Diary Form	Johnson (2020, Chapter 5) Furrow et al. (2022, Chapter 4)
Week 4	Use of macrointerventions The tango	Exercise 4: Attachment-Reframed Validation Watch: *Emotionally Focused Therapy in Action* [video; https://iceeft.com/product/emotionally-focused-therapy-in-action-individual-version/] Deliberate Practice Diary Form	Johnson (2020, Chapter 4)
Week 5	Working with emotions: Primary and secondary Deepening	Exercise 5: Deepening Emotions With RISSSSC Deliberate Practice Diary Form	Johnson (2008, pp. 3–97) Furrow et al. (2022, Chapter 3)
Week 6	Self of therapist considerations	Exercise 6: Tracking the Therapist's Inner Experience Deliberate Practice Diary Form	Johnson (2020, Chapter 10) Montagno et al. (2011) Kailanko et al. (2022) Watch: DeBruin (2019) [video]
Week 7	Research on EFCT Case studies Process studies Randomized controlled studies	Exercise 7: Providing a Rationale for EFCT Deliberate Practice Diary Form	Bradley & Furrow (2007) Sandberg et al. (2020) Spengler et al. (2024)
Week 8	Working with emotions Assembling and organizing emotional experience	Exercise 8: Gathering and Assembling Elements of Emotion Deliberate Practice Diary Form	Brubacher (2018, Chapter 5) Furrow et al. (2022, Chapter 5)
Week 9	EFCT Stage 2 change events: Withdrawer reengagement	Exercise 9: Enactments Watch: *Re-engaging Withdrawers* [video; https://iceeft.com/product/training-dvd-5-re-engaging-withdrawers-digital-download/] Deliberate Practice Diary Form	Brubacher (2018, Chapter 6) Furrow et al. (2022, Chapter 6)
Week 10	EFCT Stage 2 change events: Pursuer softening Integrating skills into the EFCT tango Stage 2	Exercise 10: Slicing the Risk Thinner Watch: *Risking, Reaching, and Responding* [video; https://iceeft.com/product/risking-reaching-and-responding/] Deliberate Practice Diary Form	Johnson (2020, Chapter 9) Furrow et al. (2022, Chapter 7) Brubacher (2018, Chapter 7)
Week 11	Bullets and other EFCT impasses in Stage 1	Exercise 11: Catching the Bullet I Watch: *Caught in the Struggle: Emotional Dysregulation in the EFT Therapist* [video; https://iceeft.com/product/caught-in-the-struggle-emotional-dysregulation-in-the-eft-therapist/] Deliberate Practice Diary Form	Furrow et al. (2022, Chapter 8)
Week 12	Culture, race, age, sexual and gender issues	Exercise 12: Catching the Bullet II Deliberate Practice Diary Form	Guillory (2022, Chapters 3 & 10) Nightingale et al. (2019) Zeytinoglu-Saydam (2018) Allan & Johnson (2017)
Week 13	Identification of EFCT skills embedded within a real session Improving emotional/verbal fluency	Exercise 13: Annotated EFCT Practice Session Transcript	Read Exercise 13 in preparation for enacting it in class Johnson (2020, Chapter 13) Review of Exercises 1–12
Week 14	Working with real sessions Improving verbal fluency	Exercise 14: Mock EFCT Sessions	Johnson (2020, Chapter 14) Mendelson (2024a)
Week 15	Putting it all together	Share final papers in class	Final paper (see possible choices) Self-evaluation

Class Format

Classes are 3 hours long. Course time is split evenly between learning EFCT and acquiring EFCT skills.

Lecture and Discussion Class: Each week for the first half of the class, there will be lecture and discussion. Students will be expected to have read the required reading assignments before class and to participate in class discussions. Instructor presentations will include lecture, recorded demonstrations of EFCT, and guided discussion.

EFCT Skills Lab: The second half of each week's class will focus on practicing one EFCT skill using the exercises in this book. The exercises use therapy simulations (structured role-plays) with the following goals:

1. Build trainees' skill and confidence for using EFCT skills with real couples.
2. Provide a safe space for learning, observing, and practicing specific EFCT therapeutic interventions, without fear of making mistakes, using deliberate practice exercises.
3. Provide opportunities to explore and "try on" this attachment-theory-based orientation to couple therapy.

Mock Session: Once in the semester, trainees will do a psychotherapy mock session in the EFCT skills lab. In contrast to highly structured and repetitive deliberate practice exercises, a psychotherapy mock session is an unstructured and improvised role-played therapy session. Mock sessions allow trainees to

1. practice the EFT tango incorporating the EFCT skills they have learned,
2. experiment with clinical attunement and decision making in an unscripted context, and
3. build endurance for working with real couples.

Homework

Homework will be assigned each week and will include reading.

Writing Assignments

Students are to write a paper due the last day of class. The instructor will choose the topic. Here are some possibilities:

1. Make up a couple (or adapt one that has appeared in a novel, movie, or TV show). Imagine their interactive cycle. Pretend you have interviewed them regarding their early attachment experiences and how they coped with those experiences. Then write a 3- to 5-page paper describing your conceptualization of the case and your plan for treating this couple using EFCT.

2. Using one of the mock therapy cases from Exercise 14, construct a partial transcript of an imagined session. The transcript must include at least nine of the 12 skills from this book identified within the transcripted material (5–10 pages).

3. Write a deliberate practice exercise on a skill not described in this book. Your write-up should include a short introduction to the skill, skill criteria, and three examples using the format outlined in this book (3–4 pages).

Multicultural Orientation

This course is taught in a multicultural context, defined as "how the cultural worldviews, values, and beliefs of the clients and therapist interact and influence one another to cocreate a relational experience that is in the spirit of healing" (Davis et al., 2018, p. 3). Core features of the multicultural orientation include cultural comfort, humility, and responding to cultural opportunities (or previously missed opportunities). Throughout this course, students are encouraged to reflect on their own cultural identity and improve their ability to attune with their clients' cultural identities (Hook et al., 2017). An important resource is the book, *Emotionally Focused Therapy With African American Couples: Love Heals* (Guillory, 2022). An in-depth case study (Mendelson, 2024a) with commentaries by Kelly (2024) and Skean and Brown (2024) is also helpful for understanding how to integrate EFCT and multicultural theory. And for specific deliberate practice exercises to improve multicultural skills, see *Deliberate Practice in Multicultural Therapy* (Harris et al., 2024).

Vulnerability, Privacy, and Boundaries

This course is aimed at developing EFCT skills, self-awareness, and interpersonal skills in an experiential framework relevant to clinical work. It is not psychotherapy or a substitute for psychotherapy. Students should interact at a level of self-disclosure that is personally comfortable and helpful to their own learning. Although becoming aware of internal emotional and psychological processes is necessary for a therapist's development, it is not necessary to reveal all that information to the instructor. It is important for students to sense their own level of safety and privacy. Students are not evaluated on the level of material that they choose to reveal in the class.

In accordance with the *Ethical Principles of Psychologists and Code of Conduct* (American Psychological Association, 2017), students are **not required to disclose personal information.** Because this class is about developing both interpersonal and EFCT competence, following are some important points so that students are fully informed as they make choices to self-disclose:

- Students choose how much, when, and what to disclose. They are not penalized for the choice not to share personal information.

- The learning environment is susceptible to group dynamics much like any other group space, and therefore students may be asked to share their observations and experiences of the class environment with the singular goal of fostering a more inclusive and productive learning environment.

Confidentiality

Due to the nature of the material covered in class, there are many occasions when personal life experience (self, friends, or family) may be pertinent for the learning environment. Although it cannot be required to share personal experiences, some trainees may be inclined to do so. To create a safe learning environment that is respectful of client and therapist information and to foster open and vulnerable conversations in class, class members are invited to discuss adhering to a confidentiality agreement within and outside of the instructional setting.

Self-Evaluation

At the end of the semester (Week 15), trainees will perform a self-evaluation. This will help trainees track their progress and identify areas for further development. The Guidance for Trainees section in Chapter 3 of this book highlights potential areas of focus for self-evaluation.

Grading Criteria

As designed, students would be accountable for the level and quality of their performance in

- Class discussion and participation (30% of grade)
- The skills lab exercises (25% of grade)
- Self-evaluation based on coaching feedback (20% of grade)
- Final paper (25% of grade)

Required Readings and Resources

Allan, R., & Johnson, S. M. (2017). Conceptual and application issues: Emotionally focused therapy with gay male couples. *Journal of Couple & Relationship Therapy, 16*(4), 286–305. https://doi.org/10.1080/15332691.2016.1238800

Bradley, B., & Furrow, J. (2007). Inside blamer softening: Maps and missteps. *Journal of Systemic Therapies, 26*(4), 25–43. https://doi.org/10.1521/jsyt.2007.26.4.25

Brubacher, L. (2018). *Stepping into emotionally focused therapy: Key ingredients for change.* Routledge. https://doi.org/10.4324/9780429480478

DeBruin, K. (2019, August 4). *Self of the therapist in EFT* [Video]. https://www.youtube.com/watch?v=ZMZjMLcMdjc

Furrow, J. L., Johnson, S. M., Bradley, B., Brubacher, L., Campbell, T. L., Kallos-Lilly, V., Palmer, G., Rheem, K., & Woolley, S. (2022). *Becoming an emotionally focused therapist: The workbook* (2nd ed.). Routledge. https://doi.org/10.4324/9781003039457

Guillory, P. (2022). *Emotionally focused therapy with African American couples: Love heals.* Routledge. https://doi.org/10.4324/9780429355127

Johnson, S. (2008). *Hold me tight: Seven conversations for a lifetime of love.* Little, Brown & Company.

Johnson, S. M. (2020). *The practice of emotionally focused couple therapy: Creating connection* (3rd ed.). Routledge.

Kailanko, S., Wiebe, S. A., Tasca, G. A., Laitila, A. A., & Allan, R. (2022). Somatic experience of emotion in emotionally focused couple therapy: Experienced trainer therapists' views and experiences. *Journal of Marital and Family Therapy, 48*(3), 677–692. https://doi.org/10.1111/jmft.12543

Mendelson, D. (2024a). "The commitment of a lifetime": The role of emotionally focused couple therapy in strengthening attachment bonds and improving relationship health in later-life couples—The teletherapy case of "Alice" and "Steve." *Pragmatic Case Studies in Psychotherapy, 20*(1), 1–80.

Mendelson, D. (2024b). Response to commentaries on "The commitment of a lifetime": The role of emotionally focused couple therapy in strengthening attachment bonds and improving relationship health in later-life couples—The teletherapy case of "Alice" and "Steve." *Pragmatic Case Studies in Psychotherapy, 20*(1), 106–116.

Montagno, M., Svatovic, M., & Levenson, H. (2011). Short-term and long-term effects of training in emotionally focused couple therapy: Professional and personal aspects. *Journal of Marital and Family Therapy, 37*(4), 380–392. https://doi.org/10.1111/j.1752-0606.2011.00250.x

Nightingale, M., Awosan, C. I., & Stavrianopoulos, K. (2019). Emotionally focused therapy: A culturally sensitive approach for African American heterosexual couples. *Journal of Family Psychotherapy, 30*(3), 221–244. https://doi.org/10.1080/08975353.2019.1666497

Sandberg, J. G., Rodríguez-González, M., Pereyra, S., Lybbert, R., Perez, L., & Willis, K. (2020). The experience of learning EFT in Spanish-speaking countries: A multinational replication study. *Journal of Marital and Family Therapy, 46*(2), 256–271. https://doi.org/10.1111/jmft.12383

Spengler, P. M., Lee, N. A., Wiebe, S. A., & Wittenborn, A. K. (2024). A comprehensive meta-analysis on the efficacy of emotionally focused couple therapy. *Couple and Family Psychology: Research and Practice, 13*(2), 81–99. https://doi.org/10.1037/cfp0000233

Zeytinoglu-Saydam, S. (2018). Cross-culturally responsive training of emotionally focused couple therapy: International experiences. In S. Poulsen & R. Allan (Eds.), *Cross-cultural responsiveness and systemic therapy* (pp. 53–67). Springer International Publishing. https://doi.org/10.1007/978-3-319-71395-3_4

Supplemental and Optional Readings

Bograd, M., & Mederos, F. (1999). Battering and couples therapy: Universal screening and selection of treatment modality. *Journal of Marital and Family Therapy, 25*(3), 291–312. https://doi.org/10.1111/j.1752-0606.1999.tb00249.x

Bradley, B., & Palmer, G. (2003). Attachment in later life-implications for intervention with older adults. In S. M. Johnson & V. Whiffen (Eds.), *Attachment processes in couple and family therapy* (pp. 281–299). Guilford Press.

Chapman, D. M., & Caldwell, B. E. (2012). Attachment injury resolution in couples when one partner is trans-identified. *Journal of Systemic Therapies, 31*(2), 36–53. https://doi.org/10.1521/jsyt.2012.31.2.36

Cozolino, L. (2014). *The neuroscience of human relationships: Attachment and the developing social brain* (2nd ed.). W. W. Norton & Co.

Edwards, C., Allan, R., Marzo, N., Wynfield, T., & Hicks, R. (2023). The use of emotionally focused therapy with polyamorous relationships. *Family Process, 62*(4), 1362–1376. https://doi.org/10.1111/famp.12934

Furrow, J. L., & Palmer, G. (2018). Emotionally focused family therapy. In J. Lebow, A. Chambers, & D. Breunlin (Eds.), *Encyclopedia of couple and family therapy* (pp. 1–5). Springer. https://doi.org/10.1007/978-3-319-15877-8_900-1

Greenman, P. S., Young, M. Y., & Johnson, S. M. (2009). Emotionally focused couple therapy with intercultural couples. In M. Rastogi & V. Thomas (Eds.), *Multicultural couple therapy* (pp. 143–166). Sage Publications. https://doi.org/10.4135/9781452275000.n8

Johnson, S. M. (2013). Facing the dragon together: Emotionally focused couples therapy with trauma survivors. In D. Catherall (Ed.), *Handbook of stress, trauma, and the family* (pp. 493–512). Routledge/Taylor & Francis Group.

Johnson, S. M. (2017). An emotionally focused approach to sex therapy. In Z. D. Peterson (Ed.), *The Wiley-Blackwell handbook of sex therapy* (pp. 250–266). Wiley-Blackwell. https://doi.org/10.1002/9781118510384.ch16

Johnson, S. M. (2019). *Attachment theory in practice: Emotionally focused therapy with individuals, couples and families.* Guilford Press.

Johnson, S. M., Burgess Moser, M., Beckes, L., Smith, A., Dalgleish, T., Halchuk, R., Hasselmo, K., Greenman, P. S., Merali, Z., & Coan, J. A. (2013). Soothing the threatened brain: Leveraging contact comfort with emotionally focused therapy [Erratum at https://doi.org/10.1371/journal.pone.0105489]. *PLOS ONE, 8*(11), e79314. https://doi.org/10.1371/journal.pone.0079314

Josephson, G. J. (2003). Using an attachment-based intervention for same-sex couples. In S. M. Johnson & V. Whiffen (Eds.), *Attachment processes in couple and family therapy* (pp. 300–320). Guilford Press.

Karakurt, G., Whiting, K., van Esch, C., Bolen, S. D., & Calabrese, J. R. (2016). Couples therapy for intimate partner violence: A systematic review and meta-analysis. *Journal of Marital and Family Therapy, 42*(4), 567–583. https://doi.org/10.1111/jmft.12178

Linhof, A. Y., & Allan, R. (2019). A narrative expansion of emotionally focused therapy with intercultural couples. *The Family Journal, 27*(1), 44–49. https://doi.org/10.1177/1066480718809426

Liu, T., & Wittenborn, A. (2011). Emotionally focused therapy with culturally diverse couples. In J. Furrow, B. Bradley, & S. Johnson (Eds.), *The emotionally focused casebook: New directions in treating couples* (pp. 295–316). Routledge.

Moors, A. C., Ryan, W. S., & Chopik, W. J. (2019). Multiple loves: The effects of attachment with multiple concurrent romantic partners on relational functioning. *Personality and Individual Differences, 147*, 102–110. https://doi.org/10.1016/j.paid.2019.04.023

Rheem, K., & Campbell, T. L. (2018). Emotionally focused couple therapy and trauma. In J. Lebow, A. Chambers, & D. Breunlin (Eds.), *Encyclopedia of couple and family therapy* (pp. 875–879). Springer. https://doi.org/10.1007/978-3-319-15877-8_898-1

Wiebe, S. A., Elliott, C., Johnson, S. M., Burgess Moser, M., Dalgleish, T. L., Lafontaine, M. F., & Tasca, G. A. (2019). Attachment change in emotionally focused couple therapy and sexual satisfaction outcomes in a two-year follow-up study. *Journal of Couple & Relationship Therapy, 18*(1), 1–21. https://doi.org/10.1080/15332691.2018.1481799

Wiebe, S. A., Johnson, S. M., Lafontaine, M. F., Burgess Moser, M., Dalgleish, T. L., & Tasca, G. A. (2017). Two-year follow-up outcomes in emotionally focused couple therapy: An investigation of relationship satisfaction and attachment trajectories. *Journal of Marital and Family Therapy, 43*(2), 227–244. https://doi.org/10.1111/jmft.12206

Zuccarini, D., & Karos, L. (2011). Emotionally focused therapy for gay and lesbian couples: Strong identities, strong bonds. In J. Furrow, B. Bradley, & S. Johnson (Eds.), *The emotionally focused casebook: New directions in treating couples* (pp. 317–342). Routledge.

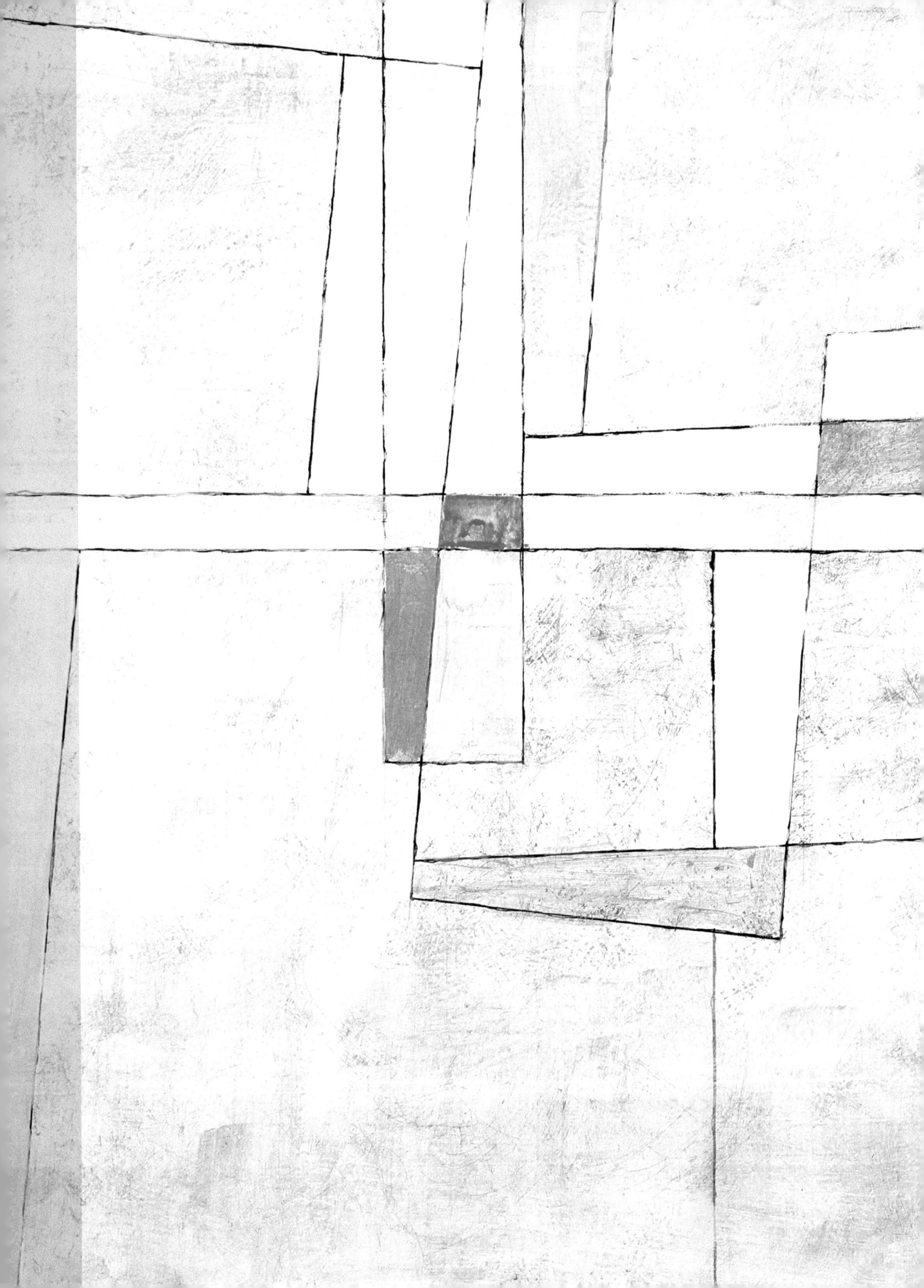

References

Ainsworth, M. D. S. (1962). The effects of maternal deprivation: A review of findings and controversy in the context of research strategy. *Public Health Papers, 14*, 97–165.

Allan, R., Edwards, C., & Lee, N. (2023). Cultural adaptations of emotionally focused therapy. *Journal of Couple & Relationship Therapy, 22*(1), 43–63. https://doi.org/10.1080/15332691.2022.2052391

Allan, R., & Johnson, S. M. (2017). Conceptual and application issues: Emotionally focused therapy with gay male couples. *Journal of Couple & Relationship Therapy, 16*(4), 286–305. https://doi.org/10.1080/15332691.2016.1238800

American Psychological Association. (2017). *Ethical principles of psychologists and code of conduct* (2002, Amended June 1, 2010, and January 1, 2017). https://www.apa.org/ethics/code/

Anderson, T., Ogles, B. M., Patterson, C. L., Lambert, M. J., & Vermeersch, D. A. (2009). Therapist effects: Facilitative interpersonal skills as a predictor of therapist success. *Journal of Clinical Psychology, 65*(7), 755–768. https://doi.org/10.1002/jclp.20583

Arnold, M. B. (1960). *Emotion and personality.* Columbia University Press.

Bailey, R. J., & Ogles, B. M. (2019). Common factors as a therapeutic approach: What is required? *Practice Innovations, 4*(4), 241–254. https://doi.org/10.1037/pri0000100

Barlow, D. H. (2010). Negative effects from psychological treatments: A perspective. *American Psychologist, 65*(1), 13–20. https://doi.org/10.1037/a0015643

Bennett-Levy, J. (2019). Why therapists should walk the talk: The theoretical and empirical case for personal practice in therapist training and professional development. *Journal of Behavior Therapy and Experimental Psychiatry, 62*, 133–145. https://doi.org/10.1016/j.jbtep.2018.08.004

Bennett-Levy, J., & Finlay-Jones, A. (2018). The role of personal practice in therapist skill development: A model to guide therapists, educators, supervisors and researchers. *Cognitive Behaviour Therapy, 47*(3), 185–205. https://doi.org/10.1080/16506073.2018.1434678

Blow, A. J., Seedall, R. B., Miller, D. L., Rousmaniere, T., & Vaz, A. (2023). *Deliberate practice in systemic family therapy.* American Psychological Association. https://doi.org/10.1037/0000301-000

Bohart, A. C., & Wade, A. G. (2013). The client in psychotherapy. In M. J. Lambert (Ed.), *Bergin and Garfield's handbook of psychotherapy and behavior change* (5th ed., pp. 13–43). John Wiley & Sons.

Bowlby, J. (1969). *Attachment: Attachment and loss* (Vol. 1). Basic Books.

Bowlby, J. (1988). *A secure base.* Routledge.

Bradley, B., & Furrow, J. (2007). Inside blamer softening: Maps and missteps. *Journal of Systemic Therapies, 26*(4), 25–43. https://doi.org/10.1521/jsyt.2007.26.4.25

Brubacher, L. (2018). *Stepping into emotionally focused therapy: Key ingredients for change.* Routledge. https://doi.org/10.4324/9780429480478

Bugatti, M., & Boswell, J. F. (2016). Clinical errors as a lack of context responsiveness. *Psychotherapy: Theory, Research, & Practice, 53*(3), 262–267. https://doi.org/10.1037/pst0000080

Burgess Moser, M., Johnson, S. M., Dalgleish, T. L., Lafontaine, M.-F., Wiebe, S. A., & Tasca, G. A. (2016). Changes in relationship-specific attachment in emotionally focused couple therapy. *Journal of Marital and Family Therapy, 42*(2), 231–245. https://doi.org/10.1111/jmft.12139

Campbell, L., Furrow, J., Johnson, S., Villodas, F., & Berhe, Z. (2022, February). Tuning in with CARE in emotionally focused therapy. *The EFT Community News* (52nd issue). International Centre for Excellence in Emotionally Focused Therapy. https://static1.squarespace.com/static/58828dd5a5790a50b9f706c0/t/6255c03c866b1925b480fced/1649786940594/CARE-Article-Feb2022.pdf

Castonguay, L. G., Goldfried, M. R., Wiser, S., Raue, P. J., & Hayes, A. M. (1996). Predicting the effect of cognitive therapy for depression: A study of unique and common factors. *Journal of Consulting and Clinical Psychology, 64*(3), 497–504. https://doi.org/10.1037/0022-006X.64.3.497

Coan, J. A. (2008). Toward a neuroscience of attachment. In J. Cassidy & P. R. Shaver (Eds.), *Handbook of attachment: Theory, research, and clinical implications* (2nd ed., pp. 241–247). Guilford Press.

Coker, J. (1990). *How to practice jazz.* Jamey Aebersold.

Cook, R. (2005). *It's about that time: Miles Davis on and off record.* Atlantic Books.

Cozolino, L. (2017). *Neuroscience of psychotherapy: Healing the social brain* (3rd ed.). W. W. Norton & Co.

Csikszentmihalyi, M. (1997). *Finding flow: The psychology of engagement with everyday life.* HarperCollins.

Davis, D. E., DeBlaere, C., Owen, J., Hook, J. N., Rivera, D. P., Choe, E., Van Tongeren, D. R., Worthington, E. L., & Placeres, V. (2018). The multicultural orientation framework: A narrative review. *Psychotherapy: Theory, Research, & Practice, 55*(1), 89–100. https://doi.org/10.1037/pst0000160

DeBruin, K. (2019, August 4). *Self of the therapist in EFT* [Video]. https://www.youtube.com/watch?v=ZMZjMLcMdjc

Duschinsky, R., Granqvist, P., & Forslund, T. (2023). *The psychology of attachment.* Routledge.

Ellis, M. V., Berger, L., Hanus, A. E., Ayala, E. E., Swords, B. A., & Siembor, M. (2014). Inadequate and harmful clinical supervision: Testing a revised framework and assessing occurrence. *The Counseling Psychologist, 42*(4), 434–472. https://doi.org/10.1177/0011000013508656

Ericsson, K. A. (2003). Development of elite performance and deliberate practice: An update from the perspective of the expert performance approach. In J. L. Starkes & K. A. Ericsson (Eds.), *Expert performance in sports: Advances in research on sport expertise* (pp. 49–83). Human Kinetics.

Ericsson, K. A. (2004). Deliberate practice and the acquisition and maintenance of expert performance in medicine and related domains: Invited address. *Academic Medicine, 79*(10), S70–S81. https://doi.org/10.1097/00001888-200410001-00022

Ericsson, K. A. (2006). The influence of experience and deliberate practice on the development of superior expert performance. In K. A. Ericsson, N. Charness, P. J. Feltovich, & R. R. Hoffman (Eds.), *The Cambridge handbook of expertise and expert performance* (pp. 683–704). Cambridge University Press. https://doi.org/10.1017/CBO9780511816796.038

Ericsson, K. A., Hoffman, R. R., Kozbelt, A., & Williams, A. M. (Eds.). (2018). *The Cambridge handbook of expertise and expert performance* (2nd ed.). Cambridge University Press. https://doi.org/10.1017/9781316480748

Ericsson, K. A., Krampe, R. T., & Tesch-Römer, C. (1993). The role of deliberate practice in the acquisition of expert performance. *Psychological Review, 100*(3), 363–406. https://doi.org/10.1037/0033-295X.100.3.363

Ericsson, K. A., & Pool, R. (2016). *Peak: Secrets from the new science of expertise.* Houghton Mifflin Harcourt.

Feuerman, M. L. (2018). Therapeutic presence in emotionally focused couples therapy. *Journal of Experiential Psychotherapy, 21*(3), 22–32.

Fischer, O., Cox, D. W., Mickelson, J. M., & Lyons, K. (2024). Bridging the multicultural orientation framework with sexual and gender minor psychotherapy: A mixed studies systematic review. *Psychotherapy*, *61*(1), 1–30. https://doi.org/10.1037/pst0000518

Fisher, R. P., & Craik, F. I. M. (1977). Interaction between encoding and retrieval operations in cued recall. *Journal of Experimental Psychology: Human Learning and Memory*, *3*(6), 701–711. https://doi.org/10.1037/0278-7393.3.6.701

Franz, D., Caffery, C., Cheng, Y., Hua, E., Capron, C. G., Allmendinger, A., & Chronister, K. (2023). Emotion focused therapy and Chinese American clients: An exploration using the cultural lens approach. *International Journal of Systemic Therapy*, *34*(3), 141–164. https://doi.org/10.1080/2692398X.2023.2183018

Furrow, J. L., Edwards, S. A., Choi, Y., & Bradley, B. (2012). Therapist's presence in emotionally focused couple therapy blamer softening events: Promoting change through emotional experience. *Journal of Marital and Family Therapy*, *38*(s1), 39–49. https://doi.org/10.1111/j.1752-0606.2012.00293.x

Furrow, J. L., Johnson, S. M., Bradley, B., Brubacher, L., Campbell, T. L., Kallos-Lilly, V., Palmer, G., Rheem, K., & Woolley, S. (2022). *Becoming an emotionally focused therapist: The workbook* (2nd ed.). Routledge. https://doi.org/10.4324/9781003039457

Furrow, J. L., Palmer, G., Johnson, S., Faller, G., & Palmer-Olsen, L. (2019). *Emotionally focused family therapy: Restoring connection and promoting resilience*. Routledge. https://doi.org/10.4324/9781315669649

Gladwell, M. (2008). *Outliers: The story of success*. Little, Brown & Company.

Goldberg, S., Rousmaniere, T. G., Miller, S. D., Whipple, J., Nielsen, S. L., Hoyt, W., & Wampold, B. E. (2016). Do psychotherapists improve with time and experience? A longitudinal analysis of outcomes in a clinical setting. *Journal of Counseling Psychology*, *63*, 1–11. https://doi.org/10.1037/cou0000131

Goldman, R. N., Vaz, A., & Rousmaniere, T. (2021). *Deliberate practice in emotion-focused therapy*. American Psychological Association. https://doi.org/10.1037/0000227-000

Goodyear, R. K. (2015). Using accountability mechanisms more intentionally: A framework and its implications for training professional psychologists. *American Psychologist*, *70*(8), 736–743. https://doi.org/10.1037/a0039828

Goodyear, R. K., & Nelson, M. L. (1997). The major formats of psychotherapy supervision. In C. E. Watkins, Jr. (Ed.), *Handbook of psychotherapy supervision* (pp. 328–334). John Wiley & Sons.

Greenberg, L. S., & Goldman, R. L. (1988). Training in experiential therapy. *Journal of Consulting and Clinical Psychology*, *56*(5), 696–702. https://doi.org/10.1037/0022-006X.56.5.696

Greenberg, L. S., & Johnson, S. M. (1988). *Emotionally focused therapy for couples*. Guilford Press.

Greenberg, L. S., & Tomescu, L. R. (2017). *Supervision essentials for emotion-focused therapy*. American Psychological Association. https://doi.org/10.1037/15966-000

Greenman, P. S., & Johnson, S. M. (2013). Process research on emotionally focused therapy (EFT) for couples: Linking theory to practice. *Family Process*, *52*(1), 46–61. https://doi.org/10.1111/famp.12015

Greenman, P. S., Young, M. Y., & Johnson, S. M. (2009). Emotionally focused couple therapy with intercultural couples. In M. Rastogi & V. Thomas (Eds.), *Multicultural couple therapy* (pp. 143–166). Sage Publications. https://doi.org/10.4135/9781452275000.n8

Guillory, P. (2022). *Emotionally focused therapy with African American couples: Love heals*. Routledge. https://doi.org/10.4324/9780429355127

Haggerty, G., & Hilsenroth, M. J. (2011). The use of video in psychotherapy supervision. *British Journal of Psychotherapy*, *27*(2), 193–210. https://doi.org/10.1111/j.1752-0118.2011.01232.x

Harris, J., Jin, J., Hoffman, S., Phan, S., Prout, T. A., Rousmaniere, T., & Vaz, A. (2024). *Deliberate practice in multicultural therapy*. American Psychological Association. https://doi.org/10.1037/0000357-000

Hatcher, R. L. (2015). Interpersonal competencies: Responsiveness, technique, and training in psychotherapy. *American Psychologist*, *70*(8), 747–757. https://doi.org/10.1037/a0039803

Henry, W. P., Strupp, H. H., Butler, S. F., Schacht, T. E., & Binder, J. L. (1993). Effects of training in time-limited dynamic psychotherapy: Changes in therapist behavior. *Journal of Consulting and Clinical Psychology*, *61*(3), 434–440. https://doi.org/10.1037/0022-006X.61.3.434

Hill, C. E., Kivlighan, D. M., III, Rousmaniere, T., Kivlighan, D. M., Jr., Gerstenblith, J., & Hillman, J. (2020). Deliberate practice for the skill of immediacy: A multiple case study of doctoral student therapists and clients. *Psychotherapy: Theory, Research, & Practice, 57*(4), 587–597. https://doi.org/10.1037/pst0000247

Hill, C. E., & Knox, S. (2013). Training and supervision in psychotherapy: Evidence for effective practice. In M. J. Lambert (Ed.), *Handbook of psychotherapy and behavior change* (6th ed., pp. 775–811). John Wiley & Sons.

Hook, J. N., Davis, D. D., Owen, J., & DeBlaere, C. (2017). *Cultural humility: Engaging diverse identities in therapy.* American Psychological Association. https://doi.org/10.1037/0000037-000

Johnson, S. (2008). *Hold me tight: Seven conversations for a lifetime of love.* Little, Brown & Company.

Johnson, S. (2016, February 4). *Love sense: From infant to adult (Sue Johnson and Ed Tronick)* [Video]. YouTube. https://www.youtube.com/watch?v=OyCHT9AbD_Y

Johnson, S., & Brubacher, L. (2016). Deepening attachment emotion in emotionally focused couple therapy (EFT). In G. R. Weeks, S. T. Fife, & C. M. Peterson (Eds.), *Techniques for the couple therapist: Essential interventions from the experts* (pp. 219–257). Routledge. https://doi.org/10.4324/9781315747330-32

Johnson, S. M. (2004). *The practice of emotionally focused couple therapy: Creating connection* (2nd ed.). Routledge.

Johnson, S. M. (2013). Facing the dragon together: Emotionally focused couples therapy with trauma survivors. In D. Catherall (Ed.), *Handbook of stress, trauma, and the family* (pp. 493–512). Routledge/Taylor & Francis Group.

Johnson, S. M. (2019). *Attachment theory in practice: Emotionally focused therapy (EFT) with individuals, couples, and families.* Guilford Press.

Johnson, S. M. (2020). *The practice of emotionally focused couple therapy: Creating connection* (3rd ed.). Routledge.

Johnson, S. M., & Campbell, T. L. (2022). *A primer for emotionally focused individual therapy (EFIT): Cultivating fitness and growth in every client.* Routledge.

Kailanko, S., Wiebe, S. A., Tasca, G. A., Laitila, A. A., & Allan, R. (2022). Somatic experience of emotion in emotionally focused couple therapy: Experienced trainer therapists' views and experiences. *Journal of Marital and Family Therapy, 48*(3), 677–692. https://doi.org/10.1111/jmft.12543

Kelly, S. (Ed.). (2017). *Diversity in couple and family therapy: Ethnicities, sexualities, and socioeconomics.* Praeger.

Kelly, S. (2024). The successful integration of emotionally focused couple therapy (EFCT) and multicultural theory: Drew Mendelson's psychotherapy with "Alice" and "Steve." *Pragmatic Case Studies in Psychotherapy, 20*(1). https://doi.org/10.55818/pcsp.v20i1.2152

Kelly, S., & Omar, Y. (2017). Cultural identity in couples and families. In J. L. Lebow, A. Chambers, & D. Breunlin (Eds.), *Encyclopedia of couple and family therapy* (pp. 1–9). Springer Science+Business Media. https://doi.org/10.1007/978-3-319-15877-8_473-1

Kendall, P. C., & Beidas, R. S. (2007). Smoothing the trail for dissemination of evidence-based practices for youth: Flexibility within fidelity. *Professional Psychology: Research and Practice, 38*(1), 13–20. https://doi.org/10.1037/0735-7028.38.1.13

Kendall, P. C., & Frank, H. E. (2018). Implementing evidence-based treatment protocols: Flexibility within fidelity. *Clinical Psychology: Science and Practice, 25*(4), Article e12271. https://doi.org/10.1111/cpsp.12271

Koren, R., Woolley, S. R., Danis, I., & Török, S. (2021). Measuring the effectiveness of the emotionally focused therapy externship training in Hungary done through translation. *Journal of Marital and Family Therapy, 47*(1), 1–17. https://doi.org/10.1111/jmft.12443

Koziol, L. F., & Budding, D. E. (2012). Procedural learning. In N. M. Seel (Ed.), *Encyclopedia of the sciences of learning* (pp. 2694–2696). Springer. https://doi.org/10.1007/978-1-4419-1428-6_670

Lambert, M. J. (2010). Yes, it is time for clinicians to monitor treatment outcome. In B. L. Duncan, S. C. Miller, B. E. Wampold, & M. A. Hubble (Eds.), *Heart and soul of change: Delivering what works in therapy* (2nd ed., pp. 239–266). American Psychological Association. https://doi.org/10.1037/12075-008

Levenson, H. (1995). *Time-limited dynamic psychotherapy: A guide to clinical practice*. Basic Books.

Levenson, H. (2017). *Brief dynamic therapy*. American Psychological Association. https://doi.org/10.1037/0000043-000

Levenson, H., Svatovic, M., & Montagno, M. (2009, October). *Knowledge and competency in emotionally focused therapy* [Paper presentation]. Annual Convention of the American Association of Marriage Family Therapists, Sacramento, CA, United States.

Markman, K. D., & Tetlock, P. E. (2000). Accountability and close-call counterfactuals: The loser who nearly won and the winner who nearly lost. *Personality and Social Psychology Bulletin, 26*(10), 1213–1224. https://doi.org/10.1177/0146167200262004

McGaghie, W. C., Issenberg, S. B., Barsuk, J. H., & Wayne, D. B. (2014). A critical review of simulation-based mastery learning with translational outcomes. *Medical Education, 48*(4), 375–385. https://doi.org/10.1111/medu.12391

McLeod, J. (2017). Qualitative methods for routine outcome measurement. In T. G. Rousmaniere, R. Goodyear, D. D. Miller, & B. E. Wampold (Eds.), *The cycle of excellence: Using deliberate practice to improve supervision and training* (pp. 99–122). John Wiley & Sons. https://doi.org/10.1002/9781119165590.ch5

Mendelson, D. (2024a). "The commitment of a lifetime": The role of emotionally focused couple therapy in strengthening attachment bonds and improving relationship health in later-life couples—The teletherapy case of "Alice" and "Steve." *Pragmatic Case Studies in Psychotherapy, 20*(1), 1–80.

Mendelson, D. (2024b). Response to commentaries on "The commitment of a lifetime": The role of emotionally focused couple therapy in strengthening attachment bonds and improving relationship health in later-life couples—The teletherapy case of "Alice" and "Steve." *Pragmatic Case Studies in Psychotherapy, 20*(1), 106–116.

Mikulincer, M., & Shaver, P. R. (2017). *Attachment in adulthood: Structure, dynamics, and change* (2nd ed.). Guilford Press.

Minuchin, S., & Fishman, H. C. (1981). *Techniques of family therapy*. Harvard University Press. https://doi.org/10.4159/9780674041110

Montagno, M., Svatovic, M., & Levenson, H. (2011). Short-term and long-term effects of training in emotionally focused couple therapy: Professional and personal aspects. *Journal of Marital and Family Therapy, 37*(4), 380–392. https://doi.org/10.1111/j.1752-0606.2011.00250.x

Nightingale, M., Awosan, C. I., & Stavrianopoulos, K. (2019). Emotionally focused therapy: A culturally sensitive approach for African American heterosexual couples. *Journal of Family Psychotherapy, 30*(3), 221–244. https://doi.org/10.1080/08975353.2019.1666497

Norcross, J. C., & Guy, J. D. (2005). The prevalence and parameters of personal therapy in the United States. In J. D. Geller, J. C. Norcross, & D. E. Orlinsky (Eds.), *The psychotherapist's own psychotherapy: Patient and clinician perspectives* (pp. 165–176). Oxford University Press.

Norcross, J. C., Lambert, M. J., & Wampold, B. E. (2019). *Psychotherapy relationships that work* (3rd ed.). Oxford University Press.

Orlinsky, D. E., Rønnestad, M. H., & Collaborative Research Network of the Society for Psychotherapy Research. (2005). *How psychotherapists develop: A study of therapeutic work and professional growth*. American Psychological Association. https://doi.org/10.1037/11157-000

Owen, J., & Hilsenroth, M. J. (2014). Treatment adherence: The importance of therapist flexibility in relation to therapy outcomes. *Journal of Counseling Psychology, 61*(2), 280–288. https://doi.org/10.1037/a0035753

Owen, J., Imel, Z., Tao, K., Wampold, B., Smith, A., & Rodolfa, E. (2011). Cultural ruptures in short-term therapy: Working alliance as a mediator between clients' perceptions of microaggressions and therapy outcomes. *Counselling & Psychotherapy Research, 11*(3), 204–212. https://doi.org/10.1080/14733145.2010.491551

Palmer-Olsen, L., Gold, L. L., & Woolley, S. R. (2011). Supervising emotionally focused therapists: A systematic research-based model. *Journal of Marital and Family Therapy, 37*(4), 411–426. https://doi.org/10.1111/j.1752-0606.2011.00253.x

PettyJohn, M. E., Tseng, C. F., & Blow, A. J. (2020). Therapeutic utility of discussing therapist/client intersectionality in treatment: When and how? *Family Process, 59*(2), 313–327. https://doi.org/10.1111/famp.12471

Prescott, D. S., Maeschalck, C. L., & Miller, S. D. (Eds.). (2017). *Feedback-informed treatment in clinical practice: Reaching for excellence.* American Psychological Association. https://doi.org/10.1037/0000039-000

Rodríguez-Gonzalez, M., Anderson, S., Osorio, A., Lafontaine, M. F., Greenman, P. S., Calatrava, M., Andrade, D., Lybbert, R., Martínez-Diaz, P., Steffen, P., de Irala, J., & Sandberg, J. (2022). Efficacy of emotionally focused therapy among Spanish-speaking couples: Study protocol of a randomized clinical trial in Argentina, Costa Rica, Guatemala, Mexico, and Spain. *Trials, 23*(1), Article 891. https://doi.org/10.1186/s13063-022-06831-7

Rodríguez-González, M., Schweer-Collins, M., Greenman, P. S., Lafontaine, M. F., Fatás, M. D., & Sandberg, J. G. (2020). Short-term and long-term effects of training in EFT: A multinational study in Spanish-speaking countries. *Journal of Marital and Family Therapy, 46*(2), 304–320. https://doi.org/10.1111/jmft.12416

Rogers, C. (1961). *On becoming a person.* Houghton Mifflin.

Rousmaniere, T. G. (2016). *Deliberate practice for psychotherapists: A guide to improving clinical effectiveness.* Routledge/Taylor & Francis Group. https://doi.org/10.4324/9781315472256

Rousmaniere, T. G. (2019). *Mastering the inner skills of psychotherapy: A deliberate practice handbook.* Gold Lantern Press.

Rousmaniere, T. G., Goodyear, R., Miller, S. D., & Wampold, B. E. (Eds.). (2017). *The cycle of excellence: Using deliberate practice to improve supervision and training.* John Wiley & Sons. https://doi.org/10.1002/9781119165590

Sandberg, J. G., & Knestel, A. (2011). The experience of learning emotionally focused couples therapy. *Journal of Marital and Family Therapy, 37*(4), 393–410. https://doi.org/10.1111/j.1752-0606.2011.00254.x

Sandberg, J. G., Rodríguez-González, M., Pereyra, S., Lybbert, R., Perez, L., & Willis, K. (2020). The experience of learning EFT in Spanish-speaking countries: A multinational replication study. *Journal of Marital and Family Therapy, 46*(2), 256–271. https://doi.org/10.1111/jmft.12383

Sexton, T., Gordon, K. C., Gurman, A., Lebow, J., Holtzworth-Munroe, A., & Johnson, S. (2011). Guidelines for classifying evidence-based treatments in couple and family therapy. *Family Process, 50*(3), 377–392.

Siegel, D. J. (2020). *The developing mind: How relationships and the brain interact to shape who we are* (3rd ed.). Guilford Press.

Skean, K. R., & Brown, E. (2024). Emotionally focused couple therapy with a late-life couple: From despair to integrity. *Pragmatic Case Studies in Psychotherapy, 20*(1). https://doi.org/10.55818/pcsp.v20i1.2151

Slootmaeckers, J., & Migerode, L. (2020). EFT and intimate partner violence: A roadmap to de-escalating violent patterns. *Family Process, 59*(2), 328–345. https://doi.org/10.1111/famp.12468

Spengler, P. M., Lee, N. A., Wiebe, S. A., & Wittenborn, A. K. (2024). A comprehensive meta-analysis on the efficacy of emotionally focused couple therapy. *Couple and Family Psychology: Research and Practice, 13*(2), 81–99. https://doi.org/10.1037/cfp0000233

Squire, L. R. (2004). Memory systems of the brain: A brief history and current perspective. *Neurobiology of Learning and Memory, 82*(3), 171–177. https://doi.org/10.1016/j.nlm.2004.06.005

Stiles, W. B., Honos-Webb, L., & Surko, M. (1998). Responsiveness in psychotherapy. *Clinical Psychology: Science and Practice, 5*(4), 439–458. https://doi.org/10.1111/j.1468-2850.1998.tb00166.x

Stiles, W. B., & Horvath, A. O. (2017). Appropriate responsiveness as a contribution to therapist effects. In L. G. Castonguay & C. E. Hill (Eds.), *How and why are some therapists better than others? Understanding therapist effects* (pp. 71–84). American Psychological Association. https://doi.org/10.1037/0000034-005

Taylor, J. M., & Neimeyer, G. J. (2017). Lifelong professional improvement: The evolution of continuing education. In T. G. Rousmaniere, R. Goodyear, S. D. Miller, & B. Wampold (Eds.), *The cycle of excellence: Using deliberate practice to improve supervision and training* (pp. 219–248). Wiley Blackwell.

Tilley, D., & Palmer, G. (2013). Enactments in emotionally focused couple therapy: Shaping moments of contact and change. *Journal of Marital and Family Therapy, 39*(3), 299–313. https://doi.org/10.1111/j.1752-0606.2012.00305.x

Tracey, T. J. G., Wampold, B. E., Goodyear, R. K., & Lichtenberg, J. W. (2015). Improving expertise in psychotherapy. *Psychotherapy Bulletin, 50*(1), 7–13.

Wass, R., & Golding, C. (2014). Sharpening a tool for teaching: The zone of proximal development. *Teaching in Higher Education, 19*(6), 671–684. https://doi.org/10.1080/13562517.2014.901958

Wiebe, S. A., & Johnson, S. M. (2016). A review of the research in emotionally focused therapy for couples. *Family Process, 55*(3), 390–407. https://doi.org/10.1111/famp.12229

Wiebe, S. A., Johnson, S. M., Lafontaine, M. F., Burgess Moser, M., Dalgleish, T. L., & Tasca, G. A. (2017). Two-year follow-up outcomes in emotionally focused couple therapy: An investigation of relationship satisfaction and attachment trajectories. *Journal of Marital and Family Therapy, 43*(2), 227–244. https://doi.org/10.1111/jmft.12206

Young, J., Tadros, E., & Gregorash, A. (2023). Cultural considerations for using emotionally focused therapy with African American couples. *International Journal of Systemic Therapy, 34*(2), 63–82. https://doi.org/10.1080/2692398X.2022.2159299

Zaretskii, V. (2009). The zone of proximal development: What Vygotsky did not have time to write. *Journal of Russian & East European Psychology, 47*(6), 70–93. https://doi.org/10.2753/RPO1061-0405470604

Zeytinoglu-Saydam, S. (2018). Cross-culturally responsive training of emotionally focused couple therapy: International experiences. In S. Poulsen & R. Allan (Eds.), *Cross-cultural responsiveness and systemic therapy* (pp. 53–67). Springer International Publishing. https://doi.org/10.1007/978-3-319-71395-3_4

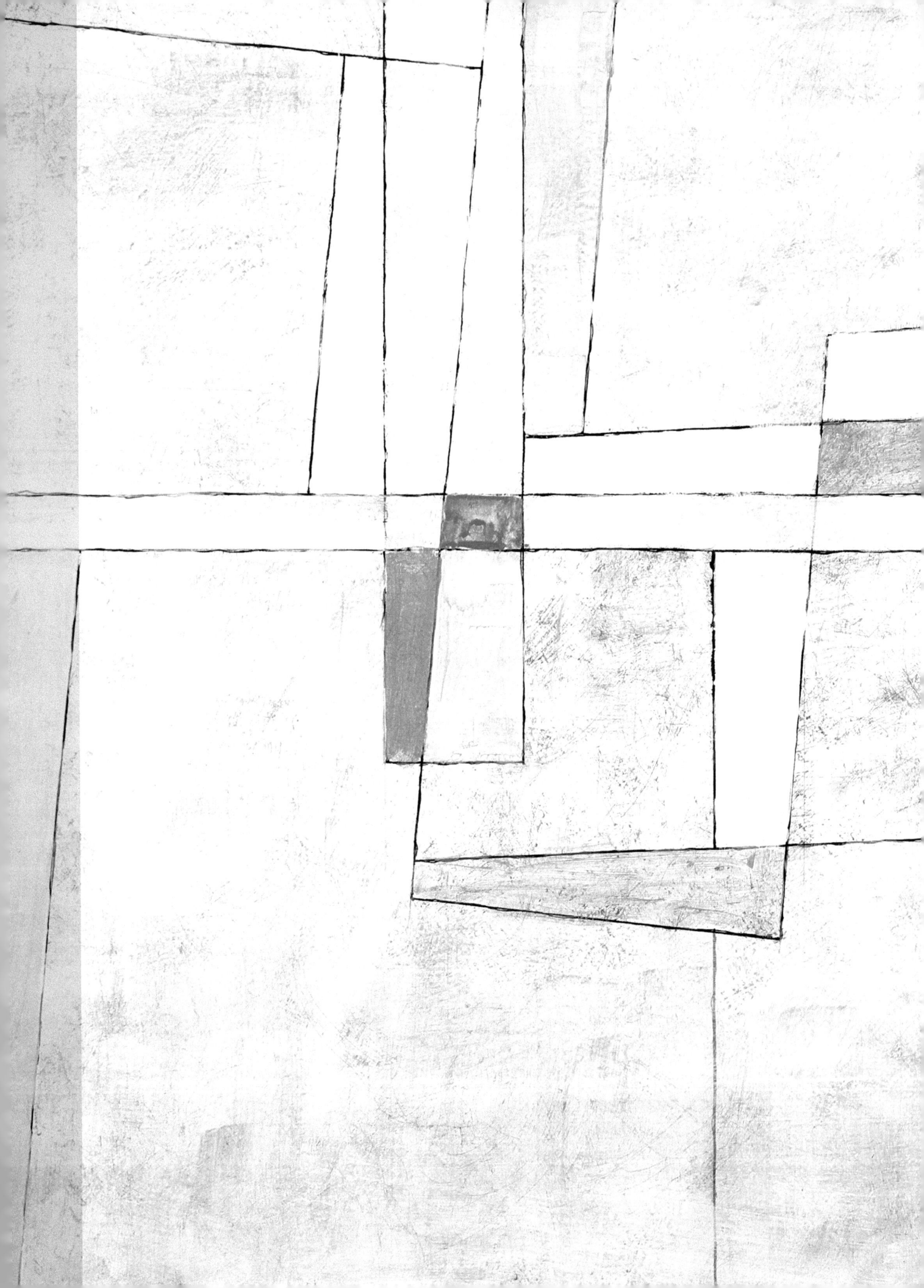

Index

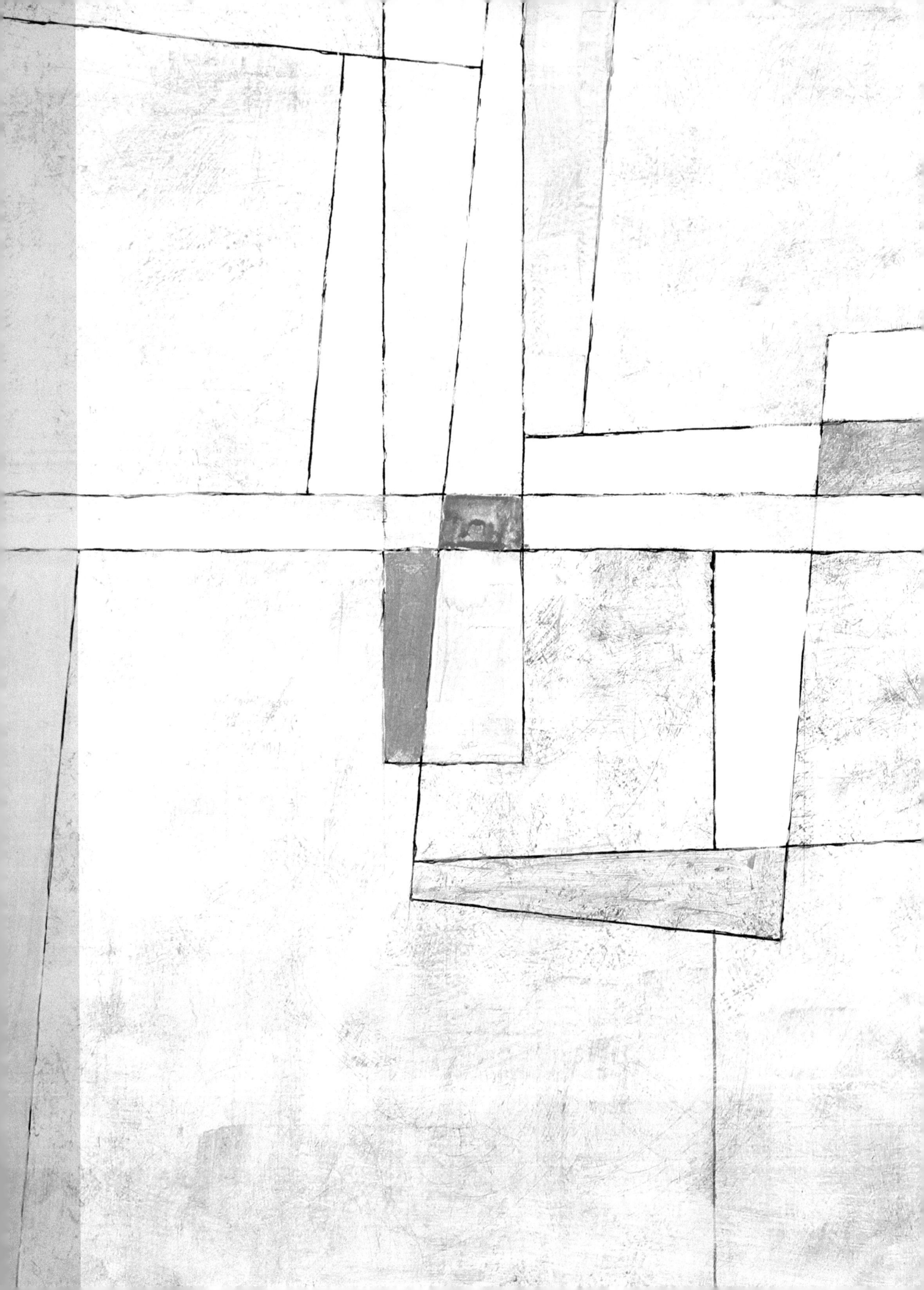

About the Authors

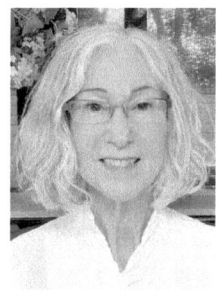

Hanna Levenson, PhD, is a certified therapist and supervisor in emotionally focused couple therapy. She is professor emerita at the Wright Institute in Berkeley, California, and a Fellow of Division 29 (Society for the Advancement of Psychotherapy) of the American Psychological Association (APA). In her private practice, she sees individuals and couples for therapy and professionals for consultation. For 20 years, Dr. Levenson was clinical professor in the Department of Psychiatry, University of California School of Medicine; director of the Brief Therapy Program at the Veterans Administration Medical Center; and director of the Brief Therapy Program at the California Pacific Medical Center, all in San Francisco. Dr. Levenson has been specializing in the areas of brief dynamic psychotherapy, supervision, and couples work for more than 40 years. She is the author or coauthor of more than 80 professional papers and six books, including *Deliberate Practice in Psychodynamic Psychotherapy* (2023) and the forthcoming *Deliberate Practice in Accelerated Experiential Dynamic Psychotherapy* (both from APA Books). In her writings and clinical work, Dr. Levenson integrates emotionally focused, experiential, and relational approaches. She is the recipient of the Distinguished Contribution to Psychology as a Profession Award from the California Psychological Association and the Certificate of Recognition Award from the National Organization of Veterans Administration Psychologists. She has provided numerous trainings to various mental health centers and universities nationally and internationally.

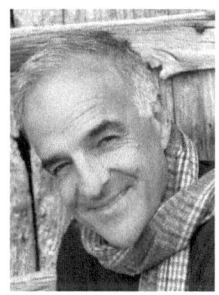

Sam Jinich, PhD, is a certified trainer in emotionally focused couple therapy (EFCT). He has been a clinical psychologist in private practice since 1995, specializing in working with couples from diverse backgrounds. Dr. Jinich was born in Mexico City and received his PhD from the University of California–San Diego State University's Joint Doctoral Program in clinical psychology, where he focused on couple and family therapy. He did his postdoctoral fellowship at the University of California, San Francisco School of Medicine's Center for AIDS Prevention Studies. In 2013, he founded the San Francisco Center for Emotionally Focused Therapy, where he is the director. More recently, he cofounded (with Natalia Gilabert) EFT Academia in Argentina, providing EFCT master classes, workshops, webinars, and supervision to clinicians around the world. As a bilingual and bicultural trainer in EFT, Dr. Jinich has been responsible for establishing EFCT in Mexico, Argentina, Costa Rica, Guatemala, Panama, Brazil, Chile, and Spain through mentoring and supervising therapists in these countries toward becoming EFCT practitioners, supervisors, and trainers. He was involved in the planning and supervision of therapists in the first-ever multinational randomized clinical trial research study in Spanish on the effectiveness of couple therapy in general, and specifically of EFCT. Dr. Jinich is particularly known for his creative and passionate presentations on EFCT.

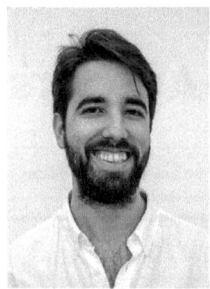

Alexandre Vaz, PhD, is cofounder and chief academic officer of Sentio University and the Sentio Counseling Center. He provides workshops, webinars, and advanced clinical training and supervision to clinicians around the world. Dr. Vaz is the author/coeditor of more than a dozen books on deliberate practice and psychotherapy training. He has held multiple committee roles for the Society for the Exploration of Psychotherapy Integration and the Society for Psychotherapy Research. Dr. Vaz is founder and host of "Psychotherapy Expert Talks," an acclaimed interview series with distinguished psychotherapists and therapy researchers.

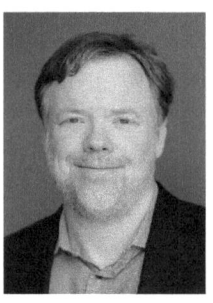

Tony Rousmaniere, PsyD, is cofounder and program director of Sentio University and the Sentio Counseling Center. He provides workshops, webinars, and advanced clinical training and supervision to clinicians around the world. Dr. Rousmaniere is the author/coeditor of more than a dozen books on deliberate practice and psychotherapy training. In 2017, he published the widely cited article "What Your Therapist Doesn't Know" in *The Atlantic*. Dr. Rousmaniere supports the open-data movement and publishes his aggregated clinical outcome data, in de-identified form, on his website (https://www.drtonyr.com). Dr. Rousmaniere is president of Division 29 of the American Psychological Association (Society for the Advancement of Psychotherapy).